Instructing Hatha Yoga

Kathy Lee Kappmeier

Diane M. Ambrosini

HUMAN KINETICS

Library of Congress Cataloging-in-Publication Data

Kappmeier, Kathy Lee, 1964-
Instructing hatha yoga / Kathy Lee Kappmeier, Diane M. Ambrosini.
    p. cm.
Includes bibliographical references.
ISBN 0-7360-5209-7 (soft cover)
1. Hatha yoga—Study and teaching. I. Ambrosini, Diane M., 1962- II. Title.
RA781.7.K36 2006
613.7'046'071—dc22
        2005011856

ISBN-10: 0-7360-5209-7
ISBN-13: 978-0-7360-5209-2

Acquisitions Editor: Gayle Kassing
Developmental Editors: Jennifer Sekosky, Ragen E. Sanner
Assistant Editor: Carmel Sielicki
Copyeditor: Amie Bell
Proofreader: Kathy Bennett
Permission Manager: Dalene Reeder
Graphic Designer: Nancy Rasmus
Graphic Artist: Angela K. Snyder
Photo Managers: Kelly J. Huff, Sarah Ritz
Cover Designer: Keith Blomburg
Photographer (cover): Kelly J. Huff
Photographer (interior): Kelly J. Huff, unless otherwise noted.
Art Manager: Kelly Hendren
Illustrator: Mic Greenberg
Printer: Versa Press

Printed in the United States of America   10   9

The paper in this book is certified under a sustainable forestry program.

Human Kinetics
Web site: www.HumanKinetics.com

United States: Human Kinetics
P.O. Box 5076
Champaign, IL 61825-5076
800-747-4457
e-mail: humank@hkusa.com

Canada: Human Kinetics
475 Devonshire Road, Unit 100
Windsor, ON N8Y 2L5
800-465-7301 (in Canada only)
e-mail: info@hkcanada.com

Europe: Human Kinetics
107 Bradford Road
Stanningley
Leeds LS28 6AT, United Kingdom
+44 (0)113 255 5665
e-mail: hk@hkeurope.com

Australia: Human Kinetics
57A Price Avenue
Lower Mitcham, South Australia 5062
08 8372 0999
e-mail: info@hkaustralia.com

New Zealand: Human Kinetics
P.O. Box 80
Torrens Park, South Australia 5062
0800 222 062
e-mail: info@hknewzealand.com

We dedicate this book to aspects of the Divine as depicted in yoga mythology and literature. To the myth of Hanuman, the magical monkey figure, that devoted his heart and actions to God. Reflecting on this dedication keeps us humble, inspired, and motivated in our work. The image of Hanuman moving mountains helped move the manuscript along! And to the essence of Durga, the warrior goddess, who rode a mighty tiger and battled many armies. We called upon that warrior energy to battle writer's block; time-management monsters; and unexpected challenges and tribulations including eight computers, two tape recorders, one broken hand, and a wrecked Harley Davidson motorcycle.

Without the *Yoga Sutras* as written by the "Father of Yoga," Patanjali, it is doubtful if many or any forms of yoga would be in practice today. Patanjali wrote the *Sutras* in a time when there was much confusion and controversy regarding how to *practice* yoga. It is our hope, in a much smaller yet progressive way, that our book will bring clarity on how to *teach* yoga.

Kathy Lee would like to personally thank:

- The staff at Café India. It was at this mom-and-pop landmark establishment that I spent many, many hours in a booth consuming chai and working on my laptop.
- The wonderful sisterhood of riders in San Diego's Women in the Wind. When I couldn't drive after my accident, Leona offered rides anywhere and everywhere, including to Café India to work on the book.
- To Lauren and Rich for their input as people who practice yoga and law. Their unique perspectives, not only as friends and students but also as experienced and creative writers, were always valuable. I'm also very grateful for my beautiful sister in meditation, Rhonda, who has always showered me with brilliant, radiant enthusiasm in all my yogic endeavors.
- And to peaceful artist Claudia, who is so supportive in many incredible ways.

Diane thanks:

The two brightest lights in my life: Dave and Ben Massey. I appreciate your patience, your love, and the balance you bring to my life. The journey wouldn't be worth traveling without the two of you! Yip! A special thanks to Suzanne and Laura for insight and encouragement. And for the support of family, students, and friends too numerous to list!

contents

Part 3   Structuring a Class

poses

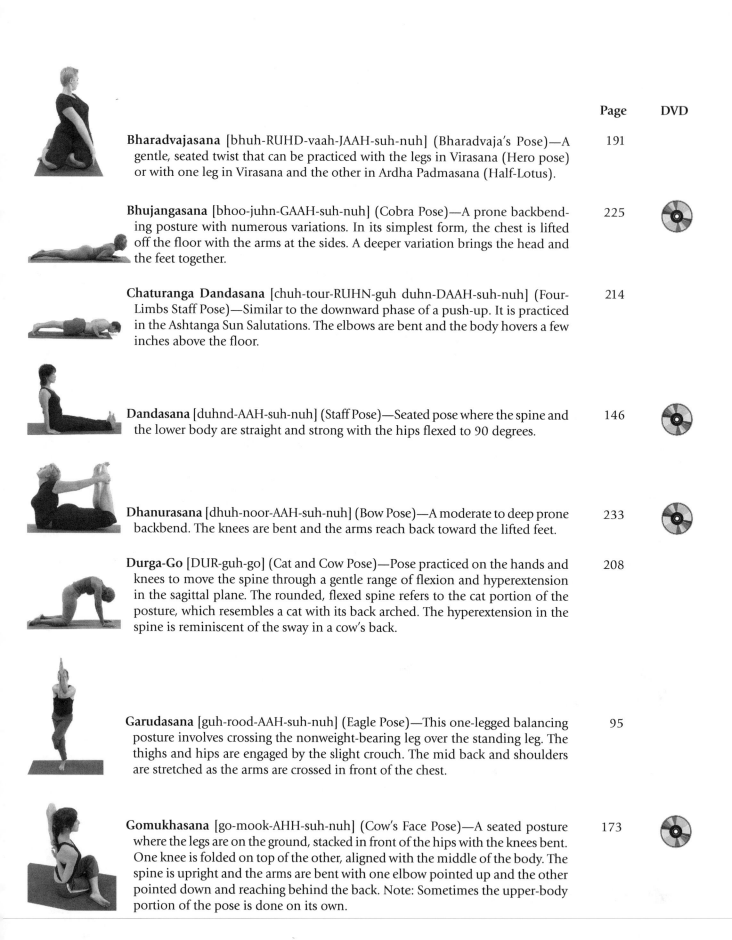

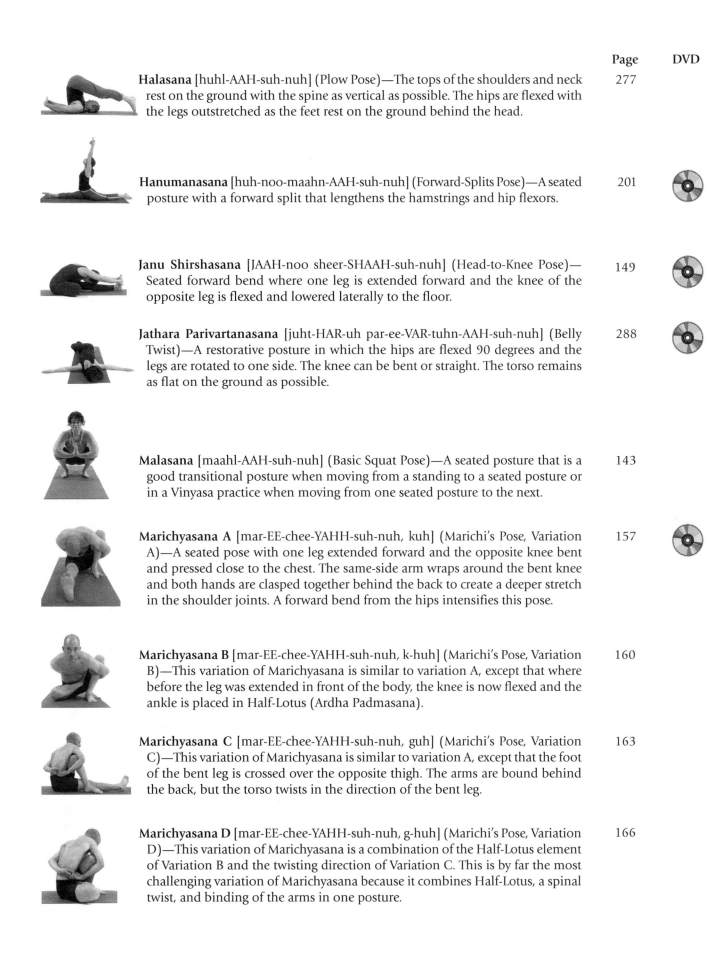

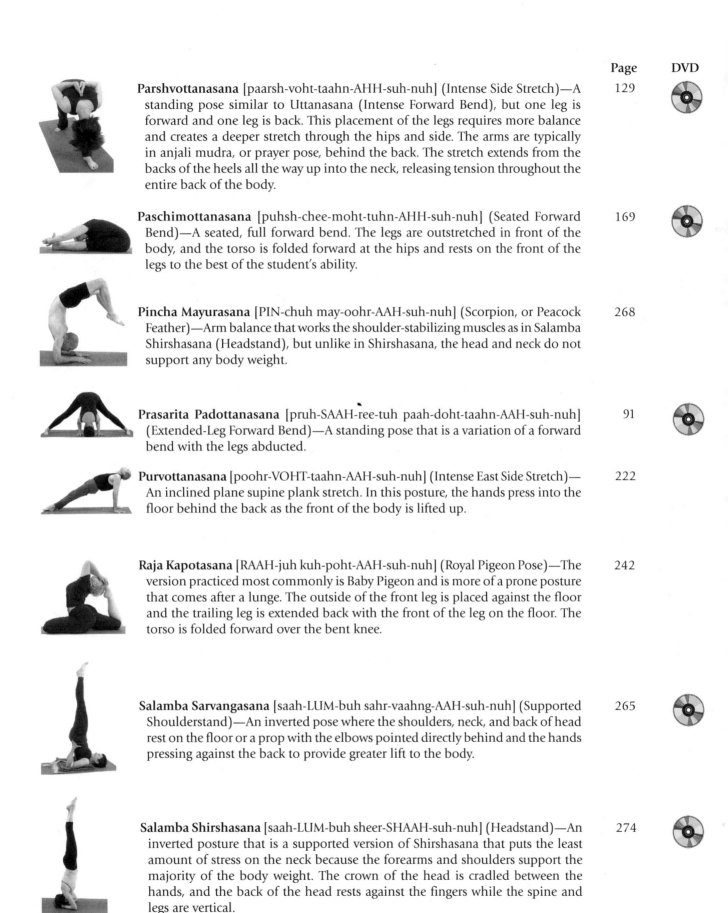

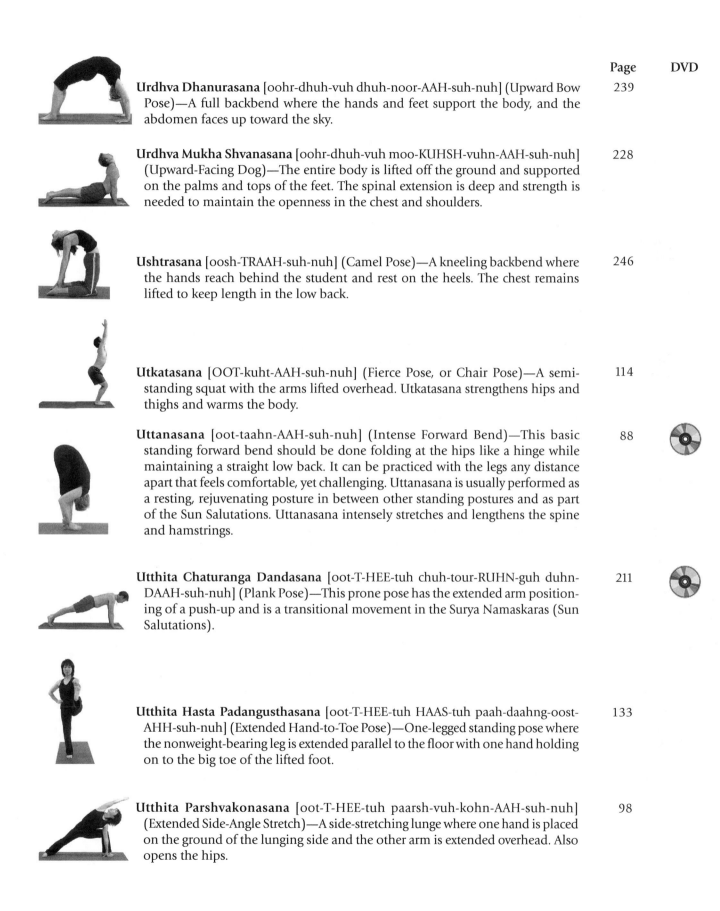

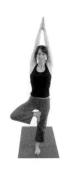
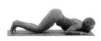

preface

On October 7th, 2002, as the camera panned the sidelines, viewers saw former San Diego Chargers' tight end Tim Dwight warming up with a number of *asanas* [AHH-suh-nuhs] (yoga postures). In the October 2003 issue of *Yogi Times*, Dwight said that yoga is a philosophy he's bonded with, and he believed that it enhances his athleticism in football as well as his everyday life.

In the September/October 2001 *Yoga Journal*, past and present professional athletes were interviewed and asked how a regular practice of *hatha* [HUH-tuh] yoga enhanced their athletic performance and general well-being. Eddie George (then with the Tennessee Titans) related that he felt that the increased range of motion and the overall flexibility he gained after practicing yoga has aided in keeping him injury free in his professional career.

Yoga is not just for East Indians and professional athletes, however. Data from the second annual "Yoga in America" survey, sponsored by *Yoga Journal* (February 2005), shows that approximately 16.5 million people in the United States practice yoga. This figure revealed a 5.6% increase from the previous year's survey and a 43% increase from 2002. In addition, the survey results indicated that approximately one out of seven nonpracticing people state that they intended to try yoga within the next 12 months.

Just by perusing the mind-body-spirit section of most bookstores and libraries you can see that yoga has become accepted by the mainstream as a means for increasing the strength and flexibility of the body and the mind. Hatha yoga is a system of mind-body exercises that was once taught only to small groups of monks. Today, the practice of yoga is constantly evolving and can be found everywhere from prisons to cruise ships!

The discipline of hatha yoga, which originated in India over 6,000 years ago, has become the focus of an evergrowing fitness and social trend in the Western world. Today, yoga is one of the fastest growing fitness activities in the United States. Yoga classes are being taught in such diverse locations as studios, fitness centers, hospitals, senior centers, prisons, community facilities, military bases, and scholastic settings from elementary school to the university level. With the rapid increase in demand for yoga classes, there is also a profound need for qualified yoga instructors.

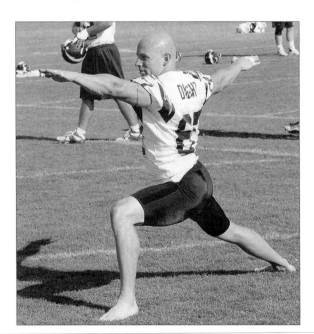

Photo courtesy of San Diego Chargers. LaFranceJ@chargers.nfl.com.

Yoga Alliance

In the past, yoga tradition was passed down orally, over many years, from guru (master teacher) to student. Unfortunately, because of the increase in demand for instructors, some individuals are now teaching who have had little or no formal training in the subject. These individuals often possess little or no knowledge of how to create a safe and effective environment for their students.

With the increase in demand for yoga classes, and the realization that instructors filling teaching positions come from vastly diverse backgrounds, Yoga

Alliance (an ad hoc organization of yoga professionals) established a set of minimum standards for teacher training programs. These standards include sections on anatomy and physiology, yoga history and philosophy, ethics, techniques, and teaching methodologies. In 1999, the Alliance formed a national Yoga Teachers' Registry with the intent of recognizing and promoting teachers whose training meets those standards. Although participation in the registry is strictly voluntary, it is a way for instructors to promote themselves as having attained a level of professional acceptance within the community at large. The registry also is a tool employers and the general public can use to determine whether an instructor has the appropriate credentials. Yoga Alliance has registered hundreds of training programs and thousands of individual instructors. Although each training program and individual may have a different focus on style or methodology, they all have a common thread, in that they have complied with the registry standards.

From Aerobics to Yoga

"Ten years ago, people hit the gym to attain the ideal body," reported Bill Howland, Director of Research for IHRSA (International Health, Racquet, & Sportsclub Association) in the August 2003 *Yoga Journal*. "Members now express a keen interest in holistic health." Howland further explained that members of fitness facilities are looking to reduce stress and gain not only physical but also emotional benefits from their exercise routines. Yoga fits that bill. In a related article, the September 2002 issue of *Yoga Journal* quotes former professional ballerina Lauren Peterson as saying, "Dance is all about what's happening on the outside. Yoga is all about what's happening on the inside" (Bauman, 2002).

Yoga not only strengthens the body but also the mind. Hatha yoga is usually much more challenging physically than most people realize. In addition, the discipline is one of the few, if not the only, activities known to develop symmetry and balance in the body and (sometimes) mind instead of creating stress as a negative side effect. The ideal is for yogis (yoga practitioners) to push themselves to the edge of their comfort level. The activity is actually relatively gentle, which might explain, in part, why yoga was not universally accepted in the 1980s era of aerobic exercise, which was characterized by the exercise philosophy "no pain, no gain."

Because so many Americans were so enthralled with aerobic classes, it took a few years to establish

that just because a person was bouncy and perky, it didn't mean that the person would make a good and effective aerobic instructor. Because of the numerous injuries occurring in aerobic classes, organizations such as American Council on Sports Medicine (ACSM), American Council on Exercise (ACE), and Aerobics and Fitness Association of America (AFFA) began to create standards to certify qualified individuals. The need became painstakingly clear (literally) to health club, gym, and recreation center coordinators that only certified instructors could be counted on to be a responsible asset instead of a major liability.

Our Experience

As a teenager, Kathy Lee Kappmeier turned to yoga when no other form of exercise or therapy helped her weak and crooked spine. She found her scoliosis was a blessing in disguise because without it she may never have discovered the benefits of yoga or her future vocation. Beginning a yoga practice as a teenager gave her insights into struggling with an ego, when she would go to class and not be able to bend forward but a few inches past her knees. In the meantime, students three to four times her age were easily placing their hands on the floor.

In the early 1980s, Kathy Lee started going through a plethora of yoga certification courses and workshops (Kundalini, Iyengar, Ashtanga, Shivananda, to name a few). She was searching for a complete curriculum that would merge the traditional essence of yoga with scientific applications, sports medicine, and stress reduction. She wanted to gain access to information that would help her modify poses so that she could responsibly coach people with injuries or other issues.

With so many styles of yoga and no set standards, it was very challenging to find any program that offered what she was looking for. At that time, it was very hard to communicate to prospective employers and convince them that yoga was a safe and effective physical and mental program. Her quest took over 25 years, during which she earned various educational degrees (physical therapy and psychology), gathered numerous certifications, and furthered her study with travel to India. While studying physical therapy, Kathy Lee noticed the similarity between the physical therapy exercise known as the "MacKenzie Press-Up" and yoga poses such as Bhujangasana [bhoo-juhn-GAAH-suh-nuh] (Cobra pose). Subsequently, Kathy Lee began applying yoga to personal training, fitness, and therapy for her clients. In addition to the physical medicine of yoga, she learned about the psychological balance possible with yoga practice. Based on her work with diverse populations in a variety of settings and with differing demands and changing attitudes, she began to create her own Yoga Teacher Training program.

In 2001, international best-selling author Jeanette Vos began taking the Yoga Teacher Training program with Kathy Lee. Dr. Vos is one of the leading experts on learning, and Kathy Lee attended some of her educational training courses. These education courses served to validate and further spark Kathy Lee's understanding. These ideas are now incorporated in the accelerated learning Yoga Teacher Training (YTT) certification program that Kathy Lee offers under the auspices of Yogawell's Institute of Progressive Therapies at the Rancho San Diego Yoga Center and at various yoga retreats and conferences. She produced a series of YTT videos to help her teacher candidates study how to adjust and teach postures. However, Kathy Lee still wanted to offer a more complete resource in the form of a manual or textbook to complement the videos, homework, and workshops. Students continued to request a text that would emphasize the materials she presented in her workshops such as biomechanics, alignment, and adjustments as well as an overview of yoga and teaching methods. This book is unique in covering all of these aspects of teaching yoga within one text. After beginning to work on a comprehensive manual, Kathy Lee started to consult with a colleague and former YTT student of hers, Diane Ambrosini.

Diane earned a masters of arts degree with an emphasis in biomechanics. She is a dedicated yoga instructor, personal trainer, and group exercise instructor who incorporates yoga postures to teach her clients core and functional strength training, as well as the aerobic conditioning possible with certain yogic styles. Due to her background in biomechanics, the proper physical alignment necessary in practicing yoga appealed to her and lead to the collaboration with Kathy Lee not only to create this text, but to design anatomically focused workshops for the YTT students. Together, Kathy Lee and Diane set out to complete this book, which meets the current needs and demands of the masses of aspiring yoga teachers and students.

Our intent in writing this book is to include information with timeless appeal (like most authors!) to the variety of people who are drawn to yoga and interested in learning how to teach it. People from all walks of life have enrolled in YogaWell's YTT programs, including airline pilots, computer workers, school teachers, massage therapists, and lawyers. Students of yoga and those studying to teach

yoga have increasingly diverse backgrounds. Until recently, yoga teachers have come from two main backgrounds: followers of New Age philosophy and group exercise instructors. It is challenging to have teacher candidates from such diverse pathways in the same workshop, so this book is directed toward people of all backgrounds who wish to teach yoga or further their own study. The book is designed to integrate information to make it understandable and intriguing for all interested in learning about the qualities and knowledge they need to become competent, well-qualified yoga teachers.

Our Approach

Countless books and videos are available covering a multitude of styles and methods of yoga practice. However, none of these media outline any specific curricula on how to *teach* yoga. And, until now, many components of teaching yoga including anatomy, physiology, kinesiology, and pathology were hidden in the oral tradition and seldom if ever written about. It is quite impractical for most people to find a guru and study the old-fashioned way (living in an "ashram" or East Indian monastery for many years) to learn how to practice and then teach yoga proficiently. These days many yoga schools are scrambling to include the physical sciences in their curriculum, and many colleges and universities are expanding their physical education programs to include yoga teacher education. A gap still remains between East and West—between the wisdom integrated in an ancient lineage and intensive Western learning. This text bridges that gap with accelerated learning concepts based on the authors' decades of education, experience, and best results in training others how to teach yoga with attention to safety and passion for the practice.

Instructing Hatha Yoga appeals to novice instructors, highlighting awareness and safety, and it contains information many experienced teachers have been searching for, such as detailed hands-on adjustments, biomechanics, and cautionary details on postures. It can take you to the next level of understanding and fill gaps in your training by familiarizing you with the most popular styles of yoga practiced today, as well as helping you learn the proper Sanskrit pronunciations of postures. Most important, this book illustrates how to safely and effectively provide students with hands-on adjustments in each posture and how to utilize the deeper nuances of teaching. *Instructing Hatha Yoga* can also be used as a guide for any physical educator because it is designed to be user friendly. Regardless of your background, this book can help you share with others the extraordinary benefits of yoga with correct and safe guidelines. The book also touches on the importance of the national registry process and options and resources for becoming a registered yoga teacher.

This book is designed to allow anyone from initiate to veteran yoga teachers, physical educators, physical therapists, physicians, psychologists, and recreation directors to understand more fully how to create and teach safe, effective, and successful yoga programs. This text also addresses, at least in part, each of the categories outlined by the Yoga Alliance's registry requirements (see table 1.2, page 12, for a copy of the Yoga Alliance grid of categories). *Instructing Hatha Yoga* includes the following information:

- The impact of yoga today and the potential evolutions for future students and teachers
- Valued and effective qualities of a teacher
- The importance of pranayama [praah-naah-YAAH-muh] (breath work) and how to teach it
- Definitions of the most popular styles of yoga and how they evolved
- 66 asanas (postures) and variations
- Verbal and visual cueing examples
- Adjustments and modifications for each posture
- Physical and energetic anatomy applied in asanas
- The problem with classifying poses and people as "beginning" or "advanced" and ways to work with many people with different capacities within one class
- A class overview, outlines, lesson plans, and sample syllabi
- Sample relaxation scripts for guiding students into a relaxed, meditative state (appendix A)

Unique features of this book include simple yet comprehensive verbal instructions that you can use to bring students into proper alignment and detailed directions on how to make safe hands-on physical adjustments and modifications. Tables are provided for each asana to illustrate the basic kinematics and muscle recruitment. You will find a Self-Inquiry Questionnaire in appendix B that complements chapter 2, which covers some provocative issues regarding personal integrity and teaching yoga. The purpose of the self-inquiry is for you to integrate the information you gain from reading this book with your answers

so you can evaluate your readiness, willingness, and ability to begin teaching yoga.

In part 1 of *Instructing Hatha Yoga*, chapters 1 through 5 include a review in the form of study questions (answers are in appendix D). These self-tests are an opportunity to practice answering the questions you as a yoga instructor will be expected to know. The questions highlight important information about practicing and teaching yoga, and they are similar to questions asked in YogaWell's YTT programs. Understanding this information will assist you in becoming a better practitioner and instructor. It is our hope that readers will use this book not only as a reference and study guide but also as a guide to teaching yoga well.

The YogaWell YTT video series has been abridged and made into a DVD to accompany this text. Together, this book and companion DVD demonstrate techniques for aspiring as well as experienced yoga instructors to physically assist and adjust people in yoga postures. The asanas are presented with descriptions on how to move toward the most accurate alignment. A deepening and expanding of your students' ability to become more fully aware and comfortable in a pose, as well as your ability to teach it, will ensue.

Throughout the entire book, teachers and prospective teachers alike should remain mindful of the fact that the job of a truly qualified yoga instructor is to direct students toward their own awareness, not to teach what many might consider "advanced" poses. An instructor cannot *give* students awareness; rather, students must learn to find it on their own. A successful teacher facilitates the student's path to finding one's own internal teacher. A connection can occur within each student; the information in this book is a guide to helping your students make such a connection.

Sanskrit Pronunciation

When referring to the asanas, *Instructing Hatha Yoga* attempts to present Sanskrit words and their pronunciations in a user-friendly format. For certain words we have added the letter "h" after an "s" when the pronunciation of the Sanskrit calls for such. Many publications leave out the "h" in transliterations even though the sound is pronounced "sh." Often, publishers do not have the capacity to include diacritical markings. In English texts, a dot under or a slant over the letter "s" indicates the "sh" sound. In texts that do not include these markings, terms such as *Ashtanga* and *Shavasana* are spelled *Astanga* and *Savasana* despite the "sh" sound in their pronunciations. One last note, in Sanskrit the letters "th" do not make the same sound they do in English, so *hatha* is pronounced HUH-tuh (sounding nothing like the English word "the").

Although it may seem unnecessary to learn the Sanskrit names or proper pronunciation of poses, it is important to have a standard way to refer to the postures so that there is continuity among classes. Because of differing translations and schools of thought, there can be many English names for the same posture. Most postures, however, have a common Sanskrit name. Also, it is believed that the Sanskrit sounds themselves have a specific vibration and when spoken actually stimulate energy balance in the body. For a more complete introduction to Sanskrit pronunciation and the alphabet see the resource list in appendix B.

Asana Text

The asanas presented in part 2 of this book are shown in an easy-to-follow lesson format that details everything from what the posture is and its benefits, to what to say and how to help students perform the asanas to their greatest ability.

Included in each of the asana sections are the following:

- Description—quick reference for teachers describing the posture.
- Benefits—list of the benefits to the mind and body for performing the posture.
- Cautions—some asanas require extra care for certain students. The caution section alerts you to these needs for each particular asana.
- Verbal Cues—point-by-point example of how to guide your class through the pose.
- Adjustments—description of what to watch for while the students work and how to guide them into a more comfortable alignment.
- Modifications—description of modifications to the pose that you can employ for the students who need a boost from a prop or are unable to perform the full posture.
- Kinematics—reference charts that describe positioning and movement of body segments and indicate muscle recruitment with the type of muscular contraction utilized throughout the postures (Muscles Active), as well as any muscles that are stretched or not active during the posture (Muscles Released).

A photo of the main posture accompanies each asana lesson. Many photos of adjustments and modifications are provided as well. These will help you to see the proper body alignment within the positions.

DISCLAIMER:

It is a teacher's responsibility to caution students that anyone with preexisting medical conditions is advised not to practice certain poses presented in this book. Please note that the book presents a variety of possible variations and modifications to poses that teachers can adapt for students with medical conditions. As with any physical activity, if a student has an existing condition, it is best for the student to check with a physician or other health-care professional before beginning a yoga program.

Summary

Get ready to dissect, discern, and deliver an extraordinary way to teach yoga. With practical instruction, this book explains many of the attributes needed to be not only a well-qualified and registered yoga instructor but also an inspirational and creative leader who guides students toward awareness and control of their own bodies and minds. As a yoga teacher, you enable people to have a euphoric release within a complete physical fitness workout. The goal of this publication is to increase the knowledge, expertise, and credibility of anyone seriously interested in practicing and teaching yoga at any level. By reading this book you will be able to use the information to design safe classes; teach students yoga according to their individual learning styles; and be able to answer questions regarding types of yoga, its history, and a yogic lifestyle. You will also develop a solid sense of yoga's controversies and ethical considerations.

As a yoga teacher you will deal with your students both physically and emotionally. You will be glorified one day and vilified the next. You have a hard road ahead of you if you think you will become a guru anytime soon. However, if you want to be a qualified instructor instead of simply a quagmire of information and exercises, then you have the right book in your hands.

We wish you peace throughout your continual journey to becoming the most successful and wise yoga instructor you can be. May your quest and acquisition of knowledge never fade, and may your heart always remain open to share that knowledge with others.

*Namaste, Om Shanti**

---

*Salutations (sometimes translated as "The light within me bows to the light within you and together we are one in that light," and "Vibrate and be peace." This phrase is a typical closing statement yoga teachers might use to end the class.

acknowledgments

We offer special thanks to the following:

- *Yogi Times* magazine (www.yogitimes.com) for running an article about yoga and athletes that featured former San Diego Charger Tim Dwight's enthusiasm about yoga.

- Jamaal LaFrance, manager for the San Diego Chargers, for giving permission to use the photo of Tim Dwight that appears in the preface.

- The entire staff at Human Kinetics for being receptive to our ideas and proposals. It was our first and foremost choice to be published by Human Kinetics.

- Our kind and supportive acquisitions editor, Gayle Kassing, PhD. Our only regret is that Gayle could not come to San Diego and meet with us in person.

- Developmental editors Jennifer Sekosky and Ragen Sanner, who continued where Gayle left off in guiding us through the journey to the end of the book. Ragen, thank you for your patience!

- The eagle eyes of assistant editor Carmel Sielicki! Thanks for catching some potentially serious errors and mix-ups. You helped to make the last edits less painful!

- Permissions manager Dalene Reeder for doing all the footwork to secure permissions for us.

- The creativity and skills of all in the art, graphics and design departments!

- Our exceptionally talented photographer, Kelly Huff, for his patience, humor, and professionalism before, during, and after our photo shoot.

- Doug Fink, videotape editor, for his guidance in transferring video clips to the DVD.

- Thanks to our wonderful models: Tara Bogota, Mary Brown, Dr. Beau Casey, Lauren Derstine, Ann Keenan, Vivienne Kennedy, Eiko Keyser, Nadège Margaria, Jon Pobst, Brandy Proppe, Brian Ruiz, Jennifer Schilder, and Jim Walther. Thank you for sharing your time and the beauty of your practice with the public and us.

- We also thank the gracious teachers who subbed for us when we needed extra time to write and rewrite.

- And, of course, we are most grateful to the students we are honored to have in our classes. For it is only with their presence that a teacher can teach, and the practice of yoga can be shared and enabled to live and grow. Namaste, Om Shanti!

part 1

The Practice of Yoga

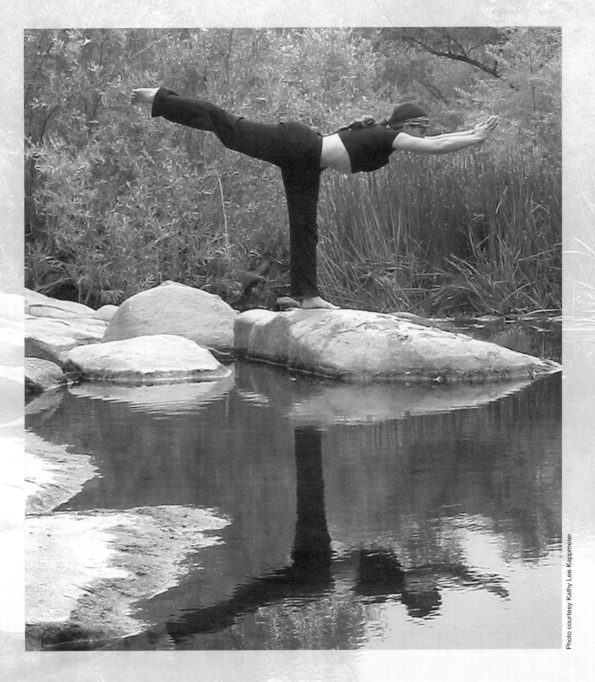

Photo courtesy Kathy Lee Kappmeier

chapter 1

Understanding Yoga

What do monks sitting in a mountain cave in East India and people sweating in a gym in the United States have in common? The practice of yoga, which was once considered nothing short of crazy, is now captivating many fitness enthusiasts. Yoga is a vehicle people can use to stretch and strengthen their bodies, minds, and spirits. Yoga is believed to have originated in India over 6,000 years ago. Evidence of the practice has also been found in pre-15th-century South American cultures such as in St. Augustine, Colombia, where statues of ancient stone depict people in yoga postures. This chapter aims at briefly defining and demystifying yoga, in particular the types of yoga you are currently practicing and teaching or will most likely practice and teach.

What does it mean when people say they practice yoga?

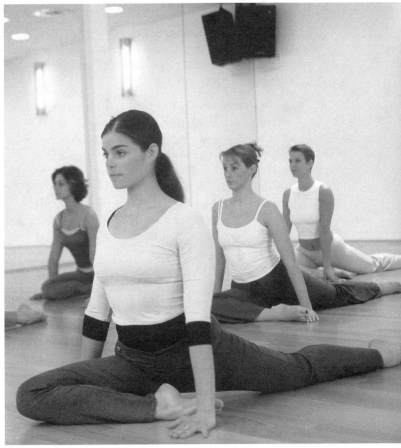

© Jumpfoto

Is it a mystic spiritual practice? Is it simply practicing postures or meditation techniques? In Sanskrit the word *yoga* means "to yoke or unite"; it can also mean "discipline." The second of the *Yoga Sutras*, a cardinal text that defines yoga, states, *Yoga chitta vritti nirodha*, which means "Yoga is the sensation of fluctuations or distractions toward evolved consciousness and being." Yoga is really *any* method by which we can become balanced and united with our own higher nature (Self) and obtain supreme bliss. Yoga is a journey of self-discovery on the path to enlightenment. For this reason, Mother Teresa and Socrates may be considered to have been *yogis* (people who practice yoga). When referring to a female yoga practitioner the term would be *yogini* [yoe-GEE-nee], whereas when speaking of a man, or of both women and men, the term *yogi* or *yogis* is applied.

Yoga is not a religion; it is a discipline without dogma. Therefore, a person of any faith or fellowship can be considered a yogi.

Types of Yoga

There truly are as many ways to practice yoga as there are ways to unite with bliss and enlightenment. However, there are essentially four primary types of yoga currently practiced:

- *Karma (KAR-muh) yoga* is the path of service through selfless action for the good of others. Mother Teresa served the poor as a way to connect the compassion of God with humanity. Unconditional service is a tradition in Hindu monasteries, or ashrams [AAHSH-ruhms], and many yoga teacher training programs require the teacher candidates to practice karma yoga by cooking and cleaning for others.
- *Bhakti (b-HUHK-tee) yoga* cultivates the expression and love of the Divine through devotional rituals. Regular prayer, chanting, singing, ceremonies, and celebration are all forms of this path.
- *Jnana (YAAH-nuh) yoga* is the path of intellect and wisdom. The study of sacred texts, intellectual debates, philosophical discussion, and introspection are all components of this path. Socrates, in this regard, was a jnana yogi.

- *Raja (RAAH-juh) yoga*, also known as the "royal path," refers to the journey toward personal enlightenment. This path consists of a balance of the three main yoga types just described—karma, bhakti, and jnana—in addition to the integration of the eight limbs, or stages, of yoga, which are discussed in the sidebar. Hatha [HUH-tuh] yoga is represented as a combination of the third and fourth limbs of the royal path, that is, asana [AAH-suh-nuh] and pranayama [praah-naah-YAAH-muh], respectively (see figure 1.1 and The Eight Limbs of the Royal Path sidebar).

The type of yoga generally practiced in modern, and especially Western, society is *hatha*. *Hatha* is usually translated from Sanskrit to mean "sun and moon," with *ha* representing the "sun energy," and *tha* representing the "moon energy." Hatha is also translated to mean "forceful" (see figure 1.2).

In *Hatha Yoga Pradipika* [praah-DEE-PEE-kuh], the text used by those who study hatha yoga, this translation is used, and some have expounded that "forceful" is applicable because hatha yoga is a discipline requiring great physical effort. On a symbolic as well as a physical level, *hatha* means a balancing of energies or forces.

Types of Hatha Yoga

Hatha yoga focuses on the path toward wellness and enlightenment through physical, mental, and spiritual means. Hatha yoga encompasses a number of popular styles of practice. Most hatha classes are generic in style, or they blend many of the popular elements of various styles that stand alone as a specific form. Iyengar and Ashtanga are among the most well-known forms of hatha, and "classical-eclectic" hatha classes often include traits from either styles, or both.

It is vital to note that although some approaches to hatha yoga differ from others, they all help practitioners achieve the goals of greater health and general well-being. This text attempts to present an overall picture of the physical discipline while bridging the gaps between East and West, ancient and progressive, physical and spiritual, science and art, flexibility and strength, and student and teacher.

Yoga is not associated with rebellion or revolution; instead, it is a practical response to our modern, hectic lives. The general practice of hatha is one that strives to be progressive while maintaining basic tradition. The

The Eight Limbs of the Royal Path

Think of the eight limbs of yoga as being a part of the great tree of yoga. Each limb connects to the trunk of the tree. Yoga is grounded and nurtured by its roots. Each limb has leaves that express the life of the limb; these leaves are the techniques of the limbs. The eight stages, or limbs, of yoga are explained in the *Yoga Sutras* by Patanjali [pa-TAHN-jah-lee], which was written around 200 to 300 B.C.

Limb 1

Yamas [YAAH-muhs]—guidelines for ethical standards and moral conduct

- Ahimsa [uh-HEEM-saah]—Nonviolence
- Satya [SUHT-yuh]—Truthfulness
- Asteya [uh-STAY-uh]—No stealing
- Brahmacharya [bruh-muh-CAHR-yuh]—Moderation
- Aparigraha [uh-PUH-reeg-ruh-huh]—Nonattachment

Limb 2

Niyamas [nee-YUH-muhs]—Observances and disciplines

- Saucha [SHOWH-chuh]—Cleanliness
- Santosha [suhn-TOH-shuh]—Contentment
- Tapas [TUH-puhs]—Austerities, translated as heat or purifying practices
- Svadhyaya [svaahd-HYAAH-yuh]—Study of spiritual scriptures
- Ishvara-Pranidhana [EEHSH-vuh-ruh Pruh-need-HAAH-nuh]—Practice of awareness and surrender to the presence and divine will of God

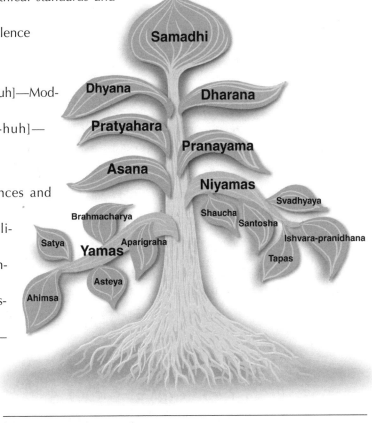

Figure 1.1 The tree of yoga.

Limb 3

Asana [AHH-suh-nuh]—body postures

Limb 4

Pranayama [praah-naah-YAAH-muh]—special breathing techniques used to control the life force, or energy, in the body

Limb 5

Pratyahara [pruht-yaah-HAAH-ruh]—withdrawal of the senses as part of the transcendence from constant nervous stimuli; the practice of sensory detachment through deep relaxation techniques

Limb 6

Dharana [dhaahr-UHN-aah]—concentration and focus

Limb 7

Dhyana [dhahy-AAH-nuh]—meditation

Limb 8

Samadhi [suh-MAAHD-hee]—the state of ecstasy, bliss, and enlightenment that transcends the self and merges with the Divine

practice venue, students, and teachers have changed considerably over the millennia; yet even as the forms and styles continue to branch out and evolve, it is important to remember that they come from the same basic roots. In fact, the founders of the two most popular styles of modern hatha, Iyengar and Ashtanga, had the very same teacher (see figure 1.3).

While yoga is ancient it is also alive.

Iyengar Yoga

World-renowned yoga master B.K.S. Iyengar created a style of hatha yoga in the early 20th century that focuses primarily on the importance of precise physical alignment during the execution of poses. At times Iyengar has been compared to a drill sergeant because his teaching style is somewhat strict with its extreme attention to positioning. Iyengar yoga students use many different types of props, which enable people at all levels of proficiency to go deeper or stay longer in postures with more accurate physical alignment. Props are becoming more common in eclectic classes as well, but Mr. Iyengar was an innovator in hatha practice because

of his insistence on precision with props and his demands on his yoga students to be consciously focused in the mind and obediently energetic in the body. Iyengar teacher trainings can take three or more years depending upon the level and focus on physical practice and the perfecting of teaching students to practice as precisely as possible.

Iyengar yoga places so much emphasis on physical alignment that Surya Namaskaras (Sun Salutations) are not performed, and pranayama (breath work) is abandoned in the asana classes. However, certain pranayamas are taught in workshops or as a separate practice altogether. Music and partner work are forbidden because they are thought to be distractions. Although some might find this hatha style intimidating, it is the safest form of physical practice because of the diligent attention to body alignment. However, it is a style that many are uncomfortable with because the instructor will not allow students to go as deeply into a posture as they might like, insisting that the students use props and move only as far into the posture as they are able while maintaining the most optimal alignment possible. Baggy clothes are not allowed in Iyengar classes because they hide too much of a student's body from view, and the

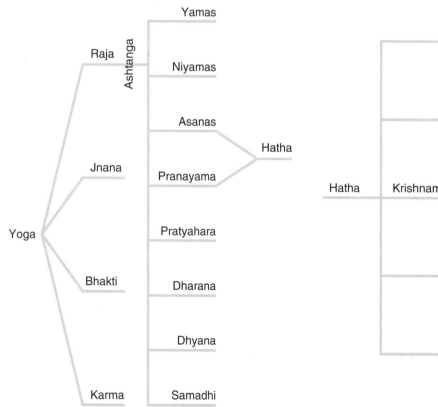

Figure 1.2   Yoga lineage.

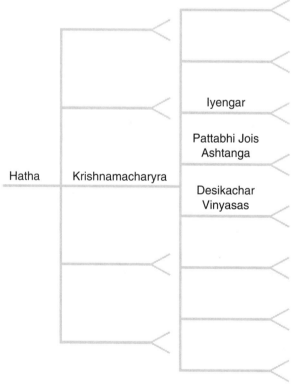

Figure 1.3   Hatha yoga lineage. The blank lines represent other lineages.

instructor might miss a detail to correct. Of course, individual teachers conduct classes in their own way, but "true-blue" Iyengar instructors tend to be stricter in their teaching style to adhere to Iyengar's exacting guidelines.

Ashtanga Yoga

Ashtanga means "eight limbs." In contemporary hatha circles there is a style of practice introduced by Pattabhi Jois that also is popularly known as Ashtanga yoga. This style is a dynamic form of hatha yoga in that there is a vigorous flow as one moves from posture to posture. Approximately six different Ashtanga series (or set combinations of postures that move from one to the next without stopping) are practiced today. Generally, however, only the first and second series are taught in class settings because the remaining four series are quite physically demanding and are only able to be practiced by those who have spent a considerable amount of time learning and accomplishing them.

Ashtanga yoga was rediscovered in the 20th century when Pattabhi Jois and his teacher Krishnamacharya worked to translate the practice they found outlined in an ancient text called the *Yoga Korunta*. In a library housing ancient texts, Krishnamacharya found the manuscript written on leaves in a form of Sanskrit that was used 5,000 years ago. The estimated date of its transcription is at minimum 1,500 years ago according to its interpreters. Pattabhi Jois called the practice *Ashtanga* because he believed it to be a lost form of yoga that was meant to accompany or append the *Yoga Sutras* by Patanjali.

Because the term *Ashtanga* either was not recognized or was misunderstood simply as raja yoga by those that did know the meaning, the term *power yoga* was in vogue for some time. Beryl Bender Birch wrote a book called *Power Yoga* that demystified the practice of Ashtanga for many, and the book serves as a great reference to the benefits of this style. Unfortunately, there is some confusion today between Ashtanga and power yoga. Ashtanga is the practice of set series of postures. Power classes generally are hybrids that use some of the postures and flow of Ashtanga, but are not true to the sequencing. In the context of this book, Ashtanga means the dynamic, set series of postures rediscovered by Pattabhi Jois and Krishnamacharya. Often a hatha class is only one hour long, or the levels of the students are so mixed that it would be impossible to go over the entire first series, so many Ashtanga yoga classes are composed of abridged versions of the original series.

In practicing either Iyengar or Ashtanga yoga one sees (and feels!) both the physical and mental differences inherent within each style. However, there is an interesting common ground between Iyengar and Ashtanga hatha yoga in that their founders, B.K.S. Iyengar and Pattabhi Jois, respectively, are contemporaries who had the same mentor, Sri Krishnamacharya. It is amazing that two styles that differ so drastically could trace back only one generation to the same root. Table 1.1 illustrates the differences in the mental focus and physical components of each style of hatha yoga.

Vinyasa Yoga

Another style of hatha yoga is the practice of linking Surya Namaskaras (Sun Salutations) or similar postures between poses. Practitioners repeat each pose in sequence before going on to the next one, and after adding each new pose, they do a vinyasa [vin-YAAH-suh] (a flowing movement, linked with the breath). The use of variations creates a flowing from pose to pose as opposed to stopping one posture and starting again. Variations of Sun Salutations are the vinyasas in Ashtanga yoga. The word *vinyasa* refers to the flow or linking together of poses.

T.K.V. Desikachar, the son of the late great Krishnamacharya who taught both Mr. Iyengar and Mr. Jois, is starting to call his style of classical-eclectic hatha "vinyoga." Mr. Desikachar is known for his emphasis on individual adaptation for therapeutic purposes and edification. Vinyasas do not have to be vigorous. They can be slow and gentle as one easy pose flows softly into another similar one.

Bikram Yoga

Once known mainly as "the yoga of the stars," this style of hatha spread throughout the United States via Beverly Hills. Bikram yoga is better known today as "Hot Yoga" because it is taught in a room kept at approximately 106 degrees Fahrenheit (41 degrees Celsius). What many people do not know is that although this style is purported to have originated with its namesake Bikram Choudhury, it actually can be traced back to Bishnu Gosh, the brother of Paramahansa Yogananda who founded the Self-Realization Fellowship in 1925. Bikram yoga has only one series consisting of 26 poses. Mr. Choudhury insists that newcomers, barring any physical limitations, come to class every day for two months before backing off their regimen. This intensity serves as an initiation and incentive

Table 1.1 Physical and Mental Comparisons of Iyengar and Ashtanga Styles of Hatha Yoga

	Class style	
	Iyengar, **founded by B.K.S. Iyengar**	**Ashtanga (power),** **founded by K. Pattabhi Jois**
Pace	Postures generally held from 30-90 seconds.	Postures are typically held for an average of 4 breaths.
Routine	No set routine. Postures often repeated with resting postures between.	Set routine. Continuous flow between postures.
Mental focus	The mind is focused on the physical form. The surrender comes from staying in the posture with great effort and attention to alignment.	The mind and body are focused on surrendering to the flow of the movement. Less attention is paid to details of alignment.
Pranayama (breathing style)	Quiet, natural	Deep, audible ujjai breath
Physical focus	Utilizing and opposing the force of gravity expands energy throughout the body and mind in the postures.	The increase in body heat, which is attained from the continuous movement between postures, allows the student to move deeper within each posture.
Name of opening posture	Tadasana (Mountain Pose)	Samasthiti (Mountain Pose)
Props	Multiple props: mats, straps, blocks, blankets, bolsters	Mats and rugs
Sun Salutations	No	Sun Salutations are the foundation for staying warm and flowing.
Partner work	No	Partner work is used to assist placement in some positions.

to this style, which promises a better body and new life through the detoxifying practice that some liken to a yoga boot camp.

Many people are leery of Bikram's extreme style. The room's heat is enhanced by the mass of body heat exuding relentlessly from the class participants as they practice one posture after another. In Ashtanga hatha, the thermal generation is created by the practitioner's own body moving through the poses linked with vigorous vinyasas; in Bikram hatha the heat originates from an artificial source. For some, the high temperature is overwhelming; yet for many the effect of the asanas done in a saunalike environment gets them hooked. Sweating alone can be very therapeutic and cleansing, but Bikram-style yoga may not be for everyone.

Kathy Lee was contacted by *Shape* magazine in 2001 to address the controversy of extreme heat in Bikram yoga. The editor expressed suspicions that this style was possibly dangerous, but she

needed some expert advice to pass along to her readers who had been inquiring about it. The editor said that enthusiasts of this method told her that the reason the temperature is turned up so high is to emulate the conditions in India. Kathy Lee explained it gets hot and humid in certain places in India during certain times of the year, but much of India is cool and has cold, harsh winters. Also, yoga was traditionally practiced outdoors or in areas with adequate ventilation instead of in stuffy rooms with closed windows and modern heating devices turned up to maximum. She explained how many people are drawn to the effects of sweating, but when students' perspiration is induced from an outside source on top of physical exercise, the situation is not right for everyone. Deconditioned students who have a tendency toward high blood pressure, or whose core body temperature tends to run high, should be very careful if they want to try this style. Some power yoga classes have adopted the routine of

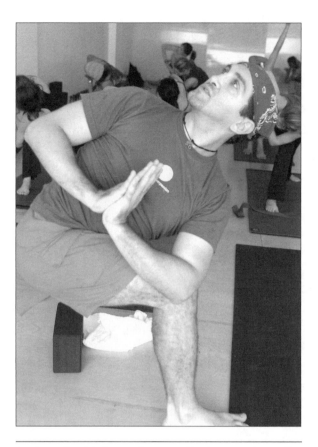

Students should choose the type of hatha yoga that will be most beneficial to their emotional and physical needs by considering the types of classes available and the environment in which they are taught.

© Levine Roberts

having the heater on in class. Many simply do not tolerate heat as well as others, and these people need to allow themselves rest periods and water breaks when they attend a class and especially when the heat is extreme.

Kundalini Hatha

Yogi Bhajan introduced a form of Sikhism to the West, and with it came a form of hatha that resembles calisthenics. Those who follow Yogi Bhajan's teachings in their entirety are the people you may have seen wearing white outfits with turbans. However, anyone can partake in the form of hatha known as Kundalini [KOOHN-duh-lee-nee]. People practicing Kundalini yoga often chant syllables and perform segments of rapid deep breathing or "breath of fire" while holding poses. It is common to practice the poses several times in a row at a fast pace of up to 108 repetitions per class or to hold certain hand gestures (mudras) for prolonged periods.

Classical-Eclectic Hatha

Together the words *classical* and *eclectic* are used to describe the generic hatha yoga that is generally taught today. Using the term *hatha* identifies this yoga as one of asana practice, and including the term *eclectic* to modify the title defines the style of hatha as blended or generic; that is, this style does not follow one strict method or consistent routine of postures. The integral yoga series as taught by Swami Sivananda and the Himalayan tradition as brought to the United States by Swami Rama belong to this category as does the style of many yoga teachers who may combine elements from various traditions and styles.

Most yoga teachers choose to teach an eclectic, or mixed, style of hatha. This method combines elements from many different styles and generally appeals to the broadest population. For example, a teacher may teach using a combination of deep breathing and background music along with attention to alignment and physical adjustments. Although one school of yoga might focus on alignment, that same school may be opposed to allowing music in class because it may be distracting (such is the case in Iyengar hatha yoga). Furthermore, a teacher's personality often colors the expression of a style, so two different teachers may present a class from the same lineage, but each class may feel completely different.

One problem in calling a yoga style *eclectic hatha* is that the term can encompass a number of different styles, and can range from gentle to vigorous. It sometimes is difficult to know what to expect if one is not familiar with the instructor. Often there is a lack of a true class description. Many brochures advertising yoga classes will list a paragraph of goals and benefits but avoid describing the style and method of the class. For example, a typical pamphlet for a class may read, "Experience the bliss of your muscles and your mind at once," or "Connect with your heart and soul for better well-being." This promise sounds great and can be a true invitation to a class; however, these words offer no hint as to how these results are achieved. The class could be a type in which the students lie on their backs resting with blankets over them the whole time almost in a sleep state (which can be highly therapeutic), or it might be a class that demands total physical challenge in a room that is kept heated over 100 degrees! Both these styles exist and offer great boons to their practitioners, but without knowing about a style by its name, reputation, or a description in a brochure, you would not know what to expect.

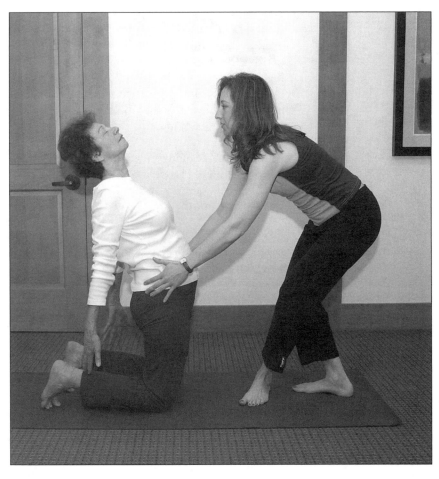

A teacher's personality can greatly influence the eclectic hatha experience.
© Dale Garvey

Classical-eclectic hatha can be found at various levels of intensity and usually has elements of the methods described earlier. For example, a Shivananda [Sheev-uhn-AAHN-duh], or integral, hatha yoga class as taught by Swami Shivananda has a nice sense of flow similar to the flow of Ashtanga classes, but postures are held longer with more resting in between (as Iyengar classes might have) and emphasis on alignment is practiced differently.

Yoga Teacher Standards

With so many different styles of hatha yoga, and each with a different emphasis on alignment, breath, and intensity, it seems impossible to develop a set of general standards for all yoga teachers. It has only been in the last few years that the Yoga Alliance (www.yogaalliance.com), an ad hoc organization of yoga instructors, formed and created standards to enable yoga teachers to be registered. These standards are generic and include all styles of yoga. The standards include a minimum of required hours in the five categories of anatomy and physiology (both gross and esoteric or energetic), philosophy, ethics, teaching methodologies, and asana practice and study. The idea of these standards is to embrace responsibility for today's diverse demands of awareness of safety issues as well as better health care and fitness while not letting go of yoga's virtuous heritage.

Many yoga instructors were skeptical that standards for yoga teachers would actually be beneficial. The fear was that standardization might make the field of teaching yoga limited to certain styles or too difficult for some people to enter into as a profession if they did not have a deep understanding of subjects such as anatomy and physiology. However, the grassroots coalition members were worried that with no set standards, no progress could be made in the status of hatha yoga and its legitimacy as a discipline. A growing number of yoga teachers had had little or no training, and veteran teachers wanted to protect the unsuspecting public from untrained teachers, superficial classes, and the possibility of injury. The Yoga Alliance now offers both the 200- and 500-hour registration level, and there is no bias

Contemporary Variations of Hatha Yoga

Classical-eclectic hatha has a growing list of specializations. The following is a brief list of some of the hybrids of classical-eclectic hatha that you can find today:

- Restorative hatha is a somewhat passive form of asana practice. This method is generally geared toward people with low energy or ability. It is appropriate for those rehabilitating from illness or injury. It is quite relaxing and therefore good for even very fit people to practice to learn how to relieve stress.

- Power hatha is a dynamic, generally flowing asana practice. Some classes mimic the postures or flow of an Ashtanga class, but rarely follow the series.

- Perinatal hatha is a practice of modified asanas for women during or after pregnancy.

- Children's hatha classes are designed specifically for children. Sometimes game playing is involved, and classes and postures are typically shorter in duration to cater to shorter attention spans.

- Chair hatha can be designed either as a corporate yoga program or as asanas adapted for those with physical challenges who are unable to move into standing postures.

- Partner hatha yoga is usually a workout done for light enjoyment. Partners can hold poses together, or one person can assist the other. Thai massage has many moves that can be practiced as partner yoga.

- Water hatha yoga is like other forms of exercise in that many asanas can be practiced in a pool.

Each type of hatha can probably be broken down further or at least overlap in styles. For example, a prenatal yoga class could consist of an Iyengar-like practice with lots of props, or it can be done in the water.

---

toward any particular style of yoga in their standards (see table 1.2 and table 1.3).

You can choose to be a registered yoga teacher and place the initials "RYT" after your name if you graduate from a school approved by the Yoga Alliance. Just as a nurse gets a diploma from an accredited school and then applies for registration as a nurse, a yoga teacher gets a diploma or certificate from an accredited school and then registers with the Yoga Alliance. The Yoga Alliance is a national registry; however, it is not against the law to teach without being registered. It is completely voluntary to be associated with them. Perhaps in the future, the education standards for yoga teachers will expand and parallel those of chiropractors and acupuncturists.

In 2003, only a few years after the inception of Yoga Alliance and the creation of initial standards, it was proposed to require continuing education hours for registered yoga teachers. To remain registered, yoga teachers must take at least 30 hours of continuing education instruction and teach a minimum of 45 hours. In 2004, more than 300 approved yoga schools and more than 8,000 instructors registered with the Alliance. Clearly, Yoga Alliance has contributed in positive ways to the professionalism of yoga teachers, and the awareness and standards of yoga classes have been raised for the benefit of teachers and the public at large.

The standards are broad, so subjects such as Sanskrit and agreed-on common names for most of the postures have been neglected. Sanskrit names of postures would be one way to preserve and honor some of the lineage of yoga (in the same way that art majors in college study art history). Also, specializations in certain types of hatha that require more knowledge or definition such as yoga therapy have yet to be addressed. Kathy Lee started a perinatal yoga committee to create some standards for registering teachers of pre- and postnatal yoga practitioners. She and her advisory board consider it important for perinatal yoga to require not only 200 to 500 hours of entry-level yoga teaching but also skills and familiarity with women's health issues in pregnancy.

Yoga itself is vast in its practice and history. Using the Sanskrit names and being familiar with the traditional and esoteric anatomy associated with yoga are some ways instructors today balance their knowledge of fitness and the postures with contemporary issues. Striving to achieve this balance allows instructors to offer a more complete mind–body education that meets Yoga Alliance standards. As the demand for hatha yoga continues to evolve, so must the qualifications of the teachers in order to keep the integrity of the growing field of yoga and all it may encompass.

Table 1.2   Yoga Alliance Hour Requirements

Category	200-hour[1] minimum required hours		500-hour[2] minimum required hours	
	Total	Contact	Total	Contact
Techniques	100	75 (50 with primary E-RYTs*)	150	100 with primary E-RYTs*
Teaching methodology	25	15 (10 with primary E-RYTs*)	30	20 with primary E-RYTs*
Anatomy and physiology	20	10	35	20
Yoga philosophy/Lifestyle and ethics for yoga teachers	30	20	60	45
Practicum	10	5 with primary E-RYTs*	40	20 (10 with primary E-RYTs*)
Electives	15		185	
Additional contact hours to be distributed among categories above to satisfy overall minimum contact hours requirements.		55		245
Total hours	200	180 (including 65 hours with primary E-RYTs*)	500	450 (including 200 hours with primary E-RYTs*, 100 of which are E-RYTs 500*)

*Primary E-RYT—In the curriculum of a RYS 200, a certain minimum numbers of contact hours must be with no more than two (2) primary E-RYTs 200 in three of the standards categories, as noted above. In a RYS 500, a certain number of contact hours in these categories must be with no more than five (5) primary E-RYTs.

*E-RYT 200 is a RYT 200 (or equivalent) who has taught yoga for at least two years and at least 1,000 hours after having met the RYT 200 standards (whether registered as a RYT 200 or not).

*E-RYT 500 is a RYT 500 (or equivalent) who has taught yoga for at least four years and at least 2,000 hours after having met the RYT standards (whether registered as a RYT or not), with at least 500 of the teaching hours after becoming a RYT 500.

*Other Faculty—In addition to the Primary Faculty, other faculty must be RYT 200s (or equivalent). Teacher trainers in Anatomy or Philosophy must have 100 hours of training or teaching experience in their respective area of expertise.

[1]Standards effective for new registrants 1/1/06; existing registrants must comply with by 1/1/07.

[2]Effective for all existing or new registrants 1/1/08. A 500 hour program is the total cumulative hours from both a 200 hour program, and 300 hours of additional advanced non-repetitive training.

© June 2005 Yoga Alliance

Adjunct Practices of Hatha Yoga

Practitioners of hatha yoga often strive to engage in lifestyle regimens of physical and mental cleanliness both on and off the mat. Although most teachers in public yoga classes do not discuss or teach much about meditation, diet specific to each body type, or philosophy, awareness of these subjects is important to yoga teachers.

Ayurveda is the medicine of ancient India and a sister science of yoga that relates to yoga lifestyle and teaching. One Ayurvedic or yoga lifestyle practice is the use of a *neti pot* [NEH-tee], which is a device used to wash the nasal passages as part of a daily ritual like brushing your teeth. Another level of yoga lifestyle practice is to discover ways to incorporate principles of the *Yoga Sutras* (in whole or part of the eight limbs) or insights from your asana sessions into the rest of your daily life. Yoga is a discipline without dogma, so every person will have different ways of incorporating aspects of their yoga practice in their daily life. Simply being more flexible in mind as well as body is one way. Strengthening your will power along with your muscles is another.

Table 1.3   Yoga Alliance Standards

Standards category	Definition
Techniques	Includes asanas, pranayamas, kriyas, chanting, mantra, meditation, and other traditional yoga techniques. These hours must be a mix between (1) analytical training in how to teach and practice the techniques, and (2) guided practice of the techniques themselves; both areas must receive substantial emphasis
Teaching methodology	Includes principles of demonstration, observation, assisting/correcting, instruction, teaching styles, qualities of a teacher, the student's process of learning, and business aspects of teaching yoga.
Anatomy and physiology	Includes both human physical anatomy and physiology (bodily systems, organs, etc.) and energy anatomy and physiology (chakras, nadis, etc.). Includes both the study of the subject and application of its principles to yoga practice (benefits, contraindications, healthy movement patterns, etc).
Yoga philosophy/ Lifestyle and ethics for yoga teachers	Includes the study of yoga philosophies, yoga lifestyle, and ethics for yoga teachers.
Practicum	Includes practice teaching, receiving feedback, observing others teaching and hearing/ giving feedback. Also includes assisting students while someone else is teaching.
Electives	Hours to be distributed among the categories above according to the school's chosen emphasis.

© June 2005 Yoga Alliance

Study Questions

1. Approximately how old is yoga?
2. How would you define yoga in just a few sentences?
3. What are the four main types of yoga, and of which type is hatha yoga?
4. What is Ashtanga yoga?
5. How did Patanjali codify yoga practice in 200 to 300 B.C.?
6. What well-known type of hatha yoga focuses on alignment, form, and the use of props?
7. What are some of the most popular styles of hatha yoga practiced today?
8. What are some issues facing modern yoga practitioners, and what are some of the ways the needs of today's students and teachers are being met?
9. What are the five categories outlined by Yoga Alliance?
10. Bonus question: Explain the meanings of the words yamas, niyamas, and neti pot.

chapter 2

Knowing Yourself and Your Students

It can be challenging to teach anything to people, but in yoga especially instructors have to take into account the bodies, minds, and emotions of their students as individuals as well as a group. Some days it may seem easier teaching yoga to a dog than to a group of diverse people! Dogs do not care if you have charisma, what you wear, if you are in good physical condition, or if you practice what you teach. People generally expect all of this and more from their yoga instructors.

Teaching yoga embodies the ancient tradition of master and pupil while meeting the complex expectations, agendas, and reactions of a modern, materialistic, and often competitive society. Awareness of your teaching inclinations and the learning styles of your students is the key factor in facilitating a successful class. To expand the potential skills of your students, you as a teacher first need to examine your perceptions

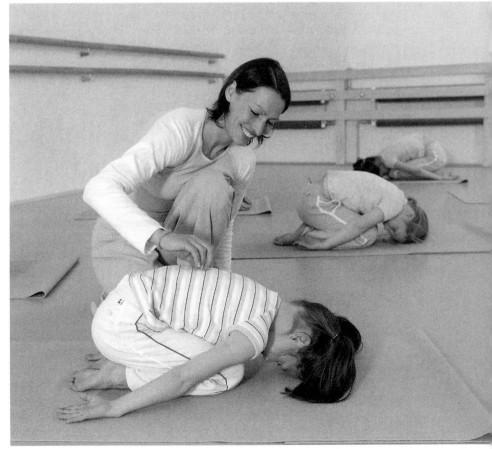

© Jumpfoto

of yourself as an example and mentor to others. It is best to explore your own moral compass and motives to gain the most understanding, tolerance, and compassion for your students. Without a balance of service and reward, which is very subjective, you will surely experience burnout.

This chapter highlights some of the most important qualities necessary for successful yoga teachers. The importance of building trust and rapport with your students is discussed. Information on how to optimize your students' yoga experience based on their learning styles is covered in this chapter, along with a listing of traits students like and dislike about instructors. This information is provided so you can recognize and expand the capacity of your students and yourself.

Often Yoga Teacher Training (YTT) programs require that you have a solid background of practicing yoga in earnest for at least one, but generally more, years before you are allowed to study how to teach. Not only does a solid practice of your own give you tremendous insight into the asanas, but also you truly appreciate the residual calm and confidence you acquire from practice during those times when you are too busy teaching to take a yoga class for yourself. Reading and applying the information contained within this book are a means to accelerate gaining wisdom that might otherwise take many years to realize. Even if you are new to yoga you can evaluate your readiness, willingness, and ability to begin teaching by reading this chapter. To help you introspect and give you thoughts to ponder as you read this chapter, and the book as a whole, we have provided a Self-Inquiry Questionnaire, located in appendix C.

Qualities of a Yoga Teacher

So, what does it take to teach people yoga, and do you have it? First, you may be relieved to know that you do not have to be able to put your foot behind your head to be a good yoga teacher. However, you do need to look deeply to find the qualities within yourself that you can use to build trust and instill confidence in your students. These qualities will also allow you to demonstrate that you have the knowledge and experience to guide students through your class. This is true for veteran as well as novice instructors.

The main responsibility of a yoga teacher is to help people "remember" themselves as they travel the path of self-awareness—to help them become whole again. As young children we explored our bodies and tested

our boundaries. Unfortunately, as adults we generally forget the joys and challenges of that exploration. People often do not pay any attention to their bodies, other than superficially critiquing them, unless they are feeling intense pain. Even athletes tend to focus on the performance of their bodies rather than the associated sensations, and they sometimes play through pain to win an event.

After years of being disassociated from bodily awareness it is not easy for people to perceive a sensation that is not painful enough to grab their attention. It is as if their mental muscles are atrophied. People who are used to paying attention to their bodies only when they can no longer ignore the pain have an atrophy of awareness. Your job is to guide them back to that awareness. Do not expect, however, to stand up in front of a group of complete strangers and miraculously send them on a path to bliss. You first need to open your heart to them and allow their hearts to open to you. To gain or enhance your ability to guide your students to their own awareness remember the four Cs of teaching yoga: connection, compassion, confidence, and commitment.

Connection

Think back on the most joyous learning you experienced with the help of a mentor. Most likely, part of the joy you felt was due to the strong connection you felt with your instructor, realizing that she or he understood you and knew just the right way to guide you to your new understanding. There was a meaningful connection between the two of you. That link of understanding created a bond of trust. As an instructor, you want to create the same connection with your students so that they are active participants in learning.

One of the simplest ways to connect with your students is to ask their names. Knowing a student's name builds rapport and lets the student know you care about her as a person. As you get to know how a student's body moves and she feels more comfortable around you, you automatically increase her sense of well-being. This connection builds trust and understanding. The more a student trusts you, the more she will follow your instructions to listen to her body instead of listening to her mental chatter.

A skilled yoga teacher directs each student to take as much responsibility for himself during class as possible. By instructing students to avoid going into a posture or to come out of a posture if they find that it hurts, you empower them and invite them to

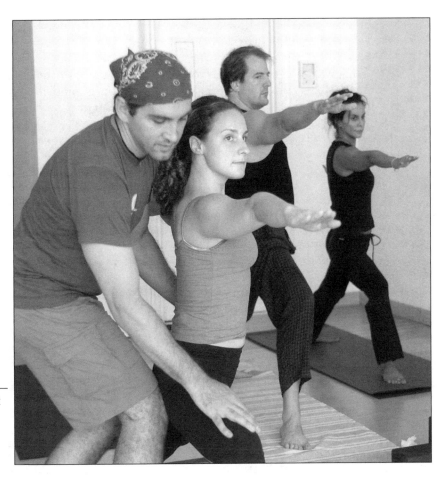

Show students that you care about them reaching their individual potential by not emphasizing that their pose is "wrong."

© Levine Roberts

explore their bodies and minds on a deeper level. By asking students how they feel in their postures, where they feel strength, weakness, tightness, or fatigue, you help them connect to their inner teacher. This inner knowledge allows them to find and expand the edge of their awareness.

In 1998, Kathy Lee was a delegate at the International Yoga Conference held in Rishikesh, India. While there she asked Swami Veda Bharati of his opinion as a traditional swami what he perceived the requirements of a yoga teacher should be in today's world. He spoke about connection and the importance of each teacher's ability to facilitate a change in the consciousness of their students. The renowned scholar and spiritual master explained that a good yoga teacher is someone who, just by his or her presence and manner, can soothe another person. He said that he worries about the hours of training focusing on the exercise and fitness aspects of asanas and wonders if this concentration perpetuates the art of yoga teaching. He questioned whether the essence of yoga itself might be lost. He said he felt that some yoga schools have lost sight of yoga's vast lineage. He wants the legacy of yoga to be protected,

and he fears that the greatest benefits of yoga will be buried if teachers do not pay attention to its roots as they endeavor to become leaf sprouts on the living tree of yoga.

With practice, the wisdom and skill of yoga science flows through you into your students. At times you may hear words coming out of your mouth and not know consciously where they came from or how you knew what to say. This experience is your reconnecting to the vast source of yoga knowledge.

Compassion

It is essential when teaching to express the compassion you have for yourself and for your students. Your heart center (the *anahata* chakra [uh-nuh-HUT-uh CHUK-ruh]) is the place compassion resides. It is an expression of your passion to nurture and provide care to others.

T.K.V. Desikachar addressed many issues to contemplate as part of the path of a yoga teacher in a book he wrote about his father, Krishnamacharya, a renowned master yoga teacher. He explained,

The qualities we seek in a teacher are a life devoted to practice: evidence that he or she, too, is ever a student of yoga; a nature that is always truthful; a commitment to the student's own awareness and possibilities, each in his own terms. And caring—above all, caring. When people arrive . . . and ask us, "Can you help me?" the only answer we can give is "I can care." (Desikachar, 1999)

Show your students that you care about them by choosing your words and actions thoughtfully. Be sure you really know what you are saying and what exactly it means. For example, some yoga teachers seem to go around correcting their students with adjustments. If you apply adjustments with the attitude that you have been given the opportunity to assist students as they experience a deeper, more relaxed posture, you provide them with an act of kindness and coaching. If you use the word *correct*, then you imply to some students that they are doing something wrong. There is no such thing as perfection. And because there should be no competition within your class, it is more thoughtful to explain to your students that if you physically adjust them it does not mean they are doing anything wrong, and, conversely, if you do not touch them that does not mean that that they have reached perfection.

In addition to caring for your students, you also must have compassion for yourself and realize that you will not have all the answers to all the questions students will ask. Yoga is too vast a field to master quickly or completely. Recognize that your teaching style will not appeal to everyone, and do not take it personally if a student finds another instructor.

Have compassion for your body and life, recognizing that they may not be perfect. This will help you relate to and help students who experience many of the same struggles you do. Keep in mind that some of the best teachers are those who have worked through physical or emotional problems; the understanding of their own problems gives them a deeper insight into their students' struggles. If asanas come easily to you then it may be difficult to work with others who have trouble understanding the postures in the beginning. When you can empathize with and nurture your students, you become a source of connection, caring, and compassion.

Confidence

It is normal to feel nervous when you are teaching, especially in a new setting or when teaching a new style. However, if you do not exude some semblance of confidence, your students will have difficulty trusting or believing in you and possibly in the benefits of practicing yoga. Even new teachers can seem extraordinary if they stick to what they know and have complete confidence in their ability to do so. Tap into the well of knowledge you have created for yourself, and your passion will shine through.

An example of how confidence can lead you through new situations successfully is illustrated by Judith Lasater, now an accomplished leader in the field of yoga in the United States. She explained that when she first taught it was because the teacher she had been studying with needed a substitute. She recalled that although she was not sure what to do, she did not want to let the class down, so she led the class through some poses and kept saying, "If it hurts, don't do it." Theoretically, you can lead a nice, relaxing yoga class just by constantly saying, "Breathe. If it hurts, don't do it. Relax. Breathe." It is possible to have a humble beginning unfold into a calling and new career. No matter what, it is crucial to maintain your humbleness.

Real confidence is not arrogance, nor is it rooted in ignorance. Confidence is part of your personal power or ego strength and might be felt in your third chakra (the *manipura* [muhn EE-poor-uh] chakra, or the solar plexus center). Being confident does not mean having a closed mind. In fact, the more confident you are in your teaching, the less you will be threatened by others who may criticize, teach differently, or appear to be more successful commercially. You need to be confident to speak clearly and loudly in front of a group. It is also important to assert yourself while not coming across as overly aggressive. Believing in yourself and your abilities gives you that confidence.

Sometimes self-doubt can creep into your psyche. Do not worry or allow yourself to think that students are coming to your class only because it is inexpensive, is close to their house, or takes place during a convenient time. Rest assured that people will not come to your class if they do not think you are good, even if you live right next door! For yourself, be the person you would like to take a class from, and for your students, be the yoga teacher they need.

Also, be sure to continually help build up your students. Encourage them throughout class, and let them know when you have seen changes in them since they began practicing with you. This builds their confidence level and gives them a feeling of self-satisfaction.

Commitment

Always take time to reflect on the scope of your knowledge and ability as an instructor. This strengthens your integrity not only as an instructor but also as a caring, compassionate human being. Regardless of your innate teaching ability, you still must know the information you are teaching well. For some, acquiring the information is the easy part, whereas learning how to impart that information is more sophisticated. Exploring your own body and its physical and mental boundaries helps you better understand the bodies and psyches of an entire class. If you are sincere and honest, then all of this is possible, regardless of where you begin.

If you commit yourself to being the best teacher you possibly can be, you will consistently look for ways to improve yourself. Stay open to learning new ways of teaching and gaining new ideas. Be the proverbial student so that you can share all of your newfound knowledge with your students. One of the most important things to keep in mind as you travel the path of a yoga instructor is that you must always keep your mind open to learning, even as you pass knowledge along to your students. Georg Feuerstein, a renowned yoga scholar, states that "Even when, after due preparation, we are called to teach others, we would be wise to remain learners—or, in traditional terms, to cultivate 'beginner's mind'...we stop growing when we think there is nothing more to learn" (Feuerstein, 37).

Becoming a Yoga Teacher

Some people begin teaching yoga because they have practiced the discipline for some time, feel that yoga has changed their lives in some meaningful way, and wish to share this gift with others. They want to be a link in the long lineage of ancient wisdom and dispense the knowledge to their students. Many in the fitness industry have discovered that practicing yoga is gentler to the body; teaching yoga has a far gentler impact on the joints, muscles, voice, and even the feet than teaching an aerobics, spin, kickboxing, or water workout. For many, teaching yoga keeps them connected to students but allows them to give their own bodies a respite from high-intensity work. And although you should not plan to get more workouts in by teaching yoga, you might be happy to find your stress suspended as you focus fully on your class. The work of your heart, head, and hands gets stronger through teaching. A well-taught class can be a peak experience not only for your students but also for you.

Long ago in India, yoga teachers never charged a fee for their services. It was considered sacrilegious to do so because teaching was considered a calling, not a job. In today's world economy there is no escaping the fact that yoga has become a fitness commodity. Unless you are officially volunteering your teaching hours, you do need to be paid. If money is your primary motivation for teaching yoga, then you either have the unusual circumstance of having a wealthy and generous client or you are sadly mistaken. However, most teachers of yoga find the satisfaction of teaching outweighs financial concerns.

Regardless of why you want to teach yoga, the important thing is that you teach well and help your students relax their minds and expand their spirits, all while protecting their bodies from physical injury. By continually focusing on your reasons and motivations for teaching, you allow yourself the space to change and grow. Remember that your greatest teachers are your own practice and your experiences with your students. Keeping these connections at the forefront of your mind brings the meaning and purpose of yoga to life within you. Both the Self-Inquiry and Yoga Class Evaluation forms in appendix C should be used on a regular basis to guide the exploration of your own yoga practice and teaching.

Education

No matter how long you have studied and practiced yoga, you can always gain deeper knowledge and insight. Retain a beginner's mind-set, and stay open to new experiences. Take classes and workshops. Doing so not only opens you to new ways of thinking, but also it keeps you energized. Interacting with other instructors as peers and as a student is rejuvenating. Use the unique and comprehensive Yoga Class Evaluation form in appendix C to evaluate your class or another teacher's approach.

Depending on your schedule, it may seem impossible for you to find the time to attend other yoga classes. However, the more you attend classes taught by others, the better off both you and your students will be. Find a good teacher who motivates you and whose class enables you to feel comfortably challenged. Try to attend these classes an average of eight hours a month, and you will be a solid example to your students. Students enjoy seeing their own instructors in other classes they attend. Again, this is a good example of practicing what you preach. If you are a new yoga teacher it is imperative that you take others' classes. If you have been teaching yoga for some time, then you might try taking a one-hour class for every 10 to 20 hours you teach.

If you are a novice instructor and cannot find the time to attend classes yourself, practicing with a video

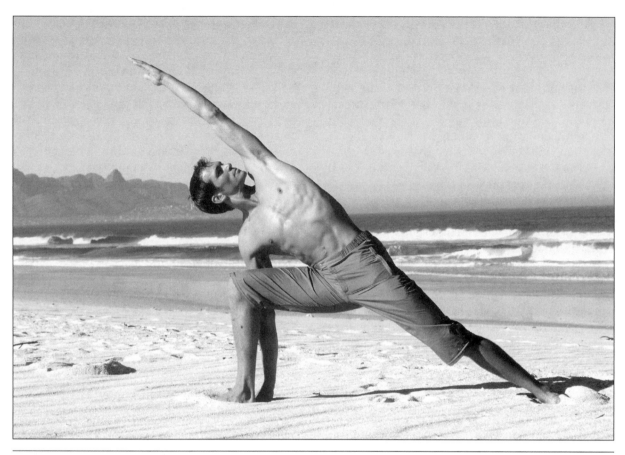

Although you may teach your class in one way, your personal practice can still reflect your own motives for wanting to participate in yoga.

© Jumpfoto

is the next best thing. You can get a taste of some well-known instructors by watching and working out with one of their videos. Although you cannot get the same feedback and teaching tailored to your needs from a video that a live instructor provides, a good video can be replayed and studied or simply enjoyed as a mini retreat from your daily grind. One student remarked that when he is tired and stressed from work he uses *30 Minute Basic Home Yoga Workout With Kathy Lee* because he finds the scenery and Kathy Lee's voice to be very relaxing.

The excitement and energy of a conference or workshop can be inspiring, and these experiences expose you to the latest trends in yoga. The more you can remain abreast of fads, research, and news that you can share with your students, the better you serve their needs and yours. Attending a conference or workshop is a good way for teachers to avoid a rut or burnout. If you go to a workshop, ask yourself how the information and experience will contribute to both your personal practice and your teaching. Usually if your personal practice is uplifted, so is your teaching.

One last caveat on education: If you have not yet studied how to provide hands-on adjustments safely, it is best not to do them until you have. Seek out the education and experience you need and in the meantime, be careful with your students as you make doing no harm (ahimsa [uh-HEEM-saah]) your top priority.

Your Personal Practice

In addition to continuing to gain knowledge through classes and workshops, it is important to have a regular, personal yoga practice so you gain firsthand experience of the benefits of yoga practice. You are an example to your students when you practice what you preach and can honestly share with students how yoga has had a positive influence on your own life. Students feel reassured when you tell them you once struggled with a posture yourself and discovered, as they will after consistent practice, that it does get easier. When students look at you as a work in progress they have more faith that they will advance in their practice as well.

Nothing can replace the wisdom you gain from the consistency of applied awareness over time. As you teach you may see yourself in some of your students, which can make it easier to explain certain aspects of an asana to them. As you answer their questions you increase your understanding of that asana as well. When you practice asanas at home, you gain insight into how to instruct an aspect of that position to others. For example, if you have tight hips and are practicing yoga sincerely, then you will become an expert on tight hips and how to work with them.

Reflect on your personal motives for practicing yoga so that when you teach you can relate honestly to your students. Learning about yourself gives you insight into the struggles and joys your students experience as you guide them through a class. You may end up teaching asanas very differently from the way you practice them. It is absolutely okay to teach a vigorous yoga class and enjoy a much gentler practice at home. No doubt there are many music teachers who teach pop music to students yet prefer to play jazz when they practice at home.

One thing people may not realize is that teaching yoga does often take away from one's own practice. As in teaching any subject or activity, gaining the knowledge and competency to teach and preparing for and facilitating classes requires a great deal of time and energy. It is important that you decide what teaching yoga is worth to you, and balance that with what you believe your personal time is worth. Unless you are a famous teacher, or you own a very popular yoga center, yoga instruction generally is a part-time job that does not reap many monetary benefits yet does bestow great karmic boons such as satisfaction in watching others heal and grow through yoga.

Ethics

As with any occupation in which one deals directly with the public, yoga instructors must follow certain guidelines, which protect students as well as instructors. The *Yoga Sutras* list *ahimsa* (nonharm) as the very first *yama* [YUH-muh] (social restraint) in the foundational limb of all of yoga. As a yoga instructor, your primary duty is to do no harm to any student.

Currently, no laws have been passed regarding behavioral interactions between yoga teachers and their students. However, many schools follow the same basic code of professional ethics that the California Yoga Teachers Association created, which state, "All forms of sexual behavior or harassment with students are unethical, even when a student invites or consents to such behavior and involvement" (www.yogateachersassoc.org).

Although Yoga Alliance has only been in existence since 1999, it has established some basic educational guidelines. One of its most current concerns is adopting an ethical standard for yoga teachers, according to Sandra Van Oosten, RYT, the executive director. In 2004, one of the hottest topics being explored was the need for a national code of conduct for yoga teachers. In a survey of *Yoga Journal* readers, 73 percent of 300 people said that they felt such a code would serve to protect both students and teachers (Barrett, 2004).

Having tea after class can be harmless, even healthy, but dating a student is definitely considered unethical. Where you draw the line of extending yourself socially or even professionally outside of class with your students is a tough call because you do not want to jeopardize the student–teacher relationship. It is very risky to blindly agree to spend time with a student alone in a nonyoga-related venture. Best friends have been known to part ways after taking a trip together or lending money to one another. It is in no one's best interest to risk the student–teacher relationship. However, if someone in your class is destined to be your best friend it will unfold in time.

One risk of having a close, personal relationship with a student is that if a student is aware of your personal issues she might have a hard time just being your student during class. She may see you and think of her friend instead of being totally present for herself during class. The student may even disagree with the way you handle a personal issue and then start thinking you do not know what you are doing in any area of your life including teaching yoga. It is a very precarious balance between being a person with faults (like everybody else) and being an authority figure who can help others. It is important therefore to strike a balance between your private and professional life.

If you feel sincerely drawn to become more intimately involved with a student, then it is best that you not continue to be that student's teacher. If the personal relationship is moving along well after a number of months, you both may feel comfortable to have the person in your class again. Keep in mind that yoga is not about being black and white with issues or guidelines, and, of course, there are always exceptions to rules. However, always be mindful of the very real and serious risks you as a yoga teacher are open to if you see students on a more than casual basis.

Discovering Your Teaching Style

When you stand in front of a room of yoga students you may feel like a performer. You may even get into a character or take on another persona when you teach. Your public teaching persona might be much different from the person you are when you are not teaching. There is nothing wrong with "acting" as you teach. The most important part of teaching is being a channel for knowledge to flow through you as you connect it to receptive students; all teachers need to find the most comfortable way to express themselves. You may slip in a little humor or some storytelling to get and keep the students tuned in; just remember that teaching is your top priority. Your purpose is to train, not entertain. If, however, you happen to mix in some entertainment as a part of stimulating some enlightenment, by all means, do it. Entertain students only as a means of enhancing their yoga education, not overshadowing it.

Keep in mind that the lessons of practicing yoga should be in the metaphysical spotlight. Even if you have a physical stage from which to teach, with the students on the floor below you, you yourself are never the actual spotlight. Rather, you shine the light on yoga, which is illuminated from within the student as much as possible.

Besides appealing to a plethora of learning persuasions and intelligences stay aware that at any given moment students may get distracted and allow their minds to focus elsewhere. If you pay close attention you can reel their attention back to your instruction by facilitating what is called a *state change*. When students appear not to listen or respond it may be because their attention span is short, your voice is monotone, or they are distracted and bored. If you suddenly, yet subtly, raise or lower your voice, walk around the room, change the pace, or alter the tone of your voice a few notches you can usually lure their attention back on track again.

Not only do you have to appeal to a broad range of learning styles and abilities, but also you must charm your class enough with the qualities they believe you should have to keep their interest. From our experience in teaching yoga in many different settings, we have composed a table of what students like and dislike about their yoga instructors (see table 2.1).

Recognizing Your Students' Needs

People come to yoga class for many different reasons. If you have 25 students in your class, most likely they will have 25 different reasons and motivations

Table 2.1   Yoga Instructor Characteristics As Enjoyed by Students

Like	Dislike
Has an engaging, nurturing personality	Seems uninterested in getting to know the students
Facilitates a feeling of "oneness" for the entire class	Is aloof or arrogant toward students
Asks students for their input before class	Has low energy or complains often
Has honest rapport with students	Uses negative words during class
Asks students' permission before giving adjustments	Dresses inappropriately; sloppy or too revealing
Exudes a positive attitude and energy	Voice is too loud or too soft
Does not share too much personal information	Is late for class or uses substitutes too often
Gives clear instructions with cues that are motivating	Uses inappropriate music for the style of class being taught
If music is used, it is appropriate to the style of class	Stops the flow of class too often
Classes have a smooth flow	Focuses too much attention on only one or two students in class
Give challenging, yet inclusive workouts	Instructs advanced asanas when it is apparent students are unable to follow
Is organized and professional	Does not provide modifications for those who need them
Has appropriate energy level for style of class	Stands in one spot, or looks at self in the mirror too often
Moves through students during class	Gives adjustments in a rough or inappropriate manner

for being there. Many of these reasons will overlap from student to student. Stress reduction, increased flexibility, and relaxation are but a few goals, and these can change from class session to class session for the same student.

Some people have some hidden agendas as to what motivates them to practice yoga. All the reasons do not have to be noble ones. If a person is motivated to practice yoga to look better, for example, that motivation is far better than not practicing yoga at all.

Sometimes people show up for yoga classes who would not dare show up in a spin or kickboxing class. An older woman with severe osteoporosis, a middle-aged man with a low back injury, a young pregnant woman—any or all of these people might be in your class. You might not be able to teach more than a few simple postures and a breathing technique, but if you do so with a soothing voice or an inspiring quote your students may leave feeling more serene than when they came.

Ask students to express their goals. Why have they come to class? Is it for stress reduction, to gain strength or flexibility, to get away from the everyday aspects of life? What do they expect to gain from their time with you? Many instructors ask their students if they have a particular area of the body that needs extra attention and structure their class to accommodate the requests.

People usually feel euphoric after a yoga class, but every once in a while emotions other than bliss surface during a class, especially during Shavasana [shuh-VAAH-suh-nuh] (Corpse Pose), the resting portion of a practice session. Many people, in their attempt to escape pain and discomfort, keep themselves busy to put off feeling the distress. Sometimes when the mind gets a chance to truly relax, emotions that were suppressed surface. Your job as the yoga teacher is to offer a safe and peaceful space for all your students.

You can empathize with your students without even saying a word. Once students begin Shavasana they should rarely be disturbed because this is their personal, private time. However, if students need your assistance you need to be there when they ask. You can reassure them that feeling emotional is not an abnormal response when practicing yoga. Let them know that sometimes part of the mental and emotional balancing process releases stored-up energy such as sadness. Reassure them that crying is a normal process of the body relieving itself. Think of it as passing gas. If something needs to be released, it needs to be released. It is unhealthy to suppress it. If a student passes gas during class you would not

call attention to it. Passing tears is another kind of gentle release in yoga.

The only caveat about dealing with an emotional student is to be careful not to take on the role of counselor. Your time with your students should not extend more than 10 minutes beyond the end of class, if that. Boundaries are important as a professional teacher. If students want to ask you a quick question, then, if you are inclined, spend a few minutes before or after class to answer them. But if the same student keeps asking you numerous questions about how he should be practicing at home, which poses are best for him and his condition, or other concerns, you should tell the student what your hourly rate is or refer him to someone else. Unless you are a professional counselor, you should direct students elsewhere for support if they ask for advice about personal issues.

As a yoga teacher you are like a parent to your students. You are a sponsor, an advocate, and a coach; maybe part friend and part drill sergeant; and a symbol of someone who can guide others to the next level of their personal awareness. Because you took the journey yourself, you understand how to guide your students along their path.

Learning Styles You Will Encounter

Just as each student has her own reasons for attending yoga classes, each person also has an individual style and capacity for learning. Many types of learning styles can exist in each person in varying degrees. Your objective is to develop your "teaching intelligence" as much as possible while utilizing the learning styles of your students for their edification.

There are three fundamental types of learning styles: visual, auditory, and kinesthetic. Visual learners need to see what they are being taught. By the same token, auditory learners conceptualize learning through hearing. Kinesthetic learners learn best through means of touch and movement. Keep in mind, however, that there are few, if any, people who learn solely with one approach. Many cues you use will overlap words, images, and touch so that your instruction can be more universal. You should use visual and verbal cues in addition to directing students' awareness to where they feel the posture in their bodies. Engaging all three of the basic learning styles allows all of your students to receive instruction in the way they can most easily understand.

Visual Learners

Students who are visual learners prefer that the instructor demonstrate poses. They also respond well to verbal cues that create imagery in their minds. For example, an appropriate cue for a visual learner might be "Imagine there is a wall behind you as you are standing in Triangle Pose, and you are becoming more flush with that wall as you press your body back." Visual learners appreciate looking at photographs of poses or handouts with illustrations. One disadvantage for visual learners is that they tend not to feel their own bodies in the asana. They have an organic need to see how to be in the pose; therefore, these learners sometimes experience a gap in feedback if you do not provide them with some visual reference. When instructing them to lower their shoulders down from their ears it is a good idea to have them peek in the mirror to see their raised shoulders first. Otherwise, they might have trouble truly grasping what you mean. Visual learners may be able to imagine and respond to such an instruction, but they usually have a learning curve to overcome when they cannot see their own backs.

Auditory Learners

Auditory learners pick up information by listening. Where visual people read music to play a song, for example, people who can play a tune after hearing it are good auditory learners. These people are receptive to good verbal cues. They learn from your words and may quickly be able to practice at home as they hear your words in their heads. If you have a nice soothing teaching voice then students often will imagine hearing your voice in their heads at home.

Invite auditory learners to close their eyes and listen to what their body says to them as they move deeper into an asana. As you move students through class, tell them the specific areas of their bodies to focus on and the types of sensations they should expect to feel.

Kinesthetic Learners

Kinesthetic learners can more easily feel places in their body that cannot be seen from the outside. They might not be sure, however, of what or where they are supposed to feel something while in an asana. To reach these learners, direct them to places to pay attention in their bodies and to notice what they feel there. In Adho Mukha Shvanasana (Downward-Facing Dog), direct the students to notice the weight of their heads stretching their spines longer and creating space between their vertebrae. The kinesthetic learner does not derive a learning connection so much from demonstration or sight but more from experiencing the posture in their own bodies, that is, feeling the sensations of their body as it moves through space.

The kinesthetic learner can more directly understand how to adjust the asana sooner because he feels the changes in his body more readily. Such learners also typically enjoy hands-on adjustments, as they are able to learn how to align more correctly based on the sensations they feel. A kinesthetic learner might have some trouble initially with a verbal direction, such as, "breathe into your lower back." But if you were to lightly place your hand on the student's lower back and tell the student to breathe into your hands, the kinesthetic learner will usually connect to the cue. You will feel the student's lower back relax and gently expand with the inhalation.

Ayurvedic Humors

Another factor in how people learn has to do with their basic dispositions. In Ayurveda [AAH-yoor-veh-duh], a holistic medical system that has been practiced in India for many centuries and a sister science to yoga, there are three basic humors, called *doshas* [DOH-shus]. Each dosha emphasizes a particular way of learning and processing information. The three doshas are *vata* [VAAH-tuh], *pitta* [PIT-tuh], and *kapha* [KUP-huh]. Everyone has all three humors but in various combinations and ratios.

The doshas are made up of the five elements: Earth, Water, Fire, Air, and Ether (sometimes referred to as Space). Vata individuals relate to the Air and Ether elements. These individuals tend to have an airy or "spacey" quality about them and are the people that can be described as "having their heads in the clouds." If a student has a mostly vata constitution, he may be easily distracted. He may seem to grasp a concept right away, such as lifting the kneecaps, but moments later will forget all about it. Repeating your directions numerous times can be helpful to such students.

Pitta people have the Fire energy or element in their humor. They tend to heat up faster than individuals with vata or kapha constitutions. Pitta students tend to stay very present and focused on their tasks. Vata learners ask questions just for the sake of exploring information, whereas pitta students gather facts with a particular goal in mind.

The kapha dosha is made up of Earth and Water. As students they may be less quick to grasp information, but once they understand a lesson they tend to remember it well. The Earth element is practically the opposite of the Air energy. Vata people can be seen fluttering around nonstop, maybe socializing with other students before and after class, whereas the kapha student is content to lie down on her mat and not stir until the teacher gives the command to begin class.

There is significantly more to the doshas than the basic behaviors and learning styles, but for purposes of teaching yoga this brief introduction is sufficient. A student can have a primary dosha that is really evident, but many times people are a combination of types. This is true of the three basic styles of learning as well. A student might learn well both visually and by auditory means, while having plenty of pitta and kapha energy. Considering that people are combinations of many variables that affect their learning process, it is clear you need to employ teaching techniques that will appeal to the three types of learners and doshas. Use table 2.2 as a guide to matching learning styles with specific teaching methods.

Classroom Management

When you teach yoga you are a channel of ancient knowledge, imparting what you know to each of your students on a level to which they can relate. You are the authority, and it is important to maintain control over your class. It is crucial, however, to temper that authority with humbleness and a realization that not every student in your class will be able to connect with you. If students start talking or people not taking your class come in and start

making noise, it is up to you to be a peace officer by asking them to be quiet. Always apply whatever rules you have equally.

Some teachers lock the door after class has begun so tardy students will not disturb the class. However, this practice is uncommon in today's hectic world. In any case, instructors cannot stop the class and make everyone wait while attending to a new or late-arriving student. Nevertheless, you do not want to incur the possible liability of the new student who does not know enough to warm up on his own and instead jumps into whatever posture the class is practicing at the moment. What many teachers do in this situation is have the class hold a pose and then attend to the new students, working with them a few moments at a time until they catch up to the rest of the group.

Part of a yoga class is not letting others distract you, and another part is not contributing to the distraction of others. Take time to explain to your students that if they come late it is disrespectful to the entire class. Try to explain this in a non-conspicuous manner so as not to bring more attention to the tardy students and disrupt the rest of the class.

Because the warm-up and resting periods are vital to the class, explain to students that if they come late they need to do a warm-up on their own. Surya Namaskara (Sun Salutation) is a good warm-up, as are most standing poses; if they leave early they need to rest in Shavasana on their own before they leave. You may wish to have a policy about being tardy and leaving early. The policy depends on where you work and the population you teach. Ideally, everyone should be there for the start and end of class, but it

Table 2.2   Learning Styles and Teaching Methods

Learning styles and Ayurvedic humors	Learning tendencies	How to best teach
Visual	Look up often, which frequently takes them off task and out of position	Physically demonstrate postures, and provide verbal imagery.
Auditory	Often feel lost when no verbal instructions are given	Give many and varied verbal cues. Use non-distracting background music.
Kinesthetic	Need to become familiar with the movement and flow of a posture to feel the effects	Provide hands-on adjustments, and remind them to breathe.
Vata	Fast, conceptual learners but quick to forget and easily distracted	Provide structure to keep their attention focused.
Pitta	Intensely focused and may be intolerant of high temperatures and teachers exuding a lack of confidence	Provide detailed descriptions, and answer questions with references.
Kapha	Slow, patient learners with good retention; can lack drive	Provide motivational feedback often.

would be prudent of you to prepare to deal with tardy and even intrusive people.

At one time or another you may have a student in your class who in some way adversely affects other members of the class. If it is a simple matter of a student wearing copious amounts of perfume (or cologne), then the solution is to ask the student to refrain from wearing scent as some students are highly sensitive to perfumes. Resolution is not as easy if a student makes inappropriate remarks, harasses other students, or constantly talks during class. In any case your responsibility is to communicate with compassion but in a way that gets the message across clearly what behaviors need to change.

You cannot always prevent hurt feelings because you cannot control someone else's emotions. To prevent hurt feelings, speak in terms of facts, not judgments. Just as a parent must sometimes say no to a child, you have to enforce certain boundaries with students. As with any position of authority, be consistent so your students know what to expect from you and the class as a whole. How strictly you control your class depends on the style of yoga taught and the people you are teaching. Although yoga has a long history steeped in tradition, it also is a living art, which means it is adaptable and constantly evolving.

Relating Information

The learning process of your students is dependent on how you deliver and relate information to them. If you are not a good conduit of yoga information, students will have difficulty learning from you. Table 2.3 serves as a checklist of things to remember to teach students well using the letters of the word *asana* as an acronym for good teaching methods: ahimsa (and ask), suggest, align, nurture, assess.

Ahimsa (and ask): Ahimsa is the practice of nonharming. Your first duty as an instructor and human being is to avoid physical or emotional injury of others at all times. Protect your students' well-being by adhering to ethical standards of honesty and good conduct. Be trustworthy as you build rapport. *Ask* permission before you touch your students, and inquire what they need from you. In addition, show compassion to yourself. Be mindful of your own body mechanics when you adjust a student, and be aware of your workload to prevent teacher burnout. Take care of yourself by setting boundaries, and make time to practice yoga on your own.

Suggest: Encourage students to take your instructions as suggestions. Invite them to explore how these suggestions affect them as they listen to their body to see if they need a rest or modification. Deliver each instruction with humble authority, compassion, and confidence. Working with a number of people of varying physical conditions and training at once demands that you give relative instructions. Even if you have only one student, or if you are teaching yourself, be open to the possibility that at any time a modification may be in order. Sometimes a student cannot muster the strength or focus to be in the posture everyone else seems to engage in easily. Because some people do not give themselves permission to be noncompetitive you need to remind them that everything but breathing is optional in yoga class. Remind them that the class is all about them as individuals.

Align: Alignment applies both to the physical adjustments you provide your students and to recognizing how connected you are to your other teaching qualities. Self-inquiry is a way to examine how much you are aligned with your path as a yoga practitioner and teacher. Keep coming back to your ideals as you progress in your practice and as a teacher.

Nurture: Nurture the evolution of your students' practice. If you have gaps in compassion for your students then start with the principle of ahimsa. Notice any empathy you have for them and whenever possible cultivate a true understanding of their needs.

Table 2.3   ASANA (Methods of a Good Instructor)

Ahimsa (and Ask)	Cause no harm to your students and yourself. --and-- Take requests, get permission to touch, and inquire about your students' conditions and goals.
Suggest	Be direct and confident with your instructions, yet let students know they can modify poses or rest at any time. Constantly redirect your students' attention back to the breath.
Align	Advocate good physical alignment to prevent injury and promote balance; become an ally with your students in battling distractions and disharmony, and be sincere and professional.
Nurture	Give specific positive reinforcement; provide a safe and soothing class that allows students to be comfortably challenged throughout their practice.
Assess	Be aware of the overall group, as well as each student's learning style and needs; progress accordingly.

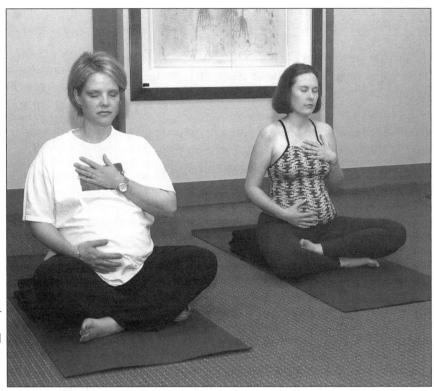

Not all of your students may be able to do all of the poses and will require suggestions for modifications.

© Dale Garvey

This idea may sound simplistic, but there are times when it is difficult not to take it personally if you have difficulty getting along with a student. A student might complain about the class in front of others. He might say negative things about you, challenge you, or mock you. If something like this occurs, remember that your job is to nurture without hurting yourself or anyone else. Conversely, if a student is stroking our ego, do your best to not give in to the temptation of encouraging this behavior. When you give feedback to your students include concrete examples (such as, "your knees are much straighter now") so the students can notice these things in themselves when you are not around. A good yoga teacher is far from being a cult leader. A good teacher guides students to find new places within themselves. If you enable a student to be dependent on you then you are nurturing your own ego.

Assess: As an instructor, it is important to continually assess and reassess your effectiveness in transmitting the essence of yoga to your students. Be aware constantly of each student's progress throughout class. By carefully watching your students you become aware of changes in the receptivity of their bodies and minds.

Summary

Looking over the information throughout this chapter, can you list the qualities of an ideal yoga instructor that are already strong in you and which ones you may wish to start cultivating more? How effective and dynamic is your voice, creativity, repertoire, and ability to build rapport? The like and dislike chart in table 2.1 is a reflection of some good professional habits. Your students want certain things from you, but you also need to ensure they are getting as many of the lessons yoga can offer. Even if students say they love having you as a teacher, it does not always mean they are learning much from you. It is good to know what they expect from you and then integrate that information into how you deliver the lessons to them effectively.

Making self-inquiries into the perceptions you have about yourself will deepen your understanding and connections to your path as a yoga practitioner and teacher. Recognizing your own obstacles and struggles will help you recognize them in your students and have empathy for people taking your classes. Knowing how your students learn best and what their motivations are can direct the compassion and instructions you give. Students will judge you consciously and unconsciously. It is more important to nurture a student's progress rather than the student's ego or your own self-interests. Your job is to present an entrancing and safe class as you embody the essence of yoga the best you can. Comparing your work habits and ethics to the qualities students reported they loved and lamented in table 2.1 could serve as a reality check for how people perceive you professionally.

Study Questions

1. What are the four Cs of teaching yoga?

2. What are the three basic types of learning styles?

3. Which dosha is made up of air?

4. Which type of student usually has trouble staying motivated?

5. List two things that students typically like and dislike about instructors.

6. How is the word *asana* used as an acronym for teaching yoga?

7. True or False? There is a very strict code of ethics you are legally required to abide by as a professional yoga teacher.

8. What aspects of your personal yoga practice will make you a better teacher?

9. Define ahimsa.

chapter 3

Creating a Class Environment

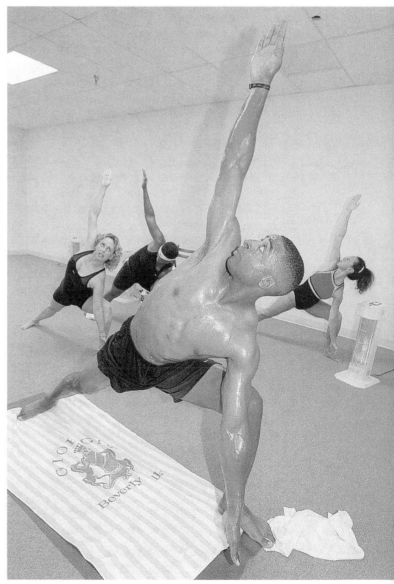

Yoga students trust that their instructor has the knowledge and ability to create a nurturing, safe, and engaging class environment for practice—an environment that can enhance each person's mental, physical, and spiritual awareness and well-being during the relatively short time they spend together. This chapter begins by discussing the types of equipment and attire typically used by students in class. A definition, in general terms, of the importance the environment plays in creating a safe, comforting practice session follows. The chapter also highlights specific environmental safety concerns instructors should be on the lookout for before, during, and after each class session. Ideas on how to create an atmosphere suitable for any practice and how to manage many of the typical distractions encountered in class are also provided.

Equipment Selection

Walking into a sporting goods store, or the retail area of any fitness club, might give one the impression that yoga requires a specific uniform and additional equipment to be practiced successfully. Western fashion sense and marketing aside, nothing could be further from the truth. Unlike many physical activities and exercise programs, yoga practice requires minimal equipment; East Indian citizens have practiced yoga for millennia with nothing more than thin reed mats, a simple loincloth or sari, and bare feet.

Although yoga instruction and practice require little in the way of equipment, certain elements can make your teaching and your students' class experience safer and more comfortable. The style of hatha yoga you teach, your student population, and the class location will generally determine what, if any, additional equipment you may wish to add to your class.

Yoga Attire

With regard to attire, and apart from personal fashion preferences, select from lightweight fabrics to allow for maximum movement and comfort. In general, comfortable shorts or leggings and a snug-fitting shirt work well for practicing yoga. Loose-fitting T-shirts, although comfortable and easy to move in, oftentimes end up over the head in inversion postures creating an annoying distraction. These clothing selections apply to students and instructors alike.

The type of yoga being practiced is another factor to consider when suggesting clothing options for students. Students in a fast-paced class may be most comfortable in a single layer of lightweight clothing to accommodate for the additional heat they will create with their bodies while in class. Students in a less-vigorous style of class might be most comfortable beginning class with additional warm-up layers, which can be peeled off as their body temperature increases and added back on as they cool down at the end of class.

Yoga instructors should follow the same guidelines in clothing for comfort and ease of movement as their students, but always dress in a professional manner. Students must be able to see how your body moves as you demonstrate, but you should avoid wearing any clothing that might be overly revealing.

Practitioners of Kundalini yoga suggest that you wear clothes made of white cotton and other natural fabrics to foster the electromagnetic field surrounding you during practice.

Yoga Mats

In addition to bare feet and comfortable clothing, the most indispensable piece of yoga equipment is a sticky yoga mat. Yoga mats provide a stable, nonslip surface and, depending on the thickness, a bit of cushion on which to practice. Mats can be found in a number of different colors, lengths, and thicknesses, all of which are really a matter of personal preference.

In some settings, yoga mats are provided on site. However, this is not always the case. If you find yourself teaching in a site where mats are not provided, and if students are reluctant or unable to purchase their own mats, you may suggest they bring a large towel or blanket. The towel or blanket should be large enough so that both hands and feet can be in contact with the mat in postures such as Adho Mukha Shvanasana (Downward-Facing Dog).

Occasionally you will encounter students who recognize that mats are beneficial to their practice, but they are under the false impression that any exercise mat will do. Mats used in Pilates floor classes can be used for yoga practice; however, these mats tend to be made of more flexible materials and do not provide the same degree of traction as do yoga mats.

Many fitness clubs provide the short, soft, and slick mats generally used for floor-exercise work. Unfortunately, these mats are designed for use as a cushion for sit-ups and exercises not requiring the traction yoga mats provide. Soft mats such as these have the potential to slide across the floor unless students pay closer attention to the mat than their own practice, which both defeats the purpose of yoga practice and increases the potential for injury. This type of mat also has too much cushion to provide stability while standing. A person would be much safer using a towel or no mat at all.

If you teach in a facility where yoga mats are provided for students, one often ignored or forgotten health and safety issue must be addressed. When multiple pairs of sweaty bare feet continually use a mat it becomes a foul-smelling, dirty habitat for germs. For this reason, the mats should be cleaned and disinfected on a regular basis and replacement mats purchased as needed. The smell factor alone should encourage students to bring their own mats! An average investment of $30 is a small price to pay for the practical protection a mat provides for a significant amount of personal use.

Props

Many hatha yoga styles utilize props to aid students as they move through and deepen their postures.

Props can be especially helpful for those new to yoga by providing additional support as they work to increase their strength, flexibility, and balance in any given posture. The many ways props can be used to modify and adjust students will be illustrated in the asana chapters later in the book. Here is a brief listing of some typical yoga props:

- Blankets or other soft bolsters can be placed beneath students with overly tight hamstrings, hips, and backs to mechanically lift and support their bodies in seated postures. If blankets or bolsters are not readily available, folded towels or mats may also be used. For those with sensitive knees, gardening kneepads can be used to comfortably settle into kneeling postures. Many studios provide blankets to keep students warm as they relax in Shavasana (Corpse Pose), the resting portion of a practice session.

- Straps or belts are used to help students extend their reach in many postures. Straps are particularly helpful in extending the stretch of the hamstrings without causing discomfort in seated or supine postures. These props also may be used to secure the limbs in certain postures.

- Blocks generally are used during standing postures to extend the arms' reach toward the ground without causing undue strain in the hamstrings and back. They also may be used in the place of bolsters or blankets to provide more stable elevation when needed. Blocks may be made of wood or a polystyrene blend. Wood

blocks tend to hold up better over prolonged use.

- Chairs or walls are used to aid those with difficulty in balance postures. Chairs also may be used as an aid in seated postural asanas for those who find it difficult to get up from the floor. In addition to balance support, a wall may be used to help students check their own alignment in many postures.

- Sandbags may be used in seated, prone, or supine postures to provide a constant yet gentle pressure to release tight muscles.

- Eye pillows are used to cover the eyes during the relaxation phase of a class. If the eye pillows are filled with herbs or essential oils, they add an aromatherapy component to aid in relaxation.

- Mirrors are included in this list of props because they may be used to visually aid both the teacher and the student in checking body alignment. Generally, wall mirrors are found in group exercise facilities and dance rooms. Depending on the style and focus, yoga studios may or may not be equipped with mirrors. Many schools of yoga feel that mirrors create too much of a distraction for the students. Depending on where and what style of yoga you teach, you may have the opportunity to use wall mirrors as an aid in aligning your students in their practice.

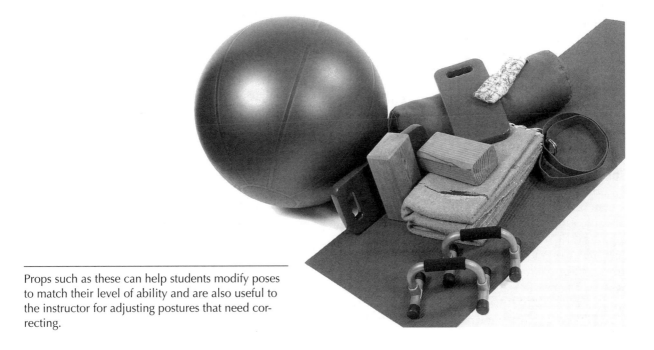

Props such as these can help students modify poses to match their level of ability and are also useful to the instructor for adjusting postures that need correcting.

Although the specific teaching methods of Iyengar-style classes are not highlighted in this text, it is important to note that Iyengar studios typically have wall-mounted equipment that is used to support students with low flexibility or injuries and guide them into postures with proper alignment.

Safety and Comfort Concerns

Most people will agree that there are inherent safety risks involved when participating in any physical activity. Because yoga practice is relatively nonimpact in nature, injury rates in students tend to be much lower than in many other activities. That is not to say that injuries cannot occur in yoga class. The following section addresses some of the most commonly identified safety and comfort issues that you and your students may face.

Student Safety

In addition to guiding your students through a blissful class practice, your primary concern as an instructor is your students' personal safety while they are in your care. At the beginning of each class, or as new students join your ongoing classes, make certain to ascertain whether anyone has any type of injury or illness that could affect his physical abilities. If so, pay particular attention to these students as you help them modify asanas as needed.

Bare Feet

Regardless of the style of yoga you are teaching, encourage students to practice in their bare feet. The foremost reason being that bare feet allow the student to feel the connection to the floor more completely in standing postures. Without the rigid constraint of shoes, the feet are strengthened and are able to move in a more natural manner, which significantly aids in balance. The bottoms of the feet also generally provide the correct amount of traction against the floor to guard against slipping in standing postures, thus increasing the student's safety. In seated postures, bare feet avoid the concern of the sole of the shoe pressing uncomfortably into the flesh or getting caught along the surface of the mat.

The traction provided between the sole of the foot and mat significantly decreases the potential for slips and falls in standing postures, thereby increasing personal safety. There are times, however, when the sole and mat connection just is not firm enough. If you have a student who is sweating profusely through the bottom of the feet, you may find that she is unable to stay stationary. In this case, you can suggest that she bring an extra towel to help absorb the sweat and provide a firmer surface.

Although rare, you may occasionally encounter a student who is opposed to practicing barefoot. If the room is chilly, or students have negative issues with their feet, it may be difficult to convince them to take their warm, and concealing, socks off during class. By gently reiterating the safety concerns presented by wearing socks, and reminding reticent students that they are free to put their socks back on during the seated portion of class, you can get most students to comply. If that still does not persuade them to remove their socks, you can assure students that classmates who are staring at others' feet instead of focusing on their own practice will not be getting full benefit from their class!

Adjustments

The most important safety issue when physically adjusting your students is to remember to respect each student's body as if it were your own. Recognize that not everyone is physically able to move the body into the picture-perfect posture. Everyone has his or her own physical and mental limitations to contend with, and it is not your decision as the instructor to dictate where each student's "perfect" position should be. Always ask your students' permission to physically touch them, and always maintain an awareness of just how far a person is willing and able to deepen the posture. Move slowly with compassion and awareness of each student's needs. With your students' permission and your gentle touch, you can significantly decrease the possibility of causing them physical and psychological injury when providing adjustments.

Also, remind students throughout the class that it is of the utmost importance that they do not take their bodies to the point of physical discomfort or pain in any of their asanas. They need to recognize the part they play in their own physical safety by respecting and accepting any immediate limitations they may feel they have as they open into any of the asanas. The mantra "No pain, no *pain*" should be recited by each student before practice begins!

Hydration and Nutrition

It is important to remember that any activity that puts a physical demand on the body requires adequate hydration and nutrition. Of course, yoga practice is no exception. For this reason, remind students to stay well hydrated before, during, and after classes. Hydration is an even more important issue in classes with high room temperatures or highly vigorous routines.

Most people who exercise on a regular basis know that it's best to exercise with a relatively empty stomach, both for comfort and for healthy digestion. However, many students new to yoga will mistakenly think that they'll "just be stretching" and will come to class having just eaten a full meal. It is important to inform your students that they will have a much more comfortable and healthful experience if they wait two to three hours after a large meal to practice yoga. The internal pressure created during certain yoga postures can cause people to feel light headed or dizzy if they are overly full. Also, when there is food in the stomach the body moves the blood and energy into digestion instead of circulating through the skeletal muscle system. So, the more empty the internal organs are during practice—this includes the bladder and bowels—the more comfortable the students will feel, thus allowing them to relax more fully into their asana practice. If a student really feels the need to charge up before class you might suggest a light, easily digestible snack (for example, yogurt or a small piece of fruit) about an hour before class.

Instructor Safety

With all the concerns about keeping your students safe and comfortable in your class, it is important not to overlook your personal well-being as you teach. Constant awareness is your best defense. Always be on the lookout for tripping hazards as you walk among students. When adjusting a student maintain your own good posture and balance. As you use your body to help a student gain or maintain balance, be sure to keep your knees slightly bent so you can make any adjustments in your own balance as needed. Stand to the side as the student performs inversions, such as a handstand, to keep from being smacked in the head as the student lifts or lowers the legs.

Environmental Safety

No matter where you find yourself teaching, from a cozy yoga studio to a wide-open school auditorium, it is imperative that you take time before each class to ensure that the practice area is clean and safe for the students and yourself. The area should be free from debris on the floor. If your yoga session follows any high-energy class where people may have been sweating a lot, a good swabbing of the floor can eliminate a significant amount of slipping potential, both on and off the mat.

Also, if possible, ask that your students store their personal possessions away from the practice area. This helps eliminate the risk of accidentally tripping and falling. As mentioned previously, this will make walking among the students a much safer task as you check their alignment and make any requested adjustments. This is especially true in larger classes where the space between students tends to be minimal.

Equipment Safety

If you use props in your class, check them regularly to make sure they are in good working order. Straps should not be frayed, blankets should be clean, and blocks should be well balanced and stable. If any props have defects, remove them from use and have them replaced.

Because one of the main objectives in this book is to teach instructors the how-to of hands-on adjustments, we must mention the importance of hand washing with regard to touching perspiring students. Although we are not advocating that instructors run out and wash their hands after touching each student (which would create quite an unacceptable break in the class flow), we want to remind instructors of the importance of good hygiene before and after class for the health of themselves as well as that of their students.

Atmosphere for Yoga Classes

If you asked the average nonyoga-practicing person what image came to his mind when he thought of a yoga class, he might describe a darkened, candlelit room, wafting with the scent of patchouli incense and filled with the sound of low-droning chants in the background. Many of these elements may be found in yoga classes; sometimes, though, quite the opposite is true. The reality of most yoga classes, however, is that wherever space is available is where the class is held. These days the most common spaces used for yoga classes are gymnasiums, group exercise rooms in fitness facilities, and community recreation centers.

Ideal Setting

Yoga classes can be, and often are, taught almost anywhere. However, some locations are more favorable for helping students achieve the release, relaxation, and body awareness they crave. Generally speaking, the most desirable space to teach and practice yoga is in an area designed specifically with yoga in mind from the onset. A spacious, warm space free from outside distractions, with good ventilation and comfortable lighting, is considered an ideal setting.

Calming music and the aromatherapy of incense burning are often associated with yoga classes and can indeed add to a soothing atmosphere. It must be must mentioned, however, that incense burning in particular is not always a welcome addition to a class. In many facilities the use of incense is strictly forbidden. If you teach in a facility that does allow incense use, it is a courtesy to first ask the students if they mind. Many individuals have severe allergies to smoke and artificial perfumes and may be adversely affected by any scent wafting through the room. For this reason, it is also advisable to have a policy stating that no one wear perfume to class.

Floor Surfaces

Yoga can be practiced almost anywhere: a beach in Hawaii, the sidelines of a football game, your living room, a mountain campground, even in the water. Although the surface can be varied, it should be as level as possible to keep from compromising a person's balance and to protect the joints when holding postures. And, as in any physical activity, some surfaces are suited more appropriately for practicing yoga. Because yoga is generally practiced indoors, floor surfaces found indoors are addressed here.

Most dance studios, high school gyms, and some older recreational facilities provide wood flooring. Newer fitness facilities outfit their group exercise rooms with wood floors as well. Wood provides a smooth, flat surface with a small amount of flexibility and is relatively forgiving to the body. Wood also provides greater warmth than concrete or other harder surfaces. Many yoga studios have wood flooring installed at the onset and to maintain the integrity of the surface do not allow outside footwear on the studio floor.

Concrete-based surfaces, which are the norm in many older fitness facilities, elementary school auditoriums, and even some newer recreation facilities, provide a smooth and generally easy-to-clean surface. In many of these settings the concrete is covered with ceramic tile or linoleum. Unfortunately, concrete does not give and provides no shock absorption for the joints. Concrete is still a viable surface for practicing yoga, however, because of the extremely low-impact nature of the activity. Mats help provide a

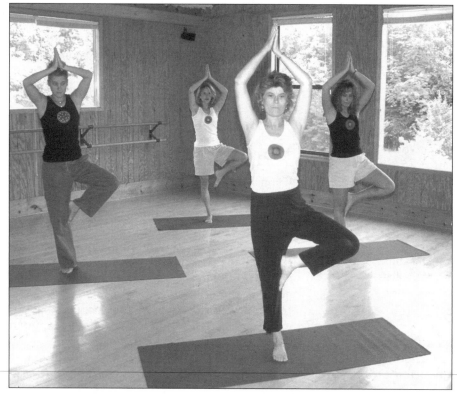

A favorable location for the instruction of yoga includes a spacious, warm space free from outside distractions, with good ventilation and comfortable lighting.

© Lynn Seldon, Inc

nice amount of cushioning and some added warmth for students to counteract the fact that concrete tends to be much cooler than wooden floors.

Some facilities have carpeted flooring. These surfaces provide the warmest floor surface and are very suitable for gentle and restorative yoga, where students spend a significant amount of time on the floor. Although carpet does provide a little extra cushioning, pay attention to what kinds of activities are preformed on the carpet. A sweat-inducing activity can create a foul-smelling and unsanitary surface if not cleaned on a regular basis.

Temperature Control

In general, the room temperature for a yoga class should be set no lower than 76 degrees Fahrenheit (about 24 degrees Celsius). This creates a comfortable environment for most students' metabolisms—not too hot, not too cold. However, room temperature should be set appropriately for the style of yoga being practiced. In some styles of yoga the room is heated from 96 to 106 degrees Fahrenheit (36 to 41 degrees Celsius), with the idea that a heated room will aid in warming the muscles for practice. In Bikram-style yoga, for example, the room is kept at a high temperature to help students release more sweat to detoxify the body.

Not all locations provide easy access to the thermostat, unfortunately, which can cause both instructor and students much consternation. An instructor teaching in a fitness club where aerobic dance was scheduled to follow her morning yoga class found that the automatic cooling fans turned on 15 minutes before class ended during cool-down and Shavasana. After much shivering and complaining by the students, the management finally was convinced to change the thermostat. In the meantime, however, many students came to class in multiple layers. In fact, one student came to class with two layers of exercise clothes, mittens, and a parka, which was remarkable considering the class was in eastern San Diego county in the summer! This anecdote may be extreme, but it is used to illustrate that it is always a good idea to remind students to dress in layers to accommodate for changing body temperatures. Also, be sure the management where you teach understands the intricacies and environmental needs of yoga practice.

Distractions

Students come to yoga for a variety of reasons. One of the most common reasons is to attain a certain level of self-awareness and focus; to clear their minds of stress and distracting thought processes. Yet, even in the most ideal yoga setting, outside distractions can seep into the class and disrupt the serene mood students crave. In less than ideal settings, such as a fitness facility where the yoga class is adjacent to a basketball court, these distractions can seem almost too much to overcome. Help to redirect students' focus to their asanas so that they can try to block out many of these distractions. Before class begins, instruct students that all cell phones and pagers must be turned off. There is nothing as distracting to both students and instructor as a phone ringing during class!

The following story illustrates how important an appropriate atmosphere is for students' yoga experience. Picture a yoga class set in a wonderfully spacious dance room situated in a quiet bungalow at an adult education center. The long-time students were delighted, and perhaps a bit spoiled, by the seclusion of the room with its warm wood floors and the whispers of wind as the only sound sneaking in from outside. Sadly, the use of the bungalow was taken away, and the class was relocated to what the administration thought was a perfect area: the cafeteria. The instructor was shown a blueprint of the school illustrating the cafeteria with a dotted line down the middle with "Yoga" written on one side and "Dance" on the other. It was explained that the line represented a dividing wall between the two classes. When she went to teach, the instructor saw that the so-called dividing wall was a mere curtain. Moreover, the dance class was a tap-dance class, wherein the instructor broadcasted show tunes over loudspeakers as the dance students stampeded on an old, warped wooden stage just a few feet from the yoga instructor's voice. As a consequence, the instructor had to shout out such phrases as "breathe" and "relax." Almost every student in that yoga class demanded their money back, and the class was canceled. This story shows that some settings may contain obstacles that are so immense they may be impossible to overcome.

Music for Atmosphere

Many yoga teachers like to use music in their classes because it can help set the mood the moment a student walks in the door. In places where distractions such as clanging weights, loud voices, or more bombastic tunes are competing for students' attention, background music helps to anchor their awareness more fully into the classroom. Although music has been proven to influence the mood or atmosphere of a class, it is possible for students to become dependent on it and have trouble getting their focus without it. Especially for students new to yoga, music can help drown out their mental distractions. After some practice, and your repeated cueing, they can use their breath to clear their minds more effectively.

Note that some traditions of yoga hold the tenet that music itself is a distraction. Iyengar hatha yoga, for example, does not allow music during practice because it is considered distracting "fluff" in the class environment. In such classes the instructor's voice and direction are most important in guiding students' minds inward to fend off outside distractions.

Music Selection

The most common style of music found playing in yoga classes is New Age music, which is characterized by soothing melodies and natural sounds. Many instructors and students are not comfortable with New Age music and prefer classical, jazz, techno-beat, or even chanting as background. Note that the pace of the music should not clash with the pace of your class. Although many people adore chants or tribal beats, some will find the rhythm of the music too distracting while also trying to listen to the instructions of a teacher.

Many yoga instructors have a naturally soft and soothing voice that in itself is almost hypnotic and can take the place of background music. If you need to speak loudly because of miscellaneous background noise, a large class size, or poor acoustics, then it is suggested you play soft New Age music to back you up. In faster-paced classes more energetic music can help move the class along quickly. Again, the tempo and style of your music should reflect your personal style and the pace of the class you are teaching.

Music As Mood Setter

If you do choose to use music in your classes, allow yourself to be creative. Do not feel you need to always stick with one style, such as New Age. Test out different pieces on your students. Remember, both you and your students will appreciate variety! If you find yourself less than enthusiastic about a piece of music you have played for the past eight class sessions, your students are likely to feel the same.

Although the objective of playing music in class is to set the mood and use it as an aid for the students, it is important the music not actually change the focus of the class. Less-than-traditional music can delightfully change the pace of a class and even express a background theme. For instance, playing Tchaikovsky's *Nutcracker Suite* could be fun while

teaching a generic yoga class in December. In a workshop that focused exclusively on more complex postures the instructor played rock-based songs with lyrics such as "have mercy." This light-hearted music created a level of levity and humor in the class that was most enjoyable, yet surprisingly undistracting. In two different ballet classes, one had a live pianist and the other was accompanied by Smokey Robinson records with the bass turned up. Students relished both classes. Why shouldn't yoga classes have the same creativity?

Summary

Although yoga practice may not require much in the way of equipment or attire, it is unique in its atmospheric needs. It is the instructor's responsibility to work with all the resources available to create a safe and comforting surrounding where students feel protected and secure enough to allow themselves to truly open their hearts and minds to your instruction.

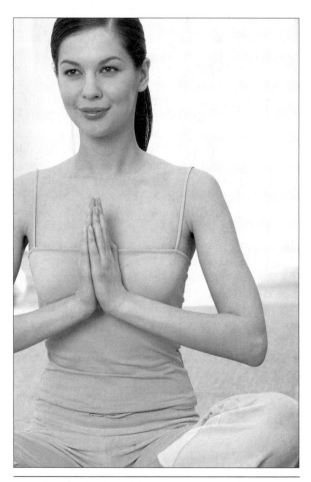

Don't be afraid to have a little fun when setting the mood for your class!

© Jumpfoto

Study Questions

1. Why would yoga practitioners choose to wear white cotton or other natural fibers?

2. What are three indispensable items used when practicing yoga?

3. How are blocks used?

4. What is the most important safety issue when physically adjusting your students?

5. How long should the average person wait after a meal before practicing yoga and why?

6. What is an ideal setting for a yoga class?

7. What temperature is generally considered the lowest acceptable for yoga practice?

8. What are some pros and cons of using music while teaching yoga?

chapter 4

Breathing and Beyond

The most important thing is your breath. These are words a good yoga teacher should say numerous times while conducting a class. Reminding students to breathe is always a good idea. Poor breathing is an epidemic bad habit in today's society, which contributes to the high anxiety and stress suffered by many. Breathing deeply and slowly allows for greater circulation with less work. Deep, slow breathing lessens stress on the heart and enhances the entire cardiovascular system. The breath can make a significant difference in ability, comfort, and awareness during asana practice.

Asanas and the practice of proper breathing are two aspects of yoga focused on by most Western practitioners. These two elements enhance each other in creating a complete awareness within the mind and body. Although other chapters focus on the asanas, this chapter focuses specifically on breath awareness, with an overview of the anatomical structures involved

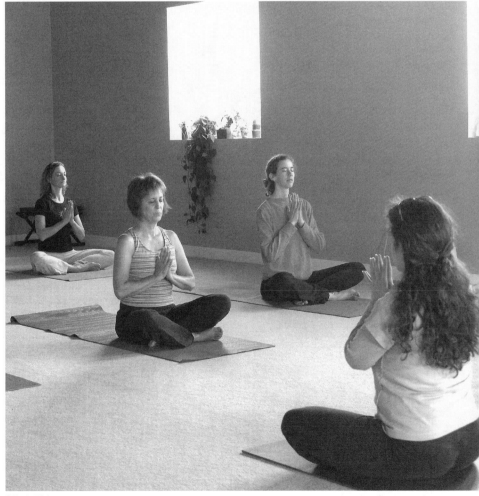

© Martha Work

in the breathing process. General guidelines on how to bring breath awareness and control to students during their asana practice, the most common yogic breathing techniques, and how they relate to asana practice also are discussed.

"Just as a lion, elephant, or tiger may be gradually brought under control, so is prana attended to. Otherwise it destroys the practitioner." — Hatha Yoga Pradipika

Pranayama

The yogis call the force behind life itself, which is inherent in the breath, *prana* [PRAAH-naah]. *Pranayama* [praah-naah-YAAH-muh] is breath work, the practice of which connects the mind and body with a shared consciousness. By focusing on the breath, a student can bypass the chatter in the mind and ego. When a student begins paying attention and controlling the breath, circulation improves in a way that brings more blood, oxygen, and fuel to the muscles as well as enhancing concentration.

Although people usually breathe "automatically," that is, with no effort or conscious thought, it does not mean that the breath cannot be controlled. For thousands of years yogis have developed ways to bring what were once considered strictly involuntary systems of the body under control. The breath is the most essential function of the body that can be regulated. It is a relatively easy and convenient mechanism to use to tune inward because the breath can be heard, felt, and counted without special equipment. Blood pressure, brain waves, immune cells, electrolytes, and digestion are much more difficult to be aware of and to control, yet these systems usually improve in function when the breath is more efficient.

Why should one be concerned with the breath? Breath can be used as an analogy to life. Not only can breathing patterns affect physiological well-being, but they also can affect and be affected by thought processes. Emotions can be triggered negatively through shallow, labored breathing or positively with smooth, flowing breaths, which stabilize our thoughts and allow relaxation to set in.

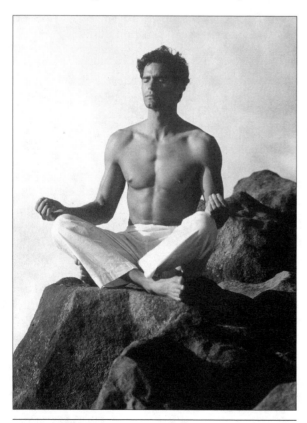

As an analogy of life, many benefits come from focusing on proper breathing.
© Jumpfoto

Process of Breathing

Most people tend to breathe too shallowly, in the uppermost region of their chests. This habit is inefficient because it leads to feeling like one has to take in more breaths to feel comfortable. This type of overbreathing is a mild form of hyperventilation and is exacerbated by stress. In fact, this chronic breathing habit actually can induce the stress response in some people. When the breaths are shallow and frequent, the heart must work much harder to bring oxygenated blood to the body. If circulation is chronically compromised, it in turn leads to many other bodily systems functioning below the level nature intended. For example, the immune system is at risk when circulation is poor because toxins cannot be eliminated as efficiently and the body's overall functional capacity becomes diminished. Pranayama plays a major role in keeping the functions of the physical and energetic body healthy, preventing the physical decay that occurs when cells do not receive adequate oxygen over a prolonged period of time. Choppy, shallow breathing occurs when the sympathetic nervous system activates the body for the fight-or-flight response in actual or perceived threatening and stressful situations. When this system stays activated over long periods it can induce *general adaptation syndrome* (GAS). The negative effects of GAS stress the body and can lead to one of many causes of early death, such as heart disease.

Anatomy of Breathing

A proper full, deep breath begins from the base of the diaphragm near the pelvic girdle. This action alone helps to relax the rest of the respiratory muscles as well as some neck muscles. The relaxation effect of deep breathing is brought about by the parasympathetic nervous system, which is concerned with allowing the body to rest and conserve energy. At the same time, this effect deactivates the sympathetic nervous system, which is concerned with bodily functions involving expending energy generally for the self-protection and nurturing of the body. According to a National Institute of Health report (September 2003 Mayo Clinic Health Letter), the regular yogic practice of deep, slow breathing through the nose produces a multitude of health benefits including reducing anxiety and high blood pressure, balancing brain waves, and improving physical endurance.

Most of the body's major organs are located within the torso, fitting closely adjacent to one another. The heart resides almost in the middle of the chest, with the bulk of its mass toward the left side. As a consequence, the fist-sized heart organ leaves the left lung room for two lobes whereas the right lung has three lobes. The diaphragm, a parachute-shaped muscle, is located below the heart and lungs and attaches to the lumbar spine, the lower six ribs, and the sternum. As this powerful muscle contracts, the diaphragm allows the lungs to fill with air, and as it relaxes it moves upward and presses the air out of the lungs (figure 4.1). Below the diaphragm to the right is the liver

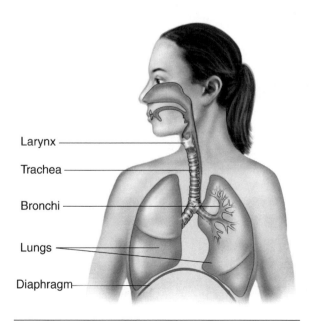

Figure 4.1 The diaphragm and lungs within the thoracic cavity.

and to the left are the stomach and spleen. The diaphragm has three openings to allow passage of the esophagus, inferior vena cava, and the aorta. As you can imagine, when the diaphragm is activated the many surrounding tissues and organs get massaged and stimulated.

When a person breathes too shallowly the lungs do not expand fully; and the air is moved only into the upper chest, which strains the neck and shoulder muscles and consequently causes more rapid and shortened breaths. A person who breathes consistently into the chest rather than into the belly creates a strain within the entire body, robbing tissues and cells of oxygen as well as creating a weakness and imbalance in the intercostal (rib) muscles and diaphragm.

Types of Pranayama

Watch a young child sleep, and you will notice the smooth, rhythmic rise and fall of the belly and the gentle expansion of the upper torso and chest. This is how all human beings begin breathing; with no worries of constantly needing to "suck in our guts" and simply allowing the fullness of prana to flow easily into and through our bodies. As a result of the stresses one picks up and begins to carry through life's journey, it is important to retrain the breathing process. The idea is to get the breath to expand below the ribcage toward the navel by engaging the diaphragm more completely.

Simply observing the breath is a type of pranayama that is often practiced during Shavasana (Corpse Pose). When breathing more efficiently, fewer breaths are needed to take in sufficient oxygen. Animals that take fewer breaths generally live the longest. For example, a tortoise breathes four times per minute and lives up to 300 years. The average human, in contrast, takes 16 to 20 breaths per minute and usually does not reach his or her 100th birthday!

It is possible for the mind to be alert while the body is resting and calm. It is also possible to be very active while breathing steadily and smoothly through the nose. Not only can we practice yoga more efficiently and easily, but also we can walk, run, and even swim at a good pace while breathing deeply and relatively slowly without taking oxygen in through the mouth, which tends to dehydrate the body.

There are many different styles and techniques of pranayama practice. The three most commonly practiced methods are outlined next: 1) deep abdominal, 2) complete yoga, and 3) *ujjayi* [oo-JAAHY-ee]

Larynx

Trachea

Bronchi

Lungs

Diaphragm

breathing. In addition, alternate nostril breathing technique (nadi shodhana [NAAH-dee SHOH-duh-nuh]) is illustrated, which can be taught at the beginning, end, or separately from a typical class setting. All methods are easily taught; however, it is best to receive hands-on training from a qualified instructor before teaching these styles with any great depth.

Deep Abdominal Breathing

Breathing deeply into the abdomen is the simplest form of pranayama practice. Teaching this breath style gives students the opportunity to become more fully aware of their current breathing patterns and shows them an easy way to begin to control the breath. One way to teach deep abdominal breathing is to have students place their hands on their lower abdomen over the navel. Instruct them to breathe slowly and deeply so that their hands gently rise up from the expansion of their breath. This exercise can be done while standing; sitting; and, most easily, lying on the floor either supine (face up) or prone (face down). Students should feel the belly expand while the ribs and chest remain relaxed (see figure 4.2).

If the students lie prone, their hands should be placed beneath their heads for comfort. They can use the feeling of their abdomen expanding against the floor for feedback. To further aid students, ask them to imagine they are a small boat drifting on the gentle sea of their breath. They can think of their torsos rising and falling like small waves. Once people are comfortable with deep abdominal breathing techniques, they will have an easier time performing other breathing styles.

Complete Yoga Breath

A full, deep breath has three parts to it. Some refer to this breathing as *durga* breathing. It is the practice of fully inflating the lungs from bottom to top. The students begin by breathing deeply into the abdominal area and continue to inhale, filling the entire torso with breath from the abdomen to the collar bones. At the end of this deep inhalation the sternum rises (from lifting the front ribs by using mid-back muscles assisted by deep breathing) and the clavicles (collar bones) expand forward and up while the shoulders remain relaxed.

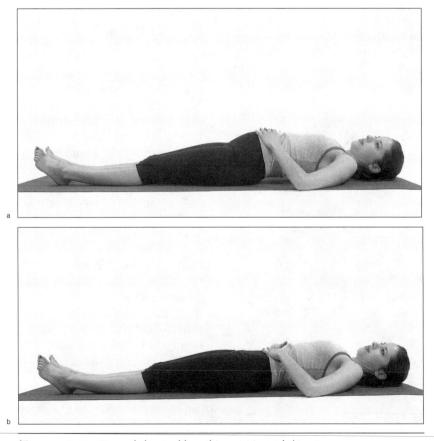

Figure 4.2 Deep abdominal breathing: (a) in and (b) out.

Repeat the cue—"Chest up, shoulders down"—when teaching this breathing technique.

The inhalation is full and deep from the abdomen, and the exhalation is equally deep and complete. When teaching this pranayama technique, direct students to release their breath from the top to the bottom of their torso, and from the chest down to the abdomen. At the end of the exhalation, instruct students to gently squeeze the abdomen in to expel as much old air as possible, thus attaining an even deeper inhalation on the next incoming breath. If students have difficulty breathing rhythmically with this technique, begin by focusing on the exhalation first.

Ujjayi Breathing

Ujjayi breathing is a more sophisticated pranayama technique and is used most often in Ashtanga yoga classes. Basic ujjayi breath expands the lungs and chest more fully and with control and can actually help to warm the body. The breath exudes a noise that resembles something like a whispering roar, producing a sound as the breath vibrates in the back of the throat and sinus areas making sibilant "ssss" on inhalation and an "hhhh" during exhalation. When an entire class synchronizes their breath it sounds like a pod of dolphins breathing together.

An easy way to introduce ujjayi breathing is to ask students to begin breathing through an open mouth while slightly tightening the backs of their throats. This action helps make the breath more audible. Instruct them to whisper as they inhale and exhale. For the more difficult inhalation sound you might have them practice making an "ash" sound while slowly breathing in. The exhalation is easier, as they can usually get a good sound if trying to whisper a prolonged "ha." Although breathing through an open mouth makes it easier to feel the breath and hear the sound, mouth breathing can be very dehydrating. As students become more comfortable with the breath pattern, instruct them to continue to breathe through their noses. As they breathe slowly and deeply through their noses, they should strive to keep and emphasize the sound vibrations.

This breathing method is very efficient and it helps students focus not only on their breathing but also on the flow of their asana movements. Because ujjayi makes such a distinct sound it automatically brings students back to the awareness of their breath. When a whole class uses this pranayama technique they become a community, much like a dolphin pod, helping each other focus through the sound they are emanating. For example, when an accomplished ujjayi breather was absent from a class one day, the other students commented on how much they missed her audible breathing to help them stay focused on their own breathing during asana practice.

Alternate Nostril Breathing

Known as nadi shodhana, alternate nostril breathing serves to increase and balance the prana flow in both nostrils and throughout the whole body. The term nadi shodhana means to clean the *nadis*, or nasal passages, which are channels for the energy, or prana, to circulate through. Chapter 5 provides more information about the energy system, but this section acquaints you with the basic technique and main benefits of alternate nostril breathing so you can practice and therefore teach it.

According to Dr. Jeanette Vos, an expert in education and brain research and best-selling author of *The Learning Revolution*, people learn five times more information when both hemispheres of the brain are active. Alternate nostril breathing engages both hemispheres of the brain as it opens up both nostrils for a better breath.

The clearing and balancing effects nadi shodhana has on both the left and right nostrils makes it easier for students to breathe through the nose overall. There are many variations and styles of the hand positions and fingering in this pranayama; however, the most traditional way is to use the ring and little finger and the thumb of the right hand to alternately close and release the nostrils. The index and middle fingers are folded inward toward the palm (see figure 4.3).

To begin, invite the students to the floor and have them find a comfortable position. Usually students are seated, but a nice way to teach this technique is to have the students supine with their legs in a comfortable cross-legged position on the floor or up against a wall. Instruct students as follows: "Begin by exhaling out the left nostril while the right thumb closes the right nostril. Then inhale through the left nostril. Use the ring and little fingers of the right hand to close the left nostril and release the right nostril. Exhale through the right nostril. Inhale through the right nostril. Close the right nostril with the thumb. Open the left nostril by releasing the ring and little fingers and exhale through the left side." This process completes one breath cycle. To start, ask the students to try 7 to 10 cycles through both nostrils.

These are simple, directed breathing techniques that can be introduced to students at all levels of yoga experience. There are many variations of hand positioning and duration of the breathing cycles. Remember: The most important concept to get across

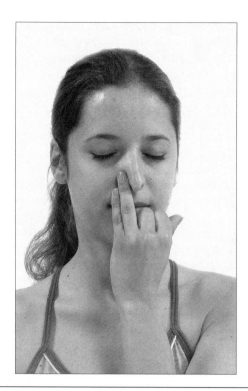

Figure 4.3 Hand positioning for nadi shodhana breathing.

to your students is how important awareness of their breathing is, not only for their asana practice but also throughout the rest of their day.

Instructing the Breathing Process

When it comes to pranayama practices, some schools of yoga instruct that pranayama should be practiced only under the tutelage of a professional yoga instructor, with a "Don't try this at home!" approach. Still others preach that students must practice these techniques every day. One reason caution exists regarding pranayama is to deter those who would abuse or exploit their shallow knowledge of such a powerful and sacred tool. Without a good foundation, a novice practitioner might hyperventilate or hold the breath when it is inappropriate to do so. A strong internal focus develops as well as a deeper awareness of the body overall when awareness is constantly brought back to the breath. Thus, the body and mind are gradually disciplined into the habit of better breathing and posture.

The breath, like the perception of the body in the asanas, should be felt and visualized from the inside out. Instruct your students to visualize the breath as white light radiating from the center of the body to expand the space of the body. The spine lengthens with the inhalation, and the spaces between each vertebra expand in all directions. The skin of the sternum subtly stretches both vertically and horizontally. When students ask you how or what they should be practicing at home between classes, educate them on the benefits of just becoming more aware of the breath and learning how to breathe more slowly and deeply.

The following are some basic guidelines to apply to pranayama practice. These guidelines may also be applied to asana and meditation practice.

- One minute fully focused is better than 20 with no focus! Quality rather than quantity is what really matters. Start off by committing to only 30 seconds or a few easy rounds of breathing to begin with. A person who decides to run a marathon would be foolish to go out and train the first day by running over 20 miles. So why approach pranayama practice in a similar manner?

- Expand according to your joy, not your clock. When the benefits of pranayama are felt and experienced, the results are a natural desire to expand the timeframe of practice. Often, this occurs without even noticing the extended time. To use the running analogy again, when one truly enjoys running, one often looks forward to taking longer runs instead of thinking of it as a chore.

- What is the meaning of pranayama practice? There should be significant meaning in every action in whatever is practiced. Instead of understanding on an intellectual level that one *should* practice pranayama, the true meaning behind the action must be addressed. The motive need not be spiritual in nature either. If students start practicing pranayama because they believe it makes the face wrinkle less, then that is an appropriate motive to begin practice and will lead to further self-exploration. In fact, many people start doing asanas to lose weight. Once the excess weight is gone, they are past the physical concerns of looks and open themselves up to feeling, eating, and thinking better as well! With the understanding of the benefits of breath awareness and its importance in overall health, the student will be able to more fully reap and appreciate the benefits of pranayama practice as its own discipline and as an aid to reaping the full benefits of the asanas.

Linking Pranayama With Asanas

Many people find it difficult to sit and focus solely on the breath. The mind constantly begs for attention or entertainment, and the body becomes numb and restless. It is common to feel more like an untamed lion than a peaceful and content yogi! For this reason, an asana session can literally jump start a pranayama practice as the calming effects of the breath help relax the mind and the movement and focus of the asanas give the body what it craves—movement.

Pranayama allows a person to achieve a more relaxed yet focused mental and physical state of being. These benefits can be achieved through practicing asanas but are enhanced by and also enhance asana practice. Asanas and pranayama work together in that the good posture created through continual asana practice allows for increased space within the torso, thus allowing for greater breath volume. The asanas help loosen the tight muscles of the ribcage and diaphragm so the breath can expand more fully. The more the breath expands, the more effectively the circulatory and muscular systems work. After years of shallow breathing the diaphragm and intercostal muscles lose functional capacity and flexibility. When a muscle is not regularly stretched and strengthened it loses both mass and function. The asanas strengthen the deep core muscles of the torso, which in turn support good spinal posture and enhance the range of motion and stability for the entire body.

Here are some general pranayama instructions for students during asanas:

- Instruct students to breathe slowly and deeply through the nose. A good duration to strive for is seven seconds for the inhalation and seven seconds for the exhalation. Also, breathing through the nose brings more oxygen directly to the brain while filtering the air and preventing dehydration.

- Keep the breath smooth and steady. If the breath becomes jerky or labored it is a sign a student is struggling and possibly overstraining. At this point the student should come out of the asana.

- Expanding and opening movements of asanas usually occur on the inhalation. For example,

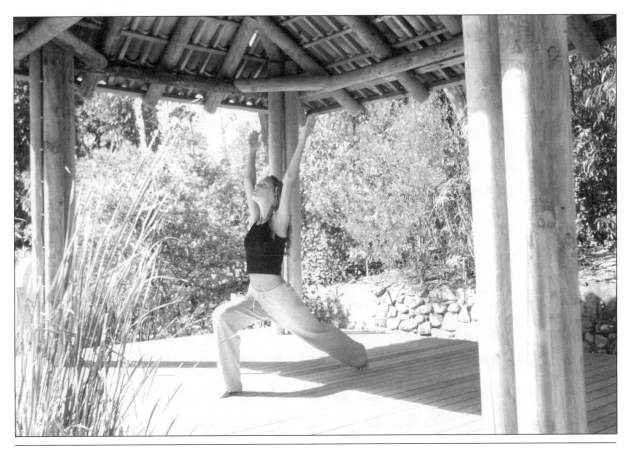

Asanas and pranayama work together when good posture helps to open the torso for better breathing.
© Jumpfoto

teachers might say, "Inhale and raise the arms overhead" and "Inhale and gently bend back."

- Releasing or relaxing movements of asanas generally occur on the exhalation: "Exhale as you bend forward from your hips."

- Direct students to visualize their breath moving into any areas of tension or resistance to release blocks and bring greater circulation and awareness to that area.

Summary

The lessons and benefits of pranayama practice take time. Give the class a chance to feel; see; and, in some instances, such as ujjayi, even hear their breath. Remember, students cannot be reminded to focus on their breath enough. Constant feedback is a necessity. Start students off with good deep and slow abdominal breathing; then, as the class progresses, begin teaching durga breathing with the asanas. If you teach a power yoga class of any kind, the ujjayi-breath techniques generally take more time when working with less experienced students. Also, because it is best to teach from experience, remember to practice these techniques yourself. If you are just starting out teaching yoga, breathing deeply and slowly will help make you feel less nervous; if you have been teaching for a while, then you already know the benefits of these pranayamas and might be ready to expand them more thoroughly in your classes.

Pranayama practice offers so many physical and mental benefits, not the least of which is to clear the mind. *Prana* signifies the breath and vital life energy. Cleaning the energy channels is also an integral component of breath work because it further aids mental focus. The rejuvenating effects of the parasympathetic nervous system are enhanced by pranayama breathing. Deep, slow breathing allows for greater circulation with less work, which reduces the stress on the entire cardiovascular system. Focused breathing makes a significant difference in ability, comfort, and awareness during asana practice.

Study Questions

1. What is an epidemic in today's society, which contributes to the high anxiety and stress suffered by many?

2. How can a student bypass the chatter in his mind and ego?

3. _____can be triggered negatively through shallow, labored breathing or positively with smooth, flowing breaths, which stabilize thoughts and allow relaxation to set in.

4. Choppy, shallow breathing is associated with which nervous system?

5. What is a type of breathing mentioned in a National Institute of Health report that when practiced can improve physical endurance?

6. How many breaths per minute does the average human take?

7. What are the three most common pranayama techniques taught in asana classes?

8. What is nadi shodhana and what effect on the brain hemispheres does it have?

9. Which is usually better, to inhale or to exhale, while entering Uttanasana (Intense Forward Bend)?

chapter 5

Energy and Anatomy

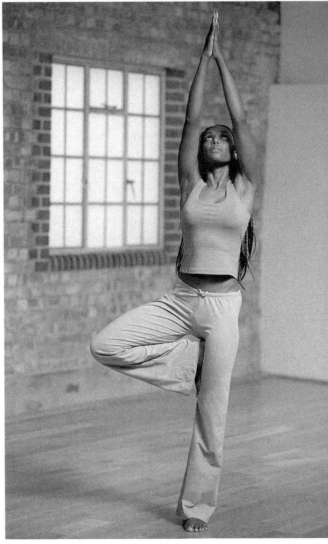

Your understanding of the skillful and safe mechanics of vertebrates and use of verbal cues are most important when adjusting students in asanas. In fact, kinesthetic and auditory instruction affords more protection to students when compared to a visual demonstration. If you teach primarily through demonstration, students tend to concentrate on imitating your movements, instead of turning their focus within—to become cognizant of their own personal edge or the boundaries of their physical and mental capabilities. A good instructor facilitates students' awareness and experience of playing the edge within a posture. They help students arrive at a place of possible discomfort, perhaps, but never pain. Students may experience some struggles both physically and mentally; however, if they surpass their personal edge in their asanas the possibility of injury ensues.

As a yoga teacher you need to have a firm grasp on the limitations of your students' knowledge of biomechanics and be aware of their physical and mental capacity and ability to focus. There are times when students, because of physical or mental imbalances, may unintentionally move their bodies in a manner that places them at physical risk of injury. It is your duty to help such a student move in a mechanically sound manner, which helps to maintain joint integrity and decrease the opportunity for injury. Because of the dynamic qualities of most styles of hatha yoga, all instructors must have at least a basic understanding of what is called energetic anatomy as well as how the human musculoskeletal system works before attempting to guide students through a class or to provide adjustments to postures.

This chapter begins with an explanation of how practicing yoga postures affects the major body systems. An introduction to and definition of terms used to describe energetic anatomy follow. An overview of basic human kinematics, movement systems, the planes of motion, and muscle mechanics illustrate the importance of describing and applying proper mechanics when observing and adjusting students in asanas. The final section of the chapter contains a list of commonly used phrases that are helpful in verbally describing positioning to students as they enter and exit poses.

Yoga Postures and Major Body Systems

The beneficial effects of yoga asanas are relative to the postures being practiced. A well-rounded program includes a number of asanas from each cat-

egory (standing, seated, supine, prone, inversions, and restorative—the chapters that make up part 2) and moves the spine through its total range of motion to bring about the most ideal results. A good yoga practice affects the person as a whole, helping eliminate stress; charge up the immune system; and ward off age-related degeneration such as arthritis, osteoporosis, and cardiovascular disease. As a yoga teacher you can educate students with some of the following information when they ask, "What can yoga do for me?"

Skeletal System

Bones make up the frame of the body, which is kept strong and aligned from yoga practice. Weight bearing stimulates osteogenesis, or bone-tissue growth. Any weight-bearing posture promotes bone strength. The standing poses, especially those that require balancing, create and maintain joint stability in the hips, knees, and ankles. Asanas that demand work of the arms, such as Adho Mukha Shvanasna (Downward-Facing Dog) or variations of plank poses, build stability in the shoulder joints, thus preventing injuries. Twists and inversions keep the spine strong and aligned. Yoga can help prevent and alleviate osteoporosis and arthritis as well as mechanical misalignments because the integrity of structural balance is maintained.

When strong, balanced muscles hold the bones in place, mechanical alignment is achieved. Chiropractors manipulate the joints of the spine to realign them, but if the muscle tissues that connect to the spine are not balanced and strengthened, then the

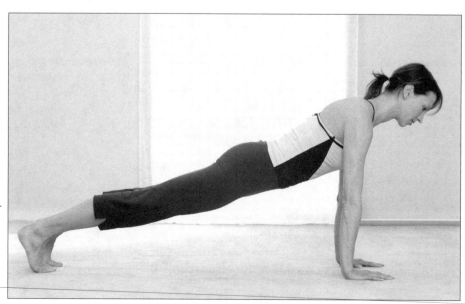

This woman is preventing the problems that stem from osteoporosis and arthritis by practicing a weight-bearing pose.

© Jumpfoto

adjustment is temporary. Likewise, many treatments can relieve the pain from a ruptured disk or pinched nerve, yet in the long run, treating the root cause of misalignments usually proves the safest and cheapest method.

Just as car tires need to be balanced and held in place with nuts and bolts, the joints of the human body are kept in alignment by strong, balanced muscles. Imagine that your car tires are misaligned. Unnecessary strain is placed on the structure of your vehicle. Not only do the tires wear out much faster, but steering is also impeded relative to the degree of imbalance. If you get your tires aligned, but the mechanic neglects to secure the tires in place, then, like your spinal joints from a chiropractic adjustment, the alignment will not hold.

Muscular System

When muscles are not used they lose mass and function. Chronic tension or scar tissue from an injury interferes with normal muscle function. Yoga is one of the few physical practices that increase functional strength and flexibility in a balanced way. Research done at the University of California at Davis demonstrated that after only eight weeks of practicing yoga, the muscular strength of people involved in the study increased by 31 percent, their muscular endurance by 57 percent, and their flexibility by 188 percent (Bauman, 2002).

An asana practice strengthens as well as deeply stretches the muscles. The effect of yoga practice on muscles and tendons can enhance fitness in addition to promoting basic healthy functioning. Both range of motion and stability are needed for optimal functioning of the structures that the muscles move. Daily living skills are preserved through regular yoga practice. If functional strength is not maintained then the ability to simply get up from a chair, walk up stairs, or open a jar becomes difficult or lost. Repetitive motion strain can be avoided as asana practice strengthens and balances opposing muscles and stretches overtense ones. A well-balanced muscular system protects the other systems of the body the muscles move or surround, such as the spine.

Digestive System

The gastrointestinal tract is toned and stretched through asana practice. Sluggishness in the digestive tract is removed as organs are stimulated. Forward bends can stimulate both digestion and hunger. Hunger is reduced in backbends as the vagus nerve is stretched. Backbends also stretch the stomach

away from the esophagus and diaphragm. Thus, with regular practice of these asanas the tendency to herniate is greatly reduced. The liver, pancreas, and other organs get a massaging effect from asanas. Yoga asanas encourage healthy digestion and elimination. Therefore, nutritional absorption increases while constipation, gas, and toxicity tend to decrease. For those suffering from digestive system disorders such as heartburn or irritable bowel syndrome (IBS), the gentle stretching and compressing of twisting yoga postures helps increase circulation to the area and soothes the entire system, thus allowing it time to heal.

Reproductive System

For women in their childbearing years, the fluctuations of hormones throughout their cycle can cause a number of unpleasant effects. Painful menstrual cramps, backaches, and irritability are just a few. The stress-reducing properties of restorative asanas can help calm the mood. Asanas that open the hips can be applied to menstrual disorders and pregnancy. Malasana (Squat Pose) is a good preparation and labor technique because the posture flushes the reproductive and urinary organs with greater circulation and the supporting musculature is strengthened. The practice of mula bandha (root lock; see later section on bandhas) can be applied to prevent or reverse prolapse in these areas.

For men, practicing pelvic-opening postures also is of benefit for the reproductive organs. The practice of mula bandha especially helps strengthen the pelvic floor muscles and increases the blood flow in these areas.

Respiratory System

The skin is the largest organ of the body, and it is part of the respiratory system. As pranayama improves the entire respiratory system, a beneficial effect will be noticed on the skin as well. The capacity of the lungs is optimized because asanas and pranayama expand the elasticity of the intercostal (inter-rib) muscles. The thoracic cage and subsequent oxygen capacity usually diminish with age as the ribs and spine stiffen, but practicing yoga provides the opposite effect. The walls of the lungs are also made stronger as the intercostal muscles are expanded in asanas. Alveoli (sacs that contain air in the lungs) are opened up more fully so that perfusion of the lung is improved. In forward-bending asanas the posterior part of the lung gets stretched and is well ventilated, which is not the case in most other forms of exercise. Poses like

Adho Mukha Shvanasana (Downward-Facing Dog) can improve vital capacity, producing the effect of having run for a prolonged period though without strain. A $\dot{V}O_2$max test is a procedure that measures the maximal oxygen uptake of a person and is used to calculate how efficiently the individual uses oxygen. In one study, regular yoga practitioners had $\dot{V}O_2$max measurements equivalent to that of moderate athletes (Bauman, 2002). Thus, the cardiovascular system also is improved by yoga. In fact, there have been documented cases of yoga masters with the ability to control their heart rate (yet this is more a function of voluntary control over so-called involuntary mechanisms of the central nervous system).

Circulatory System

Like the skeletal muscles, the heart and blood vessels are strengthened and kept flexible through yoga. The cardiac sphincter is strengthened during the movement of backbends. The anterior and lateral walls (front and sides) of the heart are completely stretched and strengthened so that the blood flow around the periphery of the organ remains healthy. Asanas enhance blood flow into the thoracic bed and improve the elasticity of the aorta. Many exercises, yoga included, improve angina tolerance. Angina is the referred chest pain that occurs when the heart muscle receives insufficient oxygen. Other forms of exercise, however, are void of the arterial-massage effect created by yoga.

Because standing poses are more static than dynamic, minimal lactic acid is formed in the muscles, so fatigue is avoided in both the circulatory system as well as the skeletal muscles. The entire circulatory system is kept healthy through yoga practice as blood vessels get relief from gravity in inversions or restorative poses where the legs are raised or the head is below the heart. The formation of varicose veins also is reduced as a result of the constant massaging effect of the asanas. Circulation to the brain is increased, which can reduce the chance of stroke. Asanas allow an increased efficiency of the circulatory system without undue strain to any systems of the body.

Endocrine System

The endocrine system monitors and produces hormonal secretions needed to regulate bodily activities. When functioning well, this system creates a healthy balance (homeostasis) within the body, thus strengthening the immune system and helping to increase the resistance to illness. Backbends stretch and stimulate the mid-sternal area where the thymus gland is located. The thymus is recognized as playing a major role in immune function. Practicing Salamba Sarvangasana (Supported Shoulderstand) bathes the thyroid gland, which is located in the neck region. It is believed that regular flushing of the gland helps with imbalances such as hypothyroidism, a condition that slows metabolism.

Psychoneuroimmunology is the study of the immune system with regard to mind and body health. More specifically, this form of study looks at how behavior and perceptions together with the endocrine system influence overall well-being. In energetic anatomy there are seven major energy centers in the body called *chakras* [CHUK-ruhs]. The centers that correspond to the endocrine system are associated with physical and mental balance. Both energetic anatomy and the chakras are discussed in more detail in the next section.

Nervous Systems

The brain and spinal cord form the central nervous system (CNS), which is the command center for the body. The CNS receives and interprets information sent from the body's many systems and, after processing the signals, sends out impulses for these systems to act on accordingly. The system of nerves that connect the CNS with the muscles and glands of the body is the peripheral nervous system (PNS). The PNS is composed of nerves, which relay information to and from the central nervous system to the body's periphery. The PNS divides further into the somatic and autonomic nervous systems. *Somatic* neurons (nerve cells) send impulses from the CNS to the skeletal muscles to produce movement. The *autonomic* neurons connect to the involuntary muscle tissues. There are two types of involuntary muscle: smooth, located in the stomach, intestines, and blood vessels, and cardiac which is located in the heart.

The autonomic nervous system divides further into the sympathetic nervous system (SNS) and the parasympathetic nervous systems (PSNS). These two branches play key roles in the stress response. When the SNS is stimulated it calls the body's systems into action. The typical response of a person who is under stress is an increase in heart rate and respiration, a redirection of blood flow away from vital organs and into the skeletal muscles, pupil dilation, and an overabundance of adrenalin and other stress hormones racing through the body.

The role of the PSNS is to bring the body's systems back to normal after a stressful event and to conserve the body's energy. As the PSNS shuts down the stress responses of the sympathetic system, the PSNS also nourishes and rebuilds the body as it brings systems back into balance. If the PSNS is unable to bring relief to the body, eventually all the systems of the body become overtaxed. In many cases, when the PSNS is unable to do its work, systems begin to fail and illness and disease are able to set in. Early death often is a result.

All the asanas promote homeostasis, or internal equilibrium, as the body strives to function without strain. Asanas that place the spine in horizontal positions are especially good because the sympathetic neurons are quieted and blood-pressure regulation occurs. Pranayama, as mentioned in chapter 4, strengthens the PSNS by bringing relaxation through rhythmic breathing. At the end of each asana workout students practice Shavasana (Corpse Pose) as a method of deep relaxation and restoration.

Energetic Anatomy

All forms of life have an essential energy flowing throughout their physical structure. To many, this energy is the essence of life itself, and as such, many world cultures base the relative health of their citizens on the health of the energy systems within each individual. Energetic, or metaphysical, anatomy refers to the systems within the body that are not necessarily observable. Energetic anatomy may or may not be consciously felt and only recently can it be measured by modern science, yet the teachings of this subtle system have existed since ancient times.

In traditional Chinese medicine the body's energy channels, or meridians, are mapped out. These maps are used to guide the practitioner in treating the patient through acupuncture. The ancient medicine of India, known as Ayurveda, also maps out the body's energy channels similar to those mapped by the meridians. The Ayurvedic term for these channels is *nadi* (NAH-dee). The nadis make up a vast network throughout the body and connect from the *chakras*, which are considered power centers located vertically alongside the spinal column. In 2000, Dr. Hiroshi Motoyama, renowned author, physiological psychologist, and founder of the California Institute for Human Science, demonstrated that the areas within the body believed to be chakras have a distinct electrical presence when compared to other locations of the body. He essentially proved the physical existence of the chakras. More information on Dr. Motoyama's research can be found at www.cihs.edu.

The nadis and chakras have corresponding psychological and physical centers. As the body moves through a variety of asanas, these centers are gently twisted, compressed, and stretched. Special techniques in hatha yoga are practiced as a means of moving and maintaining the energy of the metaphysical body while protecting the physical body. These techniques are called *bandhas* [BUHN-dhuhs]. Bandha means "lock" in Sanskrit. There are also sheaths or systems of yoga anatomy called *koshas* [KOH-shuhs], which are briefly explained later in this chapter.

Chakras

As previously explained, the chakras are the major energy centers of the physical and energetic body. Energy moves through the seven main chakras which are located from the base of the spine to the crown of the head. It is believed that each of the chakras represents a progression of stages of consciousness as we follow the path toward enlightenment. The chakras listed in figure 5.1 are also associated with a physical location within the body as well as with an emotional or psychological manifestation. Table 5.1 illustrates the connection between the chakras and their Ayurvedic elements with physical and psychological functions and associations.

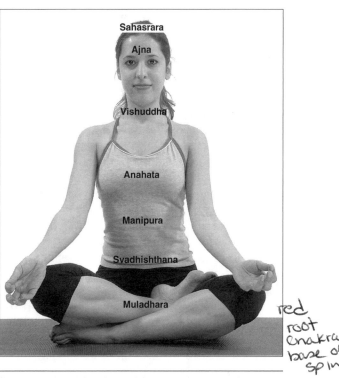

Figure 5.1 The physical locations associated with the seven chakras: Sahasrara, Ajna, Vishuddha, Anahata, Manipura, Svadhishthana, and Muladhara.

Table 5.1 Chakras

[handwritten annotations:] Chakra = wheels / spinning wheel of energy

Chakra	Chakra location	Ayurvedic element	Physical functions and associations	Psychological functions and associations
[white/violet] 7th—Sahasrara	Crown of head			
[purple indigo] 6th—Ajna	Above and between the eyebrows; "the third eye"		Medulla oblongata and pineal gland	Wisdom, intuition, and meditation
[blue] 5th—Vishuddha	Throat	Ether	Thyroid	Expression, communication, and will
[green] 4th—Anahata	Heart area	Air	Thymus, heart, and respiration	Love, compassion, and immunity
[yellow] 3rd—Manipura	Solar plexus; naval area (known as the *hara* area in Chinese medicine)	Fire	Digestive	Ambition, achievement, power, and control
[5 orange] 2nd—Svadhisthana	Sacral plexus (pelvic area)	Water	Reproductive	Sexual energy, self-esteem, and identity
[red] 1st—Muladhara	Perineum and coccyx (between genitalia and base of the spine)	Earth	Elimination	Survival and stability

Bandhas

The *bandhas* control where the internal energy moves or stays while practicing asanas. Depending on the asana, one or all of the bandhas may be activated. Just as specific muscles are activated to provide core strength or stability, the bandhas act as metaphysical or core-energy stabilizers. The energy is essentially locked within the body through the bandha by contracting certain muscles as will be described. A bandha is often applied during the asanas because it enables greater energy and stamina to work within a person on both a physical and energetic level because the energy is retained within the body.

The associations and applications of energetic anatomy are intertwined with physical, mental, and emotional effects. For example, it is advisable for women to refrain from practicing Shirsasana (Headstand) or other inversions during menstruation because during this time part of the woman's energy needs to flow downward. The term to explain downward-moving energy is *apana* (uh-PAAH-nuh). The apana is in opposition to not only a physically inverted asana but also it is in conflict with the upward promotion of energy of the root lock, or mula bandha. *Udana* [oo-DAAH-nuh], meaning upward movement, is the upward-moving energy that directs effort in the body.

A bandha generally is thought of solely in energetic terms, but it is also a physical technique with physical effects during which contraction of the muscles occurs within a particular region of the body. The body has three main bandhas: mula [MOO-luh], uddiyana [ood-dee-AH-nuh], and jalandhara [JAAH-lund-uh-ruh].

- **mula bandha**—Located in the perineum between the anus and the genitalia. The action of the lock is akin to the kegel exercise when the pubococcygeal muscles are contracted.

- **uddiyana bandha**—Located in the abdominal area. The action of this lock is the firming and lifting of the respiratory diaphragm and supporting musculature while still allowing for normal respiration.

- **jalandhara bandha**—Located at the top of the throat. The action of this lock occurs when the chest is lifted and the chin rests on the sternal notch.

By applying these physical techniques during asana practice the student is better able to retain and move energy throughout the body to increase mental and physical stability both during practice and after.

Koshas

In traditional yoga anatomy there are six koshas, which are layers or sheaths that make up a person's physical and energetic body. The six koshas are as follows:

Energy Words

bandhas [BUHN-dhuhs]—Physical techniques that lock in and prevent energy from escaping from the body.

mudras [muhd-RAAHS]—Energy-locking techniques that generally consist of hand gestures, such as prayer position, or *anjali mudra* [UHN-juh-lee muhd-RAAH].

drishti [dr-EESH-tee]—The area where your physical eyes focus while practicing asanas.

prana [PRAAH-naah]—The life force of the breath.

- **annamaya** [AAH-nuh-MAAH-yuh]—The material, or physical, sheath that requires food. All of the gross anatomy making up the physical body falls into this category.

- **pranamaya** [PRAAH-naah-MAAH-yuh]—The astral, or vital sheath, that channels prana (breath) throughout the body.

- **manomaya** [MAAH-noh-MAAH-yuh]—The emotional mind sheath, which comprises your affect, feelings, and emotional quotient (EQ).

- **jnanamaya** [YAAH-nuh-MAAH-yuh]—The sheath of knowledge, or more specifically, what one feels to be true.

- **vijnanamaya** [vih-jyuh-nuh-MAAH-yuh]—The intellectual sheath encompassing mental faculties and intelligence.

- **anandamaya** [AAH-nuhn-duh-MAAH-yuh]—The sheath of bliss. This sheath is the link to and awareness of the spirit.

The focus of this book is to give yoga instructors guidance and understanding on how to teach and adjust yoga postures appropriately. However, a basic understanding of how the ancient yogic beliefs of the interconnectedness of the physical, emotional, and spiritual realms of human existence is just as important to the well-being of your students. Table 5.1 illustrates the connection between the chakras and koshas with physical and psychological functions and associations.

A yoga class can have a positive effect on all the koshas and create a more balanced functioning of the chakras. Some people strive in yoga to integrate all their faculties, as much as possible, to experience a spiritual ecstasy. Most people in today's modern Western world simply wish to reduce stress and pain or improve their immune system through yoga practice. Many people are motivated to be in better physical shape. Regardless of the aim or the anatomy paradigm, there is a certain mindfulness that is essential in yoga practice and teaching. The more prevalent this mindfulness is, the more profound the benefits on all the anatomical systems or koshas.

Human Movement Systems

Movement of the human body occurs at many levels—from the molecular level where oxygen converts into energy within the lungs to the coordinated effort of the musculoskeletal system in intricate and complex single-limbed balance postures. The gross, or large, anatomy of the human body is described as those physical structures that can be seen with the naked eye. Although the practice of yoga postures affects the body at all levels as previously discussed, the focus of this section is on the interconnectedness of the musculoskeletal structures and how these structures are meant to move efficiently and with minimal risk of injury.

Understanding the mechanical principles of how the human body moves helps yoga instructors understand how to sequence their classes to afford students the maximum physical and mental benefits possible. Also, by applying principles of human movement, instructors are better able to recognize when students may place themselves in positions that put them at risk for physical injury and will know when and how to appropriately apply physical adjustments.

Musculoskeletal System

The human movement system is composed of bones, skeletal muscles, tendons, ligaments, and fasciae. The skeleton is the framework of bones that defines both our shape and function as human beings. Muscles attach to bones by tendons and other connective tissue and provide the means to move the bones to create specific movement patterns. A joint is formed where the ends of two bones come together. And when a muscle that crosses the joint contracts, the bone acts as a lever to create movement.

Skeletal Muscle

The contractions of the skeletal muscles create movement through the body, allowing the ability to move from posture to posture. An overview of muscle tissue illustrates how the interconnectedness of movement in one part of the body affects other, seemingly remote, areas of the body.

Each skeletal muscle consists of layers of muscle tissue bundled together and surrounded by a matrix of collagenous tissue. At the end of each muscle the connective tissues converge as tendons and connect the muscle to the bones. An extensive layer of dense connective tissue called the *deep fascia* lines the walls of the body and limbs and divides the muscles into functionally similar groupings (see figure 5.2). Another layer of connective tissue exists, the *superficial fascia*, which wraps a continuous web over the blood vessels, nerves, and lymphatics. The interstitial fluid circulating to nodes that work with the immune system and are involved in detoxifying the body are referred to as lymphatics, or lymphatic fluid.

Fascia

The fascia is a web of connective tissue throughout the entire body. On one level the fascia acts much like a stocking does when it is pulled on a leg. Imagine pulling on a long stocking, and notice what happens to the material at the toe when a tiny section of the stocking is pulled at the upper leg. The tension can be seen and felt all the way down the length of the entire stocking because all of the material in the stocking is connected. The effect is even greater in the fascia because there are more layers of fascia throughout an actual leg than just the thin, external layer of a stocking. Thus, if there is a tight spot within the body, that tightness affects the entire structure to

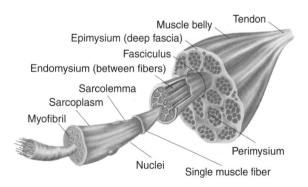

Figure 5.2 Diagram illustrating the arrangement of connective tissues within and surrounding a skeletal muscle.

Reprinted, by permission, from National Strength Training and Conditioning Association, 2000, *Essentials of strength training and conditioning,* 2nd ed. (Champaign, IL: Human Kinetics), 4.

some degree. This description illustrates how truly interconnected the physical structures of the human body are; making changes in one area affects another, even if there appears to be no direct connection. Tightness in one area of the body can manifest as pain or dysfunction in other seemingly unconnected areas of the body. Strengthening and stretching areas of the body through yoga postures can bring about a holistic balance throughout the entire system.

How Muscles Create Movement

Movement of a body segment occurs when a muscle applies some degree of force through its tendon onto its bony attachment. When muscle fibers generate sufficient tension within the muscle, a muscular contraction occurs, and the subsequent movement moves or stabilizes the body segments.

Muscles work in concert to move the body in a coordinated fashion. Because of the interconnectedness of the skeletal-system tissues and the fact that many muscles cross more than one joint, trying to isolate a single muscle in a yoga posture is like trying to isolate a single note in a chord being played. Although several muscles influence the movement of a particular body part, or segment, many times one muscle is the most responsible for the movement. These muscles are considered the *prime movers*, and the other contributing muscles are *synergistic* muscles. In addition to aiding the prime movers, the synergistic muscles are used to stabilize, or to refine, certain types of movements.

Types of Muscular Contractions

Just as it is nearly impossible to isolate one muscle to create a specific movement, most meaningful movement is created by a coordination of different types of muscular contractions. There are three primary types of muscular contractions: a concentric contraction, which shortens the muscle; an eccentric contraction, which lengthens; and an isometric contraction, which keeps the muscle held at the same length. Yoga asanas use a variety of contractions when moving into, remaining in, and moving out of any position. To illustrate how a particular asana uses all three types of contractions at specific points within the asana, the following outline highlights the action of the oblique abdominals (lateral or side) and quadratus lumborum muscles (located on each side of the spine in the lower back) when performing Utthita Trikonasana (Extended Triangle).

- An **eccentric contraction** occurs when muscle fibers lengthen from a shortened state when an external force, such as gravity, is applied. The tension within the muscles acts as a braking force, resisting the external force. In Extended Triangle, as a person extends out to the left and reaches the left hand toward the floor, the internal and external oblique muscles and the quadratus lumborum on the right side contract eccentrically to lower the torso in a controlled fashion.

- An **isometric contraction** is a contraction where the muscle length actually remains the same. As a person holds the extended position in Triangle, the same muscles (internal and external obliques and quadratus lumborum) remain essentially the same length as they hold the body in position and keep the ribcage from either collapsing or rounding.

- A **concentric contraction** occurs when muscle fibers draw together, shortening the muscle's length and bringing the two ends of the muscle toward each other. In Extended Triangle, as a person moves back into an upright position, the muscles (internal and external obliques and quadratus lumborum) contract concentrically to bring the person back to standing.

Recognize that when you are moving into and out of yoga postures, the same muscles are generally used throughout the posture. The type of contraction changes, however, as the direction of movement as well as the influence of gravity changes. This statement holds true for most yoga postures and is explained in more detail in each asana chapter in part 2.

Three-Dimensional Movement

To facilitate the proper execution of an asana with regard to spatial orientation of the body, it is important to use recognized standardized terms (see figure 5.3). The most universally accepted way to describe movement patterns is to begin with the body in what is called the *anatomical position*. To begin, picture a person standing erect, arms at the sides of the body, with the head, chest, palms, knees, and toes facing forward. Typically, movement is explained as the body deviates from the anatomical position. An action that moves a body section away from the midline of the body is called *abduction*. When a body section is moved toward the midline that action is called *adduction*. When two bones, such as the upper and lower arm bones, move closer toward each other, decreasing the angle, the joint is in *flexion*. When the segments move away from each other, thereby increasing the angle, the joint is in *extension*. *Rotation* of a body segment occurs as the segment twists about a fixed point within the joint.

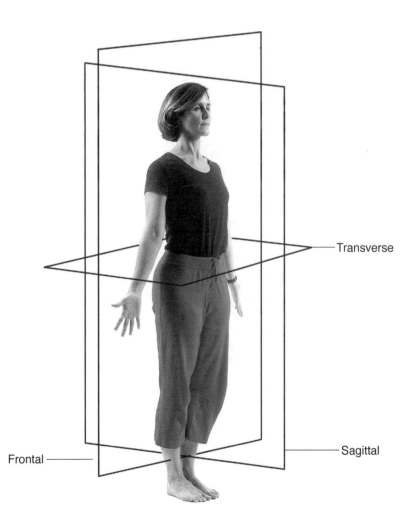

Figure 5.3 Figure in anatomical position with the body bisected into left and right (sagittal), superior and inferior (transverse), and anterior and posterior (frontal) planes.

Anatomical Planes of Motion

The body moves within the three planes of three-dimensional space: sagittal, coronal, and transverse. Each plane is perpendicular to each of the other two. By using these directional terms, one is able to describe where a body segment is in relation to another, whether standing, seated, facedown, or faceup on the floor.

The planes of motion are as follows:

- The sagittal plane is a vertical plane that passes through the body from front to back, dividing the body into left and right sides (see figure 5.4). Movements within this plane occur forward and backward, such as the typical human gait.

- The frontal, or coronal, plane passes through the body vertically, dividing the body into front (anterior) and back (posterior) parts (see figure 5.5). Movement in this plane occurs along the side.

- The transverse, or horizontal, plane is oriented horizontally and passes through the body, dividing it into upper and lower portions (see figure 5.6). Rotation of the body about the spinal axis, such as in a twist and a pirouette, occurs within this plane.

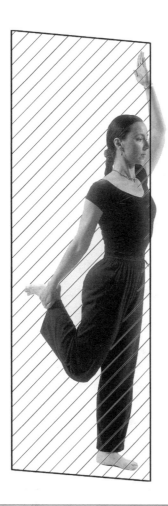

Figure 5.4 The sagittal plane.

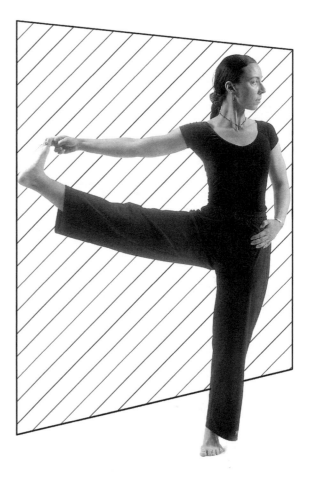

Figure 5.5 The frontal plane.

Figures 5.4 to 5.6 represent the concepts of movement and stillness in relation to the anatomical planes. Figure 5.4 illustrates the sagittal plane. The person is entering into Natarajasana (King Dancer). The bent leg is moving back, therefore it is moving in the sagittal plane.

Figure 5.5 illustrates movement in the frontal plane. The asana Utthita Hasta Padangusthasana (Extended Hand-to-Toe Pose) is depicted. When the lifted leg is out front it is in the sagittal plane. When the lifted leg is rotated out to the side it comes into the frontal plane along with the rest of the body. It rotates along the transverse plane until it is positioned in the frontal plane.

A well-crafted yoga class moves students' limbs and spines through a full range of motion, encompassing all three planes. In any given class, the spine should move in the six directions for which it is designed, which all occur in the three planes: moving forward and backward in the sagittal plane, bending laterally to the left and right in the frontal plane, and twisting (rotating) both left and right in the transverse plane.

Mechanics of Asanas

Most yoga asanas, when executed correctly, move the body fully through the anatomical planes of

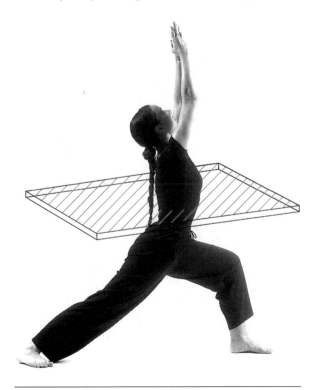

Figure 5.6   The transverse plane.

motion. For all students, especially those with limited flexibility, moving the body with the muscles properly aligned creates less strain on the stabilizing structures of the joints, allowing for greater efficiency of movement and decreased risk of injury. One of the most important areas of the human body is the spine and its surrounding structures. Generally, without mechanically sound alignment beginning in the spine, the rest of the joints and segments in any given asana can be thrown off balance. It is therefore imperative to guide your students to their best spinal alignment at the beginning of a posture before they begin to move deeper.   *tadasana*

Importance of Spinal Positioning

The ideal in human postural alignment is a flexible, strong spine with healthy curves. The spine is not meant to align perfectly straight like a pencil. A normal, healthy spine has a natural S-like shape when viewed from the right side. There is a slight concave curvature in the cervical (neck) area. The shape of the spine becomes convex in the thoracic, upper-middle area of the back, and moves into a concave curvature in the lumbar, or low back, area. A neutral position of the spine is when the natural curves are intact and not overexaggerated.

The shape of the spinal curves, in addition to the disks, provides shock absorption and allows for a greater range of motion within the spine. Stability in the range of motion and the spacing between the vertebrae allow the nerves to be free of obstruction. When standing in a semirelaxed upright position, such as Tadasana (Mountain Pose), one should strive to create as much space as possible between each vertebra. Creating this space helps lengthen the torso and allows for easier movement about the spine in yoga as well as in general everyday movement patterns.

Unfortunately, not everyone has the luxury of healthy spinal curves. A spine that curves laterally to either side or twists about the axis of the spine results in a condition known as scoliosis. If the thoracic section is in an overly pronounced convex curve, it is said to be *hyperkyphotic*. If the lower back sways far beyond a balanced neutral spine then it is considered *hyperlordodic*. A hypolordotic spine is when the lower back seems to be flat and lacking a curve. All of these conditions can create physical ailments such as general spinal pain, headaches, and compressed internal organs as well as a state in which the body overcompensates by overactivity of certain muscles as the body tries to properly align itself. Because yoga practice focuses on lengthening and strengthening the spine in all directions, those with spinal deviations can help alleviate some of the detrimental effects these conditions cause by practicing yoga regularly.

The "Perfect" Asana

Because yoga has become so popular, anyone can find a photo or videotape depicting the "perfect" positioning of a posture. Unfortunately, many people feel that even in their first attempt at a posture, they should look exactly like the people presented in a magazine or video, or like their instructor for that matter. The truth is that yoga is not solely for the svelte, flexible young models one finds most often in print media. Yoga is for everyone regardless of physical attributes, age, strength, or flexibility. Each person's body is unique, and because everyone has different imbalances in strength and flexibility it is virtually impossible to label someone as a "beginner" or "advanced" student based on the asanas they look picture perfect doing.

Advancement in hatha yoga is an extremely internal process for each student. It is much more important for students to learn how to recognize areas of tension and weakness within their body so they can work on ways to tailor an asana to their needs as opposed to striving for what they think the pose should look like. If students do not work within this principle, they are simply performing gymnastics instead of yoga.

An example of this concept is when a yogi enters a backbend. He seeks to discover how being in the posture may reveal the wisdom of his body and open the doors to peace of mind. When a gymnast enters a backbend her goal is to make her body bend backward in a certain way. A correctly executed asana is one that restores or maintains range of motion and functional postural strength. If enough awareness and control of the body and mind are engaged, not only will injuries be prevented but also the normal processes of aging can be minimized.

Everyone's ideal posture will look different. The most effective adjustments are those made from the inside out. B.K.S. Iyengar has been quoted as saying, "The brain is the hardest part of the body to

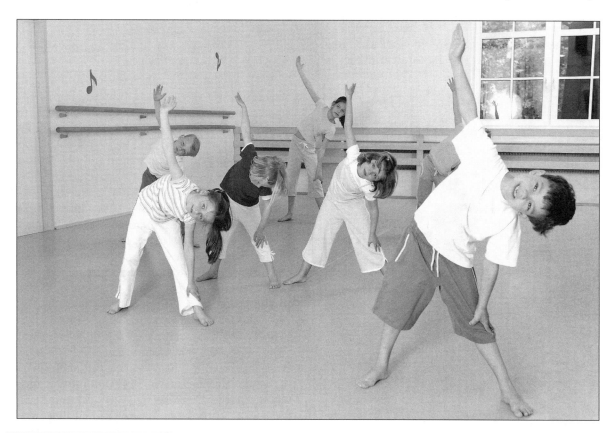

Even children can experience the life-long benefits of yoga.
© Jumpfoto

hold 5-7 breaths (handwritten)

adjust in asanas" (Iyengar, 1979). It is sometimes difficult for an instructor to change a student's attitude about the unimportance of achieving an ideal posture on one's first attempt. The skillful instructor will work to guide students into finding the perfection of a posture within themselves not outside of themselves—to help them feel the grace of their own bodies.

Holding Asanas

By focusing on the physical and mental abilities of the entire class, the instructor can decide the appropriate amount of time students should remain in postures. In some ways the length of time a posture is held can be likened to weight or endurance training. In weight training the number of repetitions and sets are modified slowly to increase muscular strength over a period of time. In endurance training the percentage of maximum heart rate and amount of time exercising increase to bring about changes in both muscular and cardiovascular endurance. No matter where a student is physically within a posture, assuming they are not in a position where they might injure themselves, one of the instructor's duties is to create an appropriate flow from one posture to the next.

In determining the amount of time students should remain in any given asana, use a scale from 1 to 10, where 1 means very little mental or physical energy is being exerted, increasing to 10 where an extreme amount of energy is put forth throughout the asana. There are actually a number of variables that the instructor and student should notice when determining the relative intensity of an asana. Ideally, the body and mind should be within the 6 to 8 range and higher on the 1 to 10 scale for each of the following variables:

- *Physical exertion.* Students should try to keep the energy level consistent in the muscles while maintaining the appropriate physical alignment. It should be noted that different body parts may need to be considered independently. For example, in Utthita Trikonasana (Extended Triangle), the legs might be strong but the neck may need to rest. The student can readjust the neck and continue on if the rest of the body remains at a 6 to 8 level. As the overall energy in the pose diminishes, they should come out of the posture.
- *Mental focus.* Students should continually ask themselves whether the mind is aware of the body, or if the mind is wandering elsewhere. Instead of noticing how the hamstrings relax

with each exhalation, one might be wondering, *How can the person next to me do this posture so much better than I can?* When these questions occur, the mental focus plummets to the lowest level on the scale, and it is time to either refocus or come out of the asana.

- *Endurance.* The postures should be held with awareness and intensity as long as breathing is steady and the mind and body do not stray from the 6 to 8 range for more than two breaths. As soon as two breaths are taken outside of the ideal range, then it is best to come out of the pose and rest or start over. Another guideline is to work up to holding the 6 to 8 plus range for each posture for 90 to 120 seconds.

In a class setting the instructor must decide on a baseline average length of time for students to hold a pose that will comfortably challenge the group as a whole. Mr. Iyengar has been quoted as saying that just when one feels one cannot hold the pose any longer is when the posture really begins. Yoga teachers must constantly observe students to assess how they are doing. A general rule of thumb is to wait until 20 percent of students have come out of the asana, and then bring the rest of the class out of the posture and move on. For example, if there are 10 students in class holding Virabhadrasana II (Warrior II), wait until two students appear to have come out of the position before moving on to the next posture. Meanwhile, if you begin to observe some minor struggles—students' breath becoming labored, faces strained, fidgeting, profuse sweating—you might quote Mr. Iyengar about how the pose may just officially be beginning for some of them. You may see smiles. You may even hear moans but probably no serious threats! If you hear sighs when you finally bring the students out of the pose, it is a good indication they were in the pose long enough to have reaped the benefits of the posture and are relieved to move on to another.

Avoiding Injury

One of the reasons students attend yoga classes is that they heard yoga makes people flexible. The consistent focus on relaxing and lengthening the muscles in asanas is a great draw. Unfortunately, because many new students have come to yoga from competitive sports or are still harboring the old-time "No pain, no gain" mentality, they have no idea just how much they can or should push themselves in class.

Muscles can stretch up to 150 percent of their resting length before tearing. Most experts agree that tendons and ligaments can stretch up to 4 percent before injury (Alter, 2004). Although there is some elasticity to tendons and ligaments, their main function is to provide stability to the joints. Recognize that stability should not be ignored or sacrificed in pursuit of greater range of motion.

The strengthening and stabilizing of many applied physical actions are fairly consistent throughout the asanas. Bending forward from the hips instead of the lower back, keeping the kneecaps lifted, but not locked, while in standing postures, rotating the shoulders externally, and rotating the thighs externally are almost universal techniques in many standing poses and make sound biomechanical sense. You can reduce the possibility of injury for each student by teaching them the importance of going into a posture with full awareness and never deepening a posture to the point of physical pain.

Spinal Stability

To properly execute both a standing or seated forward bend, the body should hinge at the hip joint while the spine remains in a lengthened position (figure 5.7*a*). However, because of decreased hamstring flexibility and weakness in the spinal muscles, many students allow their backs to relax and round while they attempt to bring the head toward the knees (figure 5.7*b*). This action causes undue stress on the weakened spinal musculature and also can exacerbate even the slightest injury or discomfort in the area.

In standing forward bends the legs help suspend the weight of the body, and because the pelvis is not resting on the floor it is able to move more freely in space. Whether gravity helps or hinders a person in forward bends is dependent on how much flexibility the person has in the hip and hamstring muscles. In general, even a person with extremely inflexible hamstrings and lower back muscles is able to bring the torso to at least 90 degrees of forward flexion. If the person is able to flex the torso more than 90 degrees, the pull of gravity encourages the spine to lengthen. To protect the lower back in students with extremely tight hamstrings, invite them to bend their knees slightly. This action loosens the hamstrings attachment at the knee joint and consequently allows for lengthening at the connection to the pelvis, which in turn allows the pelvis to rotate forward more freely. Another technique to decrease the possibility of back strain in standing forward bends is to encourage students to place their hands on their thighs for support and to concentrate on keeping the spine lengthened.

Because the legs are fixed against the ground in seated forward bends, students with limited flexibility in the hamstrings or lower back are especially affected. The gravitational force in seated forward bends encourages the spine to curl or hunch forward. The most important thing to impress on students is the need to keep their spines as straight as possible as they bend forward from the hip joint. This alignment is also the most difficult thing for many students to accomplish because they will be focused on bending forward and touching their toes at all costs!

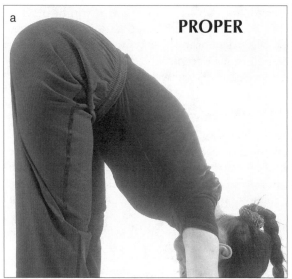 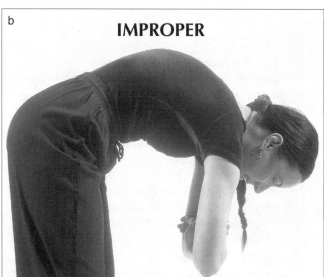

Figure 5.7   Forward bend: (a) Proper alignment of the spine and (b) **improper alignment of the spine.**

For most students in a seated forward bend, the body is placed in 90 degrees of hip flexion to begin with. The ischial tuberosities, or sits bones, are fixed against the ground making it more difficult to roll the top of the pelvis forward. Because there is less forward flexion initiated at the hip joint, more stress is placed on the lower back while bending forward. Ironically, most people think that seated poses are easier and less likely to lead to injury than standing postures, when, in fact, seated poses require greater effort and strength of the soft tissues that stabilize the spine. Seated postures have the potential to overextend the structures of the lower spine.

Given the effects just explained, be careful when physically adjusting someone in a seated forward bend, such as Janu Shirshasana (Head-to-Knee Pose) and Paschimottanasana (Seated Forward Bend). Students should avoid pressing the ribcage down toward the knees but instead lengthen the ribs away from the hips toward the toes.

Lifted Knee Caps (Not Locked)

In standing asanas, the legs provide support and stability for the entire body. Ideally, all of the lower-extremity muscles should be contracted at a moderate level to stabilize the joints and provide balance (see figure 5.8a). To extend the knee joint and keep the legs as straight as possible, the quadriceps (front thigh muscles) contract. This action slightly lifts the patellas (knee caps). If the contraction of the quadriceps is extreme, the pull

through the quadriceps tendon can bring the tibia (lower leg bone) forward of the knee joint rather than aligning the tibia with the femur (thighbone). If the hamstring muscles (back of the thigh) are relaxed, it is possible for the knee joint to move past zero degrees of extension, causing the knee to hyperextend—moving the joint in the opposite direction from which it is intended to move. The most common description for this occurrence is "locking" of the knee joint (see figure 5.8b).

You will probably find that many students make the mistake of locking the knees, especially in forward bends. If the hamstrings and quadriceps are not activated simultaneously the knees are placed in a vulnerable position. Without the balance of muscular activation between both the quadriceps and hamstrings, a person's overall posture may be adversely affected. Over time, hyperextension in the knee joint can overstretch the hamstrings tendons and can cause undue stress on the other structures within the joint. Reminding students to keep a balance of activity in the front and back of the legs can help keep them from putting the knee joint in a potentially harmful position.

External Rotation

The lifestyle of modern society is torturous on the shoulders and posture. The amount of time spent sitting and slouching in front of computers and televisions creates a tendency to allow the shoulders to roll forward and sink into the chest. Yoga practice is a wonderful way to open the chest and shoulder joint and helps to erase

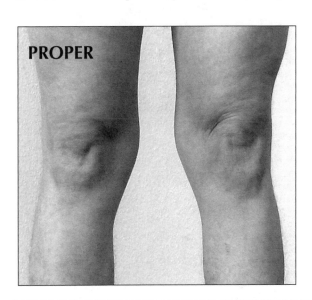
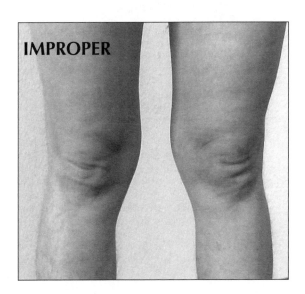

Figure 5.8 Proper leg alignment: (a) correct positioning of the knee and (b) **improper leg alignment with a locked knee.**

the effects of poor posture. In almost all the asanas, external rotation of the shoulder joint is applied to open and expand the chest.

When a student stands in the anatomical position, the humerus (upper arm bone) rests securely into the joint socket (see figure 5.9a). As the humerus is turned inward toward the chest (internal rotation), the head of the bone rolls slightly away from the secure position in the socket. In nonweight-bearing postures, this action generally does not pose much injury risk. When a student is upright with the arms by their sides, or even with the arms extended to the sides parallel to the floor, it is easy to visualize the direction needed to externally rotate the shoulders and open the chest. When a student is upside down, however, with the arms over the head, it can be somewhat disorienting for an instructor. One serious mistake inexperienced yoga instructors can make is to accidentally internally rotate the shoulders of students practicing asanas where the arms support a significant portion of the body weight (see figure 5.9b). Poses such as Adho Mukha Shvanasana (Downward-Facing Dog), Urdhva Mukha Shvanasana (Upward-Facing Dog), Utthita Chaturanga Dandasana (Plank Pose), Adho Mukha Vrkshasana (Handstand), Bakasana (Crane Pose), and Urdhva

Dhanurasana (Upward Bow Pose) all place a significant amount of bodyweight on the shoulder joint. If the shoulders are rotated internally in these asanas, the shoulder joint is placed in an unstable position, which can stress the tendons and ligaments within the shoulder. In contrast, by externally rotating the shoulder, the joint is stabilized. There have been reports of instructors seriously injuring students when adjusting them in a full backbend or Urdhva Dhanurasana. If you are not trained and experienced in physically adjusting for external rotation, it is best to stick to the verbal cues explained in this book. In addition to studying the information presented here, you can seek out a registered yoga teacher training school by contacting the Yoga Alliance (www.yogaalliance.org) and inquiring how much the program you are interested in emphasizes hands-on adjustments.

Adjustment Guidelines

An instructor's words paint a picture in students' minds, illustrating how they can best move their bodies into any given asana. The image created in their minds may or may not match the sensation

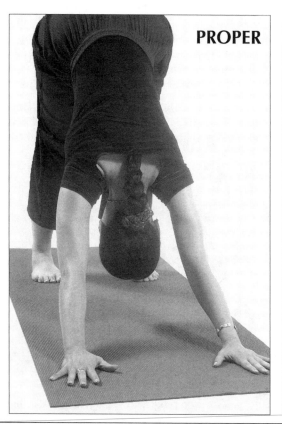 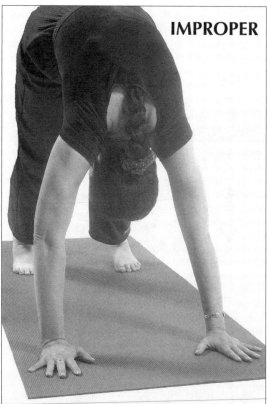

Figure 5.9 (a) Proper rotation of the shoulder and (b) **improper rotation of the shoulder.**

of their bodies. Ideally, however, the words you choose to cue a correct postural adjustment should facilitate a merger of mind and body within each student. By encouraging students to go deeper within themselves, you help them to discover an image that moves beyond a preconceived picture and experience the posture from the inside out. This integration can take place only when students locate their personal edge instead of imitating the actions of the instructor.

Imagery

As was mentioned at the beginning of this chapter, not all students are able to learn simply by watching a visual demonstration. Providing verbal instructions may help guide some students into proper alignment. However, do not be surprised if a number of your students "still don't get" your directions if you do not provide a number of different ways to verbally illustrate a concept. Even when giving verbal adjustment directions, it is necessary to address each student's learning style as discussed in chapter 2. If your students do not have even a vague understanding of anatomical terminology, they simply will not know what to do if you say, "Extend your cranium toward the ceiling." It is fine to give anatomical cues as long as you also provide a couple of other examples for students. You might say, for example, "Feel the top of your head lengthen away from your shoulders," and "Imagine that the top of your head is a magnet, and the beam above your head is metal. Notice the space you create in your neck as the magnet draws up toward the beam." These are just simple examples of how you can use different cuing methods to achieve the same adjustment by addressing the individual learning styles of each of your students. The most important aspect of auditory adjustment cuing is that you observe your class and use compassion and creativity to reach every one of them.

Physical Adjustments

At times, it is appropriate to provide further guidance to students in regard to their physical positioning in any given asana. If you see a student struggling in a posture because his body is mechanically misaligned, or if a student's positioning may place her at risk for injury, move the student into a more stable and risk-free position. In general, it is best to first try to adjust a student's posture by giving verbal cues. One reason for doing so is that if you provide continual physical adjustments the student may become dependent on

them and not be able to find his own inner instructor, the one who actually feels the appropriate place to be in the posture.

When verbal cues are not effective in realigning a student, the next possible course of action is to adjust a student physically. It is imperative, however, that you first ask for, and then receive, permission to touch a student. Adjustments made without invitation are an intrusion on students and can break down the trust students feel toward their instructor. Always ask a student's permission to touch them. Doing so lets them know that you truly honor their trust in you. And at all times when you are given permission, be sure to move each person's body as you would want another instructor to move your own: with invitation, compassion, firm support, nurturing, and receptivity to feedback.

Yoga Lexicon

Like any widely practiced discipline, yoga uses its own particular jargon to describe its philosophy and physical actions. In addition, each instructor, based on personality, devises his or her own phrases to express to students the feelings and motions the instructor wishes to relate to them.

Appropriately worded direction sets the stage for a student's ego to relax more completely while her body is engaged in the asana. Your words should create a warm, nurturing environment for your students. Allow each student to feel comforted and safe in both a physical and psychological way, and select your words with care.

Remember that your words set the tone and progress of a class. Words that imply judgment or classifications such as "advanced students" and "correct" or "perfect posture" should be avoided, as should all negative-sounding words. Appropriate descriptive words are "ideal posture," "more aware," "deeper," and "explore."

The following phrases illustrate ways to descriptively guide students through a class:

- "Extend your tailbone toward the floor." The idea to communicate to students is to lengthen the low back area without tightening the buttocks. "Extending" the tailbone downward indicates a gentle elongation of the lower back and an extension of the neutral spine, as opposed to saying, "tuck your pelvis." Many students perceive "tuck the pelvis" to mean curling the tailbone forward or under to create as much length in the spine as possible. This action moves the lower back in the opposite direction of its natural curve.

- The phrase "edge of balance" is the delicate balance point one reaches just before falling. Being at the edge of balance tests the range of motion and stability of both the body and mind.

- "Bend at the hips like a hinge" means simply to fold forward at the hips and not the waist or low back area. Bending at the hips keeps the spine long and extended and keeps stress off the spine.

- "Breathe into your _____" (any place other than your lungs). The mechanisms of breathing were introduced in the previous chapter, however, continuous focus on breathing cannot be overemphasized. When a teacher tells a student to breathe into her knees, the teacher is really asking the student to visualize and feel the breath and all the associated healing energy in the knees.

- "Stay centered" is a directive to keep students focused as internally as possible. By focusing on their breathing and on the movements, they can eliminate a number of external distractions, which can aid them in relieving stress.

- "Inhale as you expand and exhale when you release." This directive indicates how the breath should be utilized when moving into or out of postures. Typically, one should inhale when moving into postures that lengthen and extend the body. When relaxing into folding postures such as forward bends, one should exhale.

Although this list could continue, these phases were chosen because they appear to be used in yoga classes universally. It is not necessary to use these phrases constantly to express concepts; however, they are a nice way to relay directions when one is just starting out teaching.

Summary

The responsibilities of a yoga instructor are great. Students place their trust in an instructor's ability to relate physical, emotional, and spiritual concepts and that these concepts and ideals are based on a large body of knowledge. A basic understanding of how the body's major systems, both physical and metaphysical, work and how yoga practice can benefit these systems will guide students through a practice that is mechanically sound.

The adjustment information provided here should serve as a guideline in your journey as a yoga instructor. Each person is unique, and there is no one, complete formula that is right for everyone all the time. With mindful instruction and practice you will discover even more techniques along with the intuition and skill with which to apply them.

Study Questions

1. Define "safe" yoga instruction.

2. What is a nadi?

3. What is mula bandha and with which chakra is it associated?

4. Is it advisable for a woman to practice yoga while menstruating?

5. Which anatomical plane does Trikonasana move through?

6. What are the six directions the spine should move through in a balanced workout?

7. Give examples of a few asanas that stimulate osteogenesis and create joint stability.

8. What does it mean to "lift the knee caps"? Why, when, and how would you teach this?

9. Which muscles in the torso are used to move into a standing forward bend, and what type of contraction is utilized? When entering into a standing backbend?

10. What type of contraction is going on during the holding of most asanas?

11. How long should asanas be held?

12. Define what makes a yoga student more advanced.

part 2

Asanas and
Adjustments

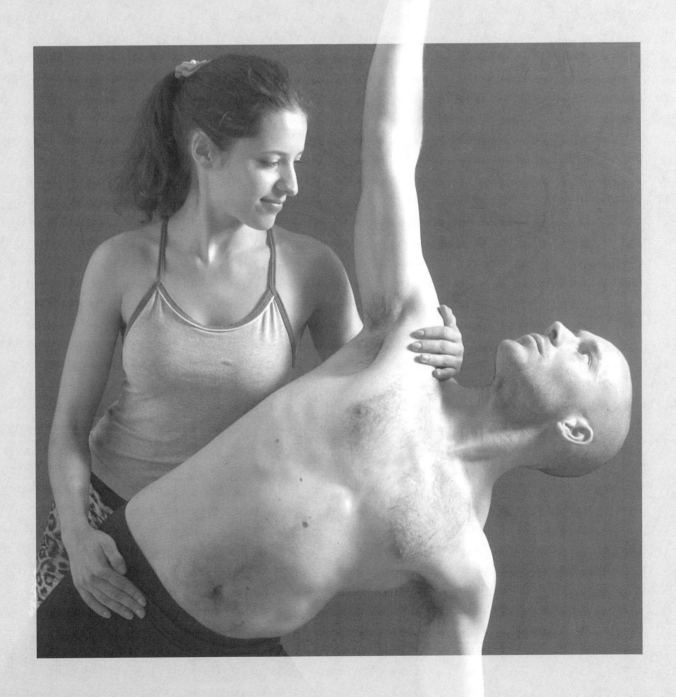

chapter 6

Sun Salutations

A small set or series of postures linked together with breath and movements make up Surya Namaskaras [SOOHR-yuh nuh-muhs-KAAH-ruhs] (Sun Salutations). *Surya* means "sun," and *Namaskara* can be translated as "salutation." The greeting "Namaste" derives from the same root.

The Classical Sun Salutation comprises a flow of postures through gentle backbends, lunges, Utthita Chaturanga Dandasana [oot-T-HEE-tuh chuh-tour-RUHN-guh duhn-DAAH-suh-nuh] (Plank Pose), and Adho Mukha Shvanasana [uhd-HOE moo-KUH SH-vuhn-AAH-suh-nuh] (Downward-Facing Dog). More vigorous salutations are practiced in Ashtanga hatha yoga called "Sun Salutations A and B" in the West and known more traditionally as *Surya Namaskara Ka* and *Kha* in Sanskrit.

The more vigorous Surya Namaskaras are usually associated with Ashtanga, but variations can be practiced in any style hatha by changing the speed or adding alternative postures to the basic form or set. For example, when cuing a lunge in a Classical

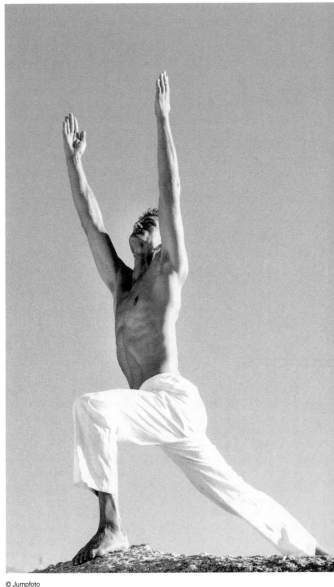

© Jumpfoto

Surya Namaskara, you can teach a variation by raising the arms overhead or clasping the hands behind the back. There are approximately 12 positions and breaths in each basic set. In addition, the sun salutations can be practiced as an entire class series. Many Vinyasa flow classes utilize the salutations to link other postures together.

Traditionally, Surya Namaskaras are practiced facing the rising sun, and the postures are linked together in a way that brings each part of the body in contact with the sun's rays. The true value of the salutations is to warm the body. You can practice one or two slowly and gently, or you can do a number of salutations quickly in a row. The momentum of practicing faster salutations warms the body, and the warmth allows a student to move into poses easier. However, going slowly builds deeper strength even though students may not warm their muscles as quickly and will not be able to rely on momentum to get into the poses.

The benefits of all the salutations are as follows:

- Warm the muscles by taking the body through a large range of motion
- Link the mind, body, and breath
- Increase overall circulation

When guiding students through the sun salutations, keep in mind that, due to the flowing nature of the sequence, each pose is held for a short time. Adjustments are generally not made unless there is a risk of student injury, but it is very important that the instructor watch for rounded backs and shoulders as the students move into and out of forward-bending poses.

The individual poses that make up the sun salutations can be found along with their specific description, cautions, verbal cues, adjustments, modifications and kinematics in chapters 7-11.

Classical Surya Namaskara

This is the traditional sun salutation practiced in many styles of hatha yoga.

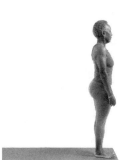 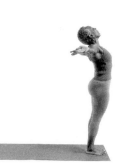 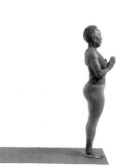 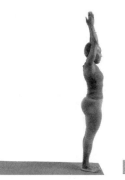 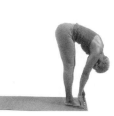

1 From Samasthiti (Mountain Pose), inhale and reach your hands up over your head, wide apart.

2 Stretch your arms and open the chest. Stretch your tailbone down toward the floor.

3 Exhale and press your palms together overhead then down to your chest.

4 Inhale and press your fingertips toward the floor, then sweep them up over your head. Arch back gently, reaching out of the lower back.

5 Exhale and fold forward from your hips into Uttanasana (Forward Bend). Bend your knees if you need to, and relax from your neck to your tailbone.

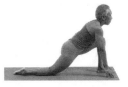 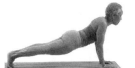 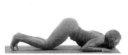 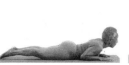 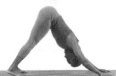

6 Inhale and take a long step back with your right leg, coming into a lunge. Roll your shoulders back. Point your tailbone toward the floor and sink your hips lower than your front knee. Open your shoulders by pressing your hands toward the floor behind you.

7 Exhale and place your hands flat against the floor, shoulder-width apart. Step your left foot back, coming into a plank position.

8 On your next exhalation, bring your knees to the floor. Hug your elbows in to your sides and slowly lower your chest and chin to the floor, resting in Zen Asana.

9 Inhale and slide your chest forward and up, coming into Bhujangasana (Cobra Pose). Roll the shoulders open.

10 Curl your toes under and as you exhale, press firmly through your hands and lift your tailbone toward the sky into Adho Mukha Shvanasana (Downward-Facing Dog). Press your chest back toward your thighs. Roll your elbows down toward the floor. Breathe in Adho Mukha Shvanasana for five to eight breaths.

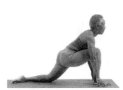 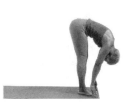 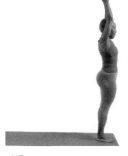 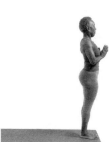

11 Inhale and step your right foot between your hands, coming back into a lunge with the left leg back. Open your shoulders by pressing your hands toward the floor behind you.

12 Exhale and step your left foot forward and fold into Uttanasana again.

13 Stretch your arms out to your sides and inhale as you lift your torso upright. Reach your hands above your head and press your palms together.

14 Exhale and bring your hands down in front of your chest.

Surya Namaskara A

This is the first salutation series done in Ashtanga-style hatha yoga.

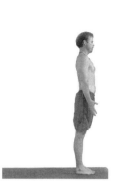 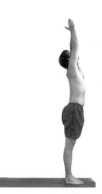 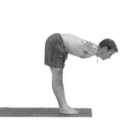 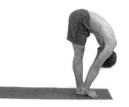 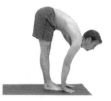

1 Start in Samasthiti, with your arms at your sides.

2 Inhale as you reach your hands above your head in anjali mudra (prayer position). Feel your ribcage lift and press your tailbone down toward the floor.

3 Exhale and bring your arms out to your sides and fold forward from your hips, leading with your chest, like a swan dive.

4 Move into Uttanasana.

5 Inhale and keeping your hands on the floor, lift your chest and chin, arching the back slightly.

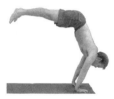 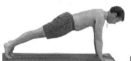 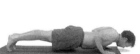 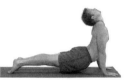 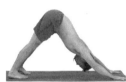

6 Exhale and step or jump back.

7 Move into Utthita Chaturanga Dandasana.

8 Slowly bend your elbows and lower the torso toward the floor into the Chaturanga Dandasana (Four-Limbs Staff Pose). Keep the elbows in toward your body and your legs straight and energized.

9 Inhale and press your hips, ribs, and chest forward and up into Urdhva Mukha Shvanasana (Upward-Facing Dog). Press firmly through the tops of your feet. Keep length in the spine.

10 Curl your toes under and as you exhale, lift your hips up and back into Adho Mukha Shvanasana. Breathe deeply for three to five breaths.

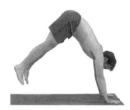 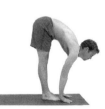 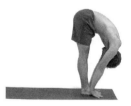 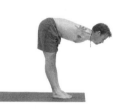 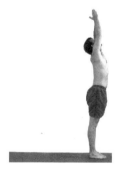

11 Inhale and either step or jump your feet forward between your hands.

12 Arch your back slightly in your forward bend.

13 Exhale and completely fold forward into Uttanasana, resting and lengthening the spine.

14 Inhale and reach your arms out to your side with your palms facing forward. Press through your feet and lift your torso upright.

15 Press your palms together overhead, making your body as long as possible.

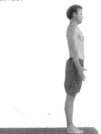

16 Exhale and bring your arms back to your sides, into Samasthiti.

Surya Namaskara B

This series is also traditionally practiced in Ashtanga hatha yoga.

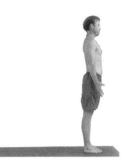 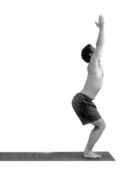 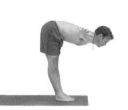 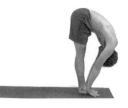 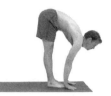

1 From Samasthiti, inhale and lift your arms over your head.

2 Simultaneously bend the knees and bring your body into Utkatasana (Chair Pose). Breathe two or three breaths. Inhale and press through your legs, straightening your body.

3 Exhale and bring your arms out to your sides and fold forward from your hips, leading with your chest, like a swan dive.

4 Move into Uttanasana.

5 Inhale and keeping your hands on the floor, lift your chest and chin, arching the back slightly.

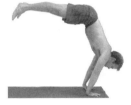 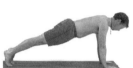 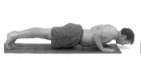 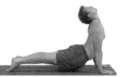 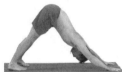

6 Exhale and step or jump back.

7 Move into Utthita Chaturanga Dandasana.

8 Slowly bend your elbows and lower the torso toward the floor into Chaturanga Dandasana. Keep the elbows in toward your body and your legs straight and energized.

9 Inhale and press your hips, ribs, and chest forward and up into Urdhva Mukha Shvanasana. Press firmly through the tops of your feet.

10 Curl your toes under and as you exhale, lift your hips up and back into Adho Mukha Shvanasana. Breathe deeply for one to three breaths.

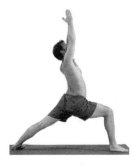 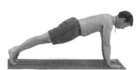 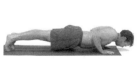 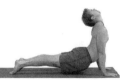 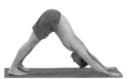

11 Turn your left foot out approximately 45 degrees. Inhale and step forward with your right foot. Bend the right knee into a lunge position, and raise your arms overhead coming into Virabhadrasana I (Warrior I).

12 Exhale and sweep your hands down to the floor as you step your right foot back, bringing your body into Utthita Chaturanga Dandasana.

13 Then down to Chaturanga Dandasana.

14 Inhale and press your hips, ribs, and chest forward and up into Urdhva Mukha Shvanasana. Press firmly through the tops of your feet.

15 Curl your toes under and as you exhale, lift your hips up and back into Adho Mukha Shvanasana. Breathe deeply one to three breaths.

(continued)

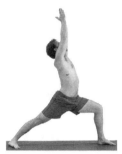

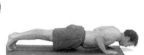

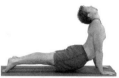

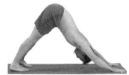

16 Turn your right foot out approximately 45 degrees. Inhale and step forward with your left foot. Bend the left knee into a lunge position and raise your arms overhead, coming into Virabhadrasana I.

17 Exhale and sweep your hands down to the floor as you step your right foot back, bringing your body into Utthita Chaturanga Dandasana.

18 Then down to Chaturanga Dandasana.

19 Inhale and press your hips, ribs, and chest forward and up into Urdhva Mukha Shvanasana. Press firmly through the tops of your feet.

20 Curl your toes under and as you exhale, lift your hips up and back into Adho Mukha Shvanasana. Breathe deeply three to five breaths.

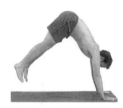

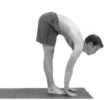

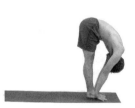

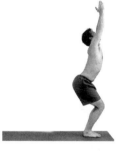

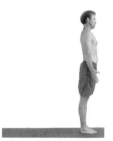

21 Inhale then exhale, and step or jump your feet forward between your hands.

22 Inhale and arch the back slightly.

23 Exhale and completely fold forward into Uttanasana, resting and lengthening the spine.

24 Inhale, bend your knees and hips. Sweep your arms overhead as you lift your torso and settle into Utkatasana.

25 Inhale and straighten your legs, stretching as tall and long as possible. Exhale and lower your arms to your sides back into Samasthiti.

chapter 7

Standing Postures

This chapter highlights 18 standing postures. Simply speaking, standing postures are asanas practiced when standing either on both feet or balanced on one leg at a time

The practice of standing asanas makes students more fully aware of their connection to the earth. Doing standing asanas helps students feel grounded, stable, and rooted. The energies of the earth draw up through the legs into the spine, creating a lightness and expansion throughout the entire body.

Standing asanas generally are sequenced at the beginning of a practice session to warm the major muscle groups and create total body and postural awareness, which continues throughout the rest of the session. In general, practicing standing postures helps to strengthen the joints of the lower extremities, thus promoting joint stabilization and integrity. Standing asanas develop the strength and stability of the feet, legs, pelvis, and spine. In addition, these asanas help students to focus on spinal alignment, develop good overall posture, and

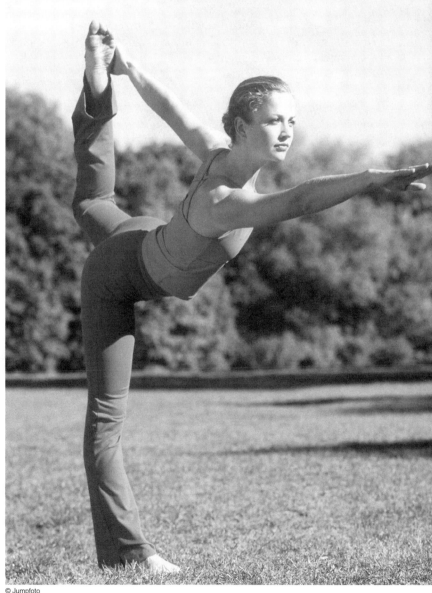

© Jumpfoto

increase balance and breath awareness. The postural awareness and strengthening of the core musculature also creates the stability needed to practice inversion asanas. Tadasana (Mountain Pose), and standing postures in general, not only build a foundation for all other postures but also are considered the safest category of poses because they draw on the entire body's strength and support. It is almost impossible to stand on one leg for very long without focusing the mind and strengthening the target muscles that increase overall balance. In yoga, without the deep awareness and good habits that arise from practicing standing postures, muscle imbalance often occurs and, over time, leads to injurious movement patterns.

The balance achieved in any standing posture can be an analogy for life's journey. It does not matter if a person actually achieves and maintains a state of being balanced. What does matter is that the person learns to recognize and become aware of where her body is in space. And, if or when the person loses her balance, she can refocus her mind and body accordingly without judgment.

The standing postures are presented here in an order so that, in general, they build from one to the next. Some classes are composed mainly of standing poses, whereas other classes include only a few. As you practice with your students in mind you will find that certain postures naturally flow into the next, based on body positioning. The first standing asana presented is Tadasana, which is considered the quintessential standing posture. For simplicity, all standing poses in this chapter begin and end in Tadasana (except for Ardha Chandrasana, which often begins from Utthita Trikonasana). Keep in mind, however, that the forward-bending postures can be interspersed throughout any standing sequencing to allow for rest and reenergizing in the mind and body. Although you can follow the order of asanas as they are listed here, you can also sequence your classes in a variety of ways depending on your personal style and class focus. Chapter 12 illustrates examples of how to sequence your class.

Mountain Pose

[taahd-AAH-suh-nuh] or [suhm-uhst-HEE-tuh-hee]

Tada in Sanskrit means mountain. *Sama* is upright, straight, unmoved; and *sthiti* is steadiness. The English translation of Tadasana is Mountain Pose. The term *tadasana* is used in Iyengar and most eclectic hatha classes. *Samasthiti* is a term used mostly by Ashtanga (power) yogis. A few yoga schools call this pose *Talasana*, which is a name for "tree" but should not be confused with *Vrkshasana,* the more common, one-legged balance pose.

DESCRIPTION

Tadasana is the foundation for all standing poses. This posture is generally performed at the beginning of a practice to direct the student's focus internally and to begin warming the muscles for further practice. We begin with the feet—the base of the body—to highlight the importance of a strong, balanced foundation.

BENEFITS

- Builds symmetry and balance in body alignment and overall posture
- Tones the lower extremities
- Improves strength in the spinal and abdominal musculature

VERBAL CUES

- As with all poses, begin by bringing your focus to your breath. Slow down and deepen your breath as you center your mind within yourself; eliminate any extraneous thoughts as you continue to breathe deeply.

- Begin with the feet parallel and as close together as comfortable, toes pointing straight ahead. Spread the toes apart and feel the length of each toe against the ground; this prevents the toes from curling under and cramping the feet.

- Press down through all four corners of each foot (big toes, little toes, inner and outer points of the heels), and balance your body weight equally between both feet. Imagine you are breathing in through your arches to help them lift slightly.

- Firm your thigh muscles as you gently lift your kneecaps upward without locking them. Your legs should remain straight, but keep your knees soft. Then, begin to roll the upper legs inward and the lower legs slightly outward. Your legs will not actually rotate in either direction, but you will become more aware of your leg muscles in the process. Continue to focus on your breath.

- Keep your pelvis in a neutral position by pulling in and up with the abdominal muscles and by keeping the hamstring muscles activated. Center your hips more directly over your heels, and find the place where you have to work to stay balanced without forcing or straining.

- Keep your chest lifted, shoulders down, and spine lengthened. With each inhale, feel your ribcage lift while you stretch your tailbone toward the ground.

- Draw your shoulder blades together slightly to allow your chest to open more fully, and extend your arms alongside your body, fingers down toward the floor; upper arms rolled out and lower arms rolled in or relaxed with the palms facing front or facing the thighs.

- Continue to focus on your breath.
- Keep your chin parallel to the floor, and imagine someone gently lifting your skull away from your shoulders.
- Keep your ears, shoulders, hips, knees, and ankles in alignment. Imagine a straight line running down the side of your body through each of these joints.
- As you continue to breathe deeply, eliminate any thoughts other than those that have to do with your alignment and your breath.
- When your awareness becomes fully present in this asana you will have the key to practicing all asanas. The extension to grow in this pose comes from deep in the mid back, and from this position the entirety of your daily posture improves.

ADJUSTMENTS

arches—Direct the student to roll the inner (medial) ankles outward to lift the arches. You can brush your hand in the direction you instruct the student to move the ankle, or you can place your fingers between the floor and the arch of the foot to create more space beneath the arch.

hips—Center a student's hips over the heels by holding the student's hips at the iliac crest (top of pelvis) as you stand behind the student and gently guide the hips into alignment.

shoulders—Check shoulder position and cue the student to drop the shoulders by placing your hands between the lifted shoulder blades (mid trapezius). You can also touch the mid chest (mid sternum) area to encourage the chest to lift.

head and neck—Place your fingertips under the student's chin or on the forehead and your thumbs at the base of the skull behind the ears; lightly suggest more length in the neck by gently lifting the head. Gently guide the ears to align over the shoulders.

MODIFICATIONS

pregnancy—Students stand with their feet as wide as needed and comfortable enough to accommodate their bellies and help them to balance.

lordosis—Students with lordosis (extreme forward spinal curvature) may need tangible feedback to move into Tadasana. It helps to have them stand against a wall and press their low backs flatter to feel the action of neutralizing the pelvis.

kyphosis—For students with kyphosis (extreme backward spinal curvature), place their backs against a wall with a pillow at the posterior bottom ribs while assisting them in pushing their shoulders back to the wall.

weakness, fatigue, paralysis—Students may place their hands on the back of a chair for support while standing or may sit instead of standing, and focus on lengthening the spine.

severe balance problems—Students stand in front of a wall and use it like a child who is learning how to ride a bike uses a training wheel. They can push against the wall with their hands for leverage. Eventually, as their balance improves, the rest of the body works more and the hands and arms work less.

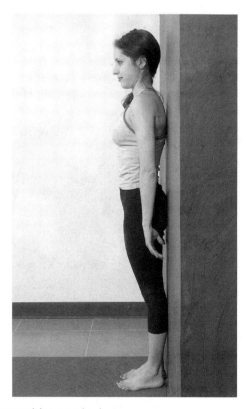

Modification: lordosis.

KINEMATICS

To the outside observer, Tadasana may appear to be nothing more than relaxed standing in the anatomical position, when in actuality it is slightly more active. Electromyographic studies on standing posture have indicated that human beings produce a rather minimal amount of muscular activity while standing in a relaxed, upright posture. In Tadasana, the muscular activity is focused on consciously attaining and maintaining length in the entire body and is generally isometric in nature.

Mechanically, if the base of the body is not aligned properly, compensations must then be made higher up the body to achieve proper balance. For example, if you stand with your shoulders rolling forward and toward each other, your neck tends to hyperextend to keep your head in a more upright posture. These compensatory changes create poor posture, which, in the long term, may lead to many physical and emotional problems.

Tadasana

Body segment	Kinematics	Muscles active
Foot and toes	Toe abduction, stability	Dorsal interossei, abductor digiti minimi brevis, abductor hallucis (C, I)
	Toe flexion (pressure into ground)	Flexor digitorum longus and brevis, flexor hallucis longus (C, I)
Lower leg	Slight external rotation of lower leg	Peroneus longus, brevis, and tertius (I)
	Stability to counter body sway (muscles relax and contract as necessary to maintain balance)	Gastrocnemius, anterior and posterior tibialis, flexor digitorum longus, flexor hallucis longus (C, E, I)
Thigh	Knee extension and patellar elevation	Quadriceps (C, I)
	Thigh extension	Hamstrings, gluteus maximus (I)
	Slight internal rotation of femur	Adductors, gluteus medius, gluteus minimus (C, I)
Hip and pelvis	Pelvic stability	Rectus abdominis, quadratus lumborum, hamstrings (I)
	Hip stability	Gluteus medius and minimus, deep external rotators (I)*
Torso	Trunk stability	Internal and external obliques, rectus abdominis, transverse abdominis, quadratus lumborum, erector spinae (I)
	Spinal extension and stability	Erector spinae (C, I)
	Rib and chest elevation	Pectoralis minor (C, I)
Shoulder	External rotation of humerus	Infraspinatus and teres minor, posterior deltoid (C, I)
Upper arm	Elbow extension	Triceps brachii (C, I)
Lower arm	Forearm supination	Supinator (C, I)
Hand and fingers	Finger extension	Extensor digitorum, indicis, and digiti minimi; lumbricales manus; interossei dorsales (C, I)
Neck	Neck extension and stability	Splenius capitis and cervicis, suboccipitals, semispinalis (I)

*Obturator externus and internus, gemellus superior and inferior, quadratus femoris, and piriformis.

C = concentric contraction, E = eccentric contraction, I = isometric contraction.

Vrkshasana

Tree Pose

[vrick-SHAAH-suh-nuh]

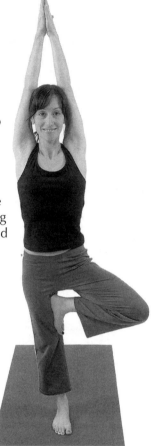

Vrksha is the Sanskrit word for tree. In Vrkshasana, the one-legged balance is reminiscent of the strength and energy of the trunk of a tree. The roots, or the standing foot, press down into the earth for support while the branches, or hands, extend up ever taller toward the sun.

Standing as a tree, you are strategically balanced so that you have energy coming up from your standing foot from the earth and are using gravity to your advantage as you push down, like roots push down into the ground. Many trees seemingly have roots on top of the earth, but the roots actually anchor into the ground. So the part of vrkshasana that represents the roots going into the ground would be the force, tension, or energy exerted by the standing foot and the reciprocal drawing of energy upward through the long alignment of the upper body. The trunk of your body, the spine and ribcage, is lifting up and your arms stretch overhead like branches reaching for the sun. As the arms extend upward, the diaphragm lifts, expanding up, and allows for more breath.

DESCRIPTION

Vrkshasana, as in all single-legged balance postures, should be practiced equally on both legs. Vrkshasana and Utthita Trikonasana (Extended Triangle) complement each other because of the work needed to stabilize and open the hips.

BENEFITS

- Builds concentration and focus
- Reduces stress—it is nearly impossible to worry and remain balanced at the same time
- Develops strength and stability in the feet and ankles
- Stabilizes and strengthens both the superficial and deep hip muscles
- Said to balance pituitary gland because of the added pressure on the first metatarsal for balance (in reflexology, pressure to the first metatarsal is said to affect the structures in the neck and head)
- Increases overall body strength

VERBAL CUES

- In Tadasana (Mountain Pose), find a point somewhere in front of you to focus on. Soften your gaze and remain fixed on that area. Breathe deeply and feel your body come into alignment.
- Slowly and smoothly, shift your body weight onto the right leg and begin to pull your left knee up toward your chest. Find the balance on your right foot from front to back. Be sure not to let the left side of your hip drop down.
- Keep your right hip pressing back; it should almost feel as if you are overcompensating. Keep your pelvis square while you bring the left knee out to the left side. Feel the front of your right hip and the inside of your left knee reaching away from each other.
- As you extend your tailbone down toward the floor place the sole of your left foot on the inside of your right leg anywhere that you feel you are comfortably, yet challengingly, balanced. Press firmly.
- Moving slowly, place your hands in *namaskara* (greeting position) with your palms pressed together at the level of your heart.
- Continue to focus on your breath.
- As you breathe in, raise your arms overhead and feel your chest and ribs lift higher away from your hips. Remain here for two to three more breaths.
- Slowly release your arms and legs and loosen up the joints of your right leg. Come back to Tadasana to prepare for the other side.

ADJUSTMENTS

toes—Remind students to spread their toes for balance and to focus on keeping the balance between the front and back of their foot. Point to or lightly brush the tops of their toes for a kinesthetic reminder. You can also push down into their first metatarsal (big toe) so that they work front to back instead of wobbling on the foot from side to side.

hip of nonweight-bearing leg—Stand behind the student and place your hands lightly on the hips as you level them. Move slowly so you do not throw them off balance. Move the hip of the straight leg back into alignment over the knee.

spine—Encourage length in the low spine by reminding students to extend the tailbone toward the floor. You can lightly brush or tap the sacrum.

chest and ribs—Stand behind the student and gently hold the ribs up, or hold the arms so you can support the student as your keep the spine and arms long and extended. Keep the pinky fingers touching to maintain external rotation at the shoulders. Standing behind the student works best because it requires little physical effort on your part.

shoulders—Place your hands lightly on top of the student's shoulders and press down gently.

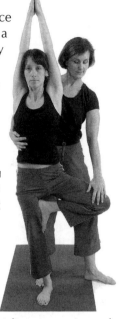

Adjustment: spine and hip alignment.

MODIFICATIONS

hip replacements—To avoid creating stress on the hip joint with its limited range of motion, have the student focus solely on balancing on one leg without much external rotation of the bent leg.

balance difficulties—Have students keep the toes of the bent leg on the floor with the heel pressed against the straight leg. Using a chair or a wall, have the students use the prop as a "training wheel" that they use only to regain their balance when they lose it.

severe balance difficulties—Have the student place the bent leg on a step stool. This technique helps students to work on opening the hips without compromising balance.

deepening the pose—Instead of placing the foot of the bent knee against the standing leg, reach the foot across to the opposite hip into Ardha Padmasana (Half Lotus) and reach the same side hand behind the back to grab the foot. If the student cannot quite reach their foot, they can use a strap.

KINEMATICS

Many times students complain that the inside of the standing thigh is "too slippery" and they are unable to hold the foot against it. Generally, the problem is not about having slippery pants or skin, it is a matter of the student not pressing the sole of the foot firmly into the opposite thigh. If the students have enough flexibility and openness in the inner thigh to enable them to place the heel of the foot into the groin, they will gain a significant amount of stability in the posture.

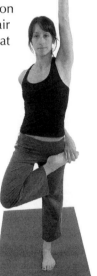

Modification: deepening the pose.

Vrkshasana (Standing on Right Leg)

Body segment	Kinematics	Muscles active	Muscles released
Foot and toes (R)	Toe abduction, stability	Dorsal interossei, abductor digiti minimi brevis, abductor hallucis (C, I)	
	Toe flexion (pressure into ground)	Flexor digitorum longus and brevis, flexor hallucis longus (C, I)	
Foot and toes (L)	Toe extension	Extensor digitorum longus, hallucis longus (C, I)	
Lower leg (R)	Stability to counter body sway (muscles relax and contract as necessary to maintain balance)	Gastrocnemius, anterior and posterior tibialis, flexor digitorum longus, flexor hallucis longus (C, E, I)	
	Knee extension	Gastrocnemius, stability (I)	
Lower leg (L)	Ankle dorsiflexion	Anterior tibialis, extensor digitorum longus, hallucis longus (C, I)	Gastrocnemius, soleus
Thigh (R)	Knee extension and patellar elevation	Quadriceps (C, I)	
	Stability and adduction (adductor magnus also helps to extend knee)	Adductors (C, I)	
Thigh (L)	Knee flexion	Hamstrings (C, I)	
Hip and pelvis (R)	Hip extension, stability	Hamstrings (C, I)	
	Hip stability	Gluteus maximus, medius, and minimus; deep external rotators* (C, I)	
	Pelvic stability	Rectus abdominis, quadratus lumborum, hamstrings (I)	
Hip and pelvis (L)	Hip flexion	Iliopsoas, rectus femoris (C, I)	Adductors
	Hip external rotation	Deep external rotators,* gluteus maximus (C, I)	
Torso	Spinal extension and stability	Erector spinae, quadratus lumborum (I)	
	Rib and chest elevation	Pectoralis minor (C, I)	
	Trunk stability	Internal and external obliques, rectus abdominis, transverse abdominis, quadratus lumborum (I)	
Shoulder	Adduction of scapulae	Rhomboids major and minor, mid trapezius (C, I)	
	Postural support in mid back and downward pull of scapulae	Lower trapezius (C, I)	
	External rotation of humerus	Infraspinatus, teres minor, posterior deltoid (C, I)	
Upper arm	Abduction of humerus	Deltoids (C, I)	
	Depression of humeral head	Infraspinatus, teres minor, subscapularis (C, I)	
Lower arm	Pronation	Pronator teres, pronator quadratus (C, I)	
	Elbow flexion	Biceps brachii, brachialis, brachioradialis (C, I)	
	Wrist hyperextension	Extensor carpi radialis brevis and longus, extensor carpi ulnaris (C, I)	Flexor carpi radialis and ulnaris, palmaris longus
Hand and fingers	Finger extension	Extensor digitorum, indicis, and digiti minimi; lumbricales manus; interossei dorsales (C, I)	
	Finger adduction	Interossei palmaris, adductor pollicis (C, I)	
Neck	Neck extension, stability	Splenius capitus and cervicis, suboccipitals, simispinals (I)	

*Obturator externus and internus, gemellus superior and inferior, quadratus femoris, and piriformis.
C = concentric contraction, E = eccentric contraction, I = isometric contraction.

Utthita Trikonasana

Extended Triangle

[oot-T-HEE-tuh tree-kohn-AAH-suh-nuh]

In Sanskrit, *utthita* means extended or stretched. *Tri* means three, and *kona* means angle. The posture is named for the triangle formed by the extended legs and the side bend in the body.

DESCRIPTION

From Tadasana, the legs are extended out as far apart as is comfortable, preferably between three and four feet (about one meter). Arms are extended out to the sides and perpendicular to the floor.

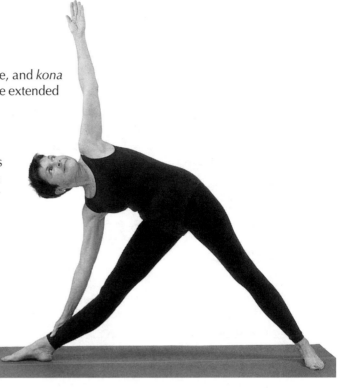

BENEFITS

- Tones the legs and strengthens the ankles
- Loosens the hip joints as well as the groin and hamstrings
- Stabilizes and opens the hips when the torso is aligned properly
- Helps release spinal musculature
- Opens the chest and shoulders
- Strengthens and aligns the neck
- Stimulates abdominal organs and improves digestion as it tones abdominals
- Aids in stress relief

CAUTIONS

heart conditions, high blood pressure—Have the student turn the gaze downward.

neck pain or injury—Direct the student to continue to gaze forward without turning the neck.

shoulder problems—Student should keep the top hand on the hip, and continue to rotate the shoulder back.

VERBAL CUES

- From Tadasana (Mountain Pose), extend your arms out to your sides with your palms facing downward.
- Continue to focus on your breath.
- Move your legs apart while trying to bring your feet as far apart as your outstretched hands.
- Rotate the right leg out 90 degrees and then turn the left foot in slightly toward the right approximately 45 degrees. Imagine a straight line drawn back from your right heel. That line should pass through the middle of your left arch.
- Keep the front thigh muscles (quadriceps) active by gently drawing the kneecaps up.
- Imagine that your back is pressed against a wall. Work to keep the right leg rolling out (externally rotate). At the same time, keep your left hip from rolling forward by pressing it back toward the imaginary wall. This action opens the front pelvis. Keep your tailbone lengthened toward the floor.
- With your arms extending out as far as possible, exhale as you reach your right fingers out to the right side by extending your trunk from your left hip joint. Create more length in your torso by imagining your tailbone and right ribcage are moving farther apart from each other.
- Continue to focus on your breath.

- Feel the left side of your torso stretch so that your left shoulder and left hip move farther away from each other. Keep your left ribcage as parallel to the floor as possible.
- Work to keep your upper and lower body in the same plane. Continue to imagine you are standing against a wall with your left shoulder and hip rotating back.
- When you have reached as far to the right as you can comfortably, begin to lower your right hand toward the floor and reach your left fingertips toward the sky. Keep your upper and lower body in alignment.
- Feel the crown of your head reaching toward your right hand, creating as much length in your spine as possible.
- Turn and look up toward your left fingers.
- Focus on balancing yourself equally over both feet as you work to keep your chest and pelvis open.
- Continue to focus on your breath.
- To come out of the posture, inhale and continue to press down through your legs as you bring your upper body into an upright standing position and prepare for the other side.

ADJUSTMENTS

arches—Encourage students to roll the inner (medial) ankles outward to lift the arches. You can brush your hand in the direction you instruct the student to move the ankle, or you can place your fingers between the floor and the student's arch to create more space beneath the arch.

legs—Remind students to pull up the front thigh muscles (quadriceps) to help them keep their kneecaps lifted. You can gently brush the mid-thigh muscles toward the hips. If the knees are hyperextending, remind students to relax the knees slightly and engage the hamstrings.

hips—Stand behind the student, using your thigh as a brace, and place your hand on the iliac crest of the student's top hip and gently press the hip toward you.

ribcage—Place the palm of your hand lightly on top of the student's upper ribcage, halfway between the shoulder and hip. Instruct the student to lengthen the spine and move the ribcage away from your hand so it does not curve toward the ceiling. Also, you may stand facing the student's outstretched arm and hold on to the wrist as you pull it toward you. While doing this, place your toes against the bend in the student's hip crease and gently press the student's pelvis away from you.

shoulders—Direct students to rotate both shoulders externally to keep the chest open and expanded. If a student's torso is extending either in front of or behind the plane of the hips, gently move the shoulders back into alignment. Be sure to hold students securely while you move them and to let go slowly, making certain they maintain their balance.

hand placement—If the student's lower hand is placed against the shin or anywhere close to the knee joint, instruct the student to be conscientious by *not* pressing against the front of the leg. Pressing back on the leg increases the risk of hyperextending the knee. If the student continues to press on the top of the leg, modify the posture by placing a block under the lower hand and instructing the student to utilize the back muscles to help support the upper body.

head and neck—Cue the student to lengthen the neck and extend the head away from the shoulders.

Adjustment: hips.

MODIFICATIONS

extreme stiffness—If a student has trouble reaching for the floor without rotating the chest toward the ground, place a block under their bottom hand to elevate it slightly. The student may also need to decrease the distance between the legs.

balance and alignment difficulty—Place the student against a wall to work on alignment. Also, the student may need to decrease the distance between the legs.

neck weakness—Suggest the student turn the gaze toward the floor. This action continues to build strength but lessens the strain on the neck.

KINEMATICS

Utthita Trikonasana employs both balance and strength. Eccentric contractions of the top lateral torso are employed to get into position. Once in position, most of the muscle activity shifts to isometric contractions to keep the body in position with balance. With the exception of the rotation of the legs and the neck turning in the transverse plane, all other movement in this asana occurs in the frontal plane, keeping the upper body aligned over the legs.

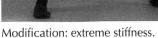

Modification: extreme stiffness.

Utthita Trikonasana (Flexing to the Right)

Body segment	Kinematics	Muscles active	Muscles released
Foot and toes	Toe abduction, foot stability	Dorsal interossei, abductor digiti minimi brevis, abductor hallucis (C, I)	
	Toe flexion (pressure into ground)	Flexor digitorum longus and brevis, flexor hallucis longus (C, I)	
Lower leg (R)	Stability to counter body sway (muscles relax and contract as necessary to maintain balance)	Peroneals, posterior tibialis, flexor digitorum longus, gastrocnemius, soleus, flexor hallucis longus (C, E, I)	
Lower leg (L)	Internal rotation of foot, stability	Anterior tibialis, posterior tibialis, flexor hallucis longus (C, I)	Gastrocnemius, soleus, peroneals
Thigh (R)	Knee extension and patella elevation	Quadriceps (C, I)	Adductors, medial hamstrings
	Hip stability	Hamstrings, gluteus maximus (I)	
	External rotation of femur, stability	Deep external rotators* (C, I)	Gluteus medius, minimus
Thigh (L)	Stability	Adductor longus, magnus (I)	Adductors
	External rotation of femur, stability	Deep external rotators* (I)	
Hip and pelvis (R)	Abduction, stability	Tensor fascia lata (I)	
	Hip stability	Gluteus medius, gluteus minimus (I)	
	Pelvic stability	Hamstrings (E, I)	
	External rotation of femur, stability	Deep external rotators,* gluteus maximus (C, I)	

(continued)

Utthita Trikonasana (Flexing to the Right) *continued*

Body segment	Kinematics	Muscles active	Muscles released
Hip and pelvis (L)	External rotation of femur, lateral flexion, stability	Deep external rotators,* gluteus maximus (C, I)	Iliopsoas, gluteus medius, tensor fascia lata
	Hip extension, stability	Hamstrings, gluteus maximus (C, E, I)	
	Lateral flexion to right, stability	Tensor fascia lata (E, I)	
	Pelvic stability	Rectus abdominis, quadratus lumborum, hamstrings (I)	
Torso (R and L)	Spinal stability	Erector spinae (C, I)	
	Rib and chest elevation	Pectoralis minor (C, I)	
	Trunk stability	Internal and external obliques, rectus abdominis, transverse abdominis, quadratus lumborum (I)	
Torso (L)	Lateral flexion to right, stability	Internal and external obliques, quadratus lumborum, latissimus dorsi, erector spinae (E, I)	Internal and external obliques, quadratus lumborum, latissimus dorsi, erector spinae
Shoulder	Abduction of humerus and joint stability	Deltoids, supraspinatus, teres minor (C, I)	Pectoralis major
	Depression and stability of humerus	Subscapularis, infraspinatus (C, I), teres minor	
	Scapular rotation	Serratus anterior, mid and lower trapeazius (C, I)	
	Scapular adduction	Rhomboids major and minor, mid trapezius (C, I)	
	Postural support in mid back and downward pull on scapulae	Lower trapezius (C, I)	
	External rotation of humerus	Infraspinatus and teres minor with some posterior deltoid (C, I)	
Upper arm	Elbow extension	Triceps brachii (C, I)	Biceps brachii, brachialis, brachioradialis
Lower arm	Forearm supination	Supinator (C, I)	
	Elbow extension	Anconeus (C, I)	
Hand and fingers	Wrist and finger extension	Extensor digitorum, indicis, and digiti minimi; lumbricales manus; interossei dorsales (C, I)	
	Finger adduction	Interossei palmaris, adductor pollicis (C, I)	
Neck (R)	Head rotation, neck stability	Sternocleidomastoid (C, I)	
Neck (L)	Head rotation, neck stability	Splenius capitus and cervicis, occipitals, cervical erector spinae (C, I)	Sternocleidomastoid

*Obturator externus and internus, gemellus superior and inferior, quadratus femoris, and piriformis.

C = concentric contraction, E = eccentric contraction, I = isometric contraction.

Parivrtta Trikonasana

Revolving Triangle Pose

[par-ee-VRT-tuh tree-kohn-AAH-suh-nuh]

Parivrtta means the other side. It is often translated as meaning to revolve, or revolving. Trikonasana is Triangle Pose, so this asana is Revolving Triangle Pose.

DESCRIPTION

Parivrtta Trikonasana is similar to Utthita Trikonasana but shifts the front of the pelvis from the frontal plane to being almost parallel to the ground, causing the upper body to twist around the spine. The twist through the mid-thoracic spine makes the posture more challenging to most students because it requires greater strength, flexibility, and balance than that required by Utthita Trikonasana.

BENEFITS

- Energizes the entire body
- Massages the internal organs and stretches supporting spinal musculature

CAUTION

back injuries—As with any twisting posture, those with acute back injuries should be cautious practicing this asana.

VERBAL CUES

- Moving from Tadasana (Mountain Pose), step the left leg back far enough so that your feet are a challenging distance apart for balance, but be sure to keep your left foot firmly on the ground. Face the right foot forward, and turn out the left foot approximately 10 to 15 degrees.
- Make sure hips are square and you face the direction of your right foot. Press your left hip forward as you pull your right hip back.
- Inhale and lengthen out of the low spine and extend your left arm forward with your right arm back.
- Exhale and fold forward from your hips like a hinge, keeping the right hip pulled back.
- Place your left hand as far down the outside of the right leg as possible without extending past your comfort range and the edge of your balance.
- Reopen the space between your hips and ribs by extending your torso away from your hips. Continue to lengthen your entire spine all the way through your neck. Inhale.
- Next, exhale as you turn your head to look at your right hand as it extends above you. Keep your left hand extending down toward the ground.
- Roll your shoulders open so that both palms face forward.
- Continue to pull your ribs and right hip away from each other, keeping length in the spine.
- Remember to press your feet into the floor and feel the revolving action through the spine, hands, and head with each inhalation.
- Exhale, drawing your shoulders away from your ears. Align your chin with your right shoulder as much as possible.
- Continue to focus on your breath.
- To exit the posture, bring both hands to either side of your front foot. Slowly bring your hands to your hips and as you inhale, raise yourself upright. Prepare for your next posture.

ADJUSTMENTS

feet—If the back foot lifts off the floor, cue the student to press down on the outside of the back heel and on the outer edge of the foot. You can lightly press on the outer aspect of the back foot with your hands or toes.

spine—If a student is rounding the spine, stand behind the student's upper back. Place your closest hand on the front of the far hip. Using your hip to support the student's balance, pull the student's hip back and use your opposite hand to open the student's top shoulder. Use your hand to roll the shoulder down, away from the ear.

MODIFICATIONS

balance difficulties—Have the student bend the front knee. This action also allows for more leverage to open the hips and straighten the spine.

tight hips or hamstrings—Place a block under the hand reaching down. The use of the block helps to maintain a straight spine.

balance or weakness—Have the student stand with the outside of the front leg against a wall. Instruct the student to lean into the wall for balance and to stretch the hand reaching down against the wall.

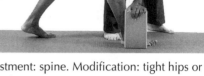

Adjustment: spine. Modification: tight hips or hamstrings.

KINEMATICS

One of the most important aspects of this posture is to keep the spine as straight as possible. For this reason, those with tightness in the hamstrings or low back should utilize a block under the bottom hand to keep the upper back from rounding.

Parivrtta Trikonasana (Rotating to the Right)

Body segment	Kinematics	Muscles active	Muscles released
Foot and toes	Toe abduction, foot stability	Dorsal interossei, abductor digiti minimi brevis, abductor hallucis (C, I)	
	Toe flexion (pressure into ground)	Flexor digitorum longus and brevis, flexor hallucis longus (C, I)	
Lower leg (R)	Plantar flexion for foot and ankle stability	Gastrocnemius, soleus (C, I)	
	Stability to counter body sway (muscles relax and contract as necessary to maintain balance)	Peroneals, anterior and posterior tibialis, flexor digitorum longus, flexor hallucis longus (C, E, I)	
Lower leg (L)	Ankle stability	Peroneals (E, I)	Gastrocnemius, soleus, peroneals
Thigh (R and L)	Knee extension and patellar elevation	Quadriceps (C, I)	
	Hip stability	Hamstrings, gluteus maximus, adductors (I)	
Hip and pelvis (R)	Hip flexion	Hamstrings (E, I)	Hamstrings, tensor fascia lata, gluteus medius and minimus, deep external rotators*

Body segment	Kinematics	Muscles active	Muscles released
Hip and pelvis (L)	Hip extension	Hamstrings (E, I)	Adductors
	Slight external rotation and stability	Deep external rotators* (I)	
Torso (R and L)	Trunk stability	Erector spinae, quadratus lumborum, rectus abdominis, transverse abdominis (I)	Erector spinae
	Rib and chest elevation	Pectoralis minor (C, I)	
Torso (R)	Rotation to right	Internal obliques, quadratus lumborum (C, I)	External obliques
Torso (L)	Rotation to right	External obliques (C, I)	Quadratus lumborum, latissimus dorsi, internal obliques
Shoulder	Humerus abduction and shoulder stability	Deltoids, infraspinatus, teres minor (C, I)	Pectoralis major
	Scapular adduction	Rhomboids major and minor and mid trapezius (C, I)	
	Postural support in mid back and downward pull of scapulae	Lower trapezius (C, I)	
	External rotation of humerus	Infraspinatus and teres minor with some posterior deltoid (C, I)	
Upper arm	Elbow	Triceps brachii (C, I)	Biceps brachii, brachialis, brachioradialis
Lower arm (R)	Forearm supination	Supinator (C, I)	
Lower arm (R and L)	Elbow	Anconeus (C, I)	
Lower arm (L)	Pronation	Pronator teres (C, I)	
	Wrist hyperextension	Extensor carpi radialis, longus, and brevis; extensor carpi ulnaris (C, I)	Flexor carpi radialis and ulnaris, palmaris longus
Hand and fingers	Finger extension	Extensor digitorum, indicis, and digiti minimi; lumbricales manus; interossei dorsales (C, I)	
	Finger adduction	Interossei palmaris, adductor pollicis (C, I)	
Neck (R)	Head rotation, neck stability	Splenius capitus and cervicis, occipitals, cervical erector spinae (C, I)	Sternocleidomastoid
Neck (L)	Head rotation	Sternocleidomastoid (C, I)	

*Obturator externus and internus, gemellus superior and inferior, quadratus femoris, and piriformis.

C = concentric contraction, E = eccentric contraction, I = isometric contraction.

Intense Forward Bend

[oot-taahn-AAH-suh-nuh]

Ut indicates intensity. *Tan* means to stretch or lengthen.

DESCRIPTION

Uttanasana intensely stretches and lengthens the spine and hamstrings. This basic standing forward bend should be done folding at the hips like a hinge while maintaining a straight low back. It can be practiced with the legs any distance apart that feels comfortable, yet challenging. Uttanasana is usually performed as a resting, rejuvenating posture in between other standing postures and as part of the Sun Salutations.

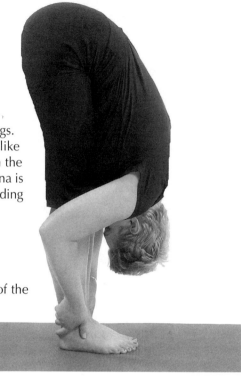

BENEFITS

- Strengthens and stretches the spinal muscles
- Lengthens and stretches the hamstrings and opens the posterior of the hips
- Relaxes and rejuvenates the whole body
- Said to improve functioning of the liver, spleen, and kidneys
- Takes pressure off the heart by placing the head below the heart
- Simulates digestive system
- Stretches and tones the backs of the legs

CAUTIONS

back problems—Anyone with low back problems should be extremely mindful of bending at the hips only as far as is comfortable. Instruct students to be careful when exiting from Uttanasana to avoid straining the low back by focusing on lifting from the crown of the head.

late pregnancy—Practice with modifications, or skip this posture.

glaucoma—As with all postures where the head is below the heart, this pose is not recommended without modification.

VERBAL CUES

- Start in Tadasana (Mountain Pose) with your feet a comfortable yet challenging distance apart. Firm the front thigh muscles, exhale and begin to fold forward at the hip joint. Keep the length of the spine intact. You can fold your arms in front of your chest or place your hands on your hips. Relax your shoulders.
- Reach out of the low back to keep length in the entire spine. Relax and sink the spine forward. If you feel any discomfort in your low back, bend your knees slightly.
- Continue to focus on your breath.
- Relax your neck so that the crown of your head sinks toward the floor.
- If your hands can touch the floor comfortably, place them near your heels and move your body weight slightly more forward so your hips align directly over your ankle joints. This action challenges your balance slightly.
- If your hands do not touch the floor, allow them to hang down or place them against your legs.
- Picture your tailbone and sits bones reaching up to the sky as the crown of your head reaches toward the floor. Press through your heels as you breathe in, and let your tailbone reach up farther. As you exhale, allow your spine to relax even deeper, suspending your upper body forward.

- Soften the belly and let the abdomen release back toward the front of the spine. Breathe into the low back, and allow the ribs to expand out to the sides, creating more space for the breath. Pull the shoulders away from your ears.
- To come out of the posture, place your hands on your hips and roll your shoulders open by gently squeezing your shoulder blades and elbows together behind you. Keep the front of the ribcage elevated, and as you inhale press through your legs. Lift through the crown of the head, and begin to raise yourself up to a standing position.

ADJUSTMENTS

feet—Be sure students' feet are parallel with big toes as close together as possible so that the knees and hips maintain alignment.

lower body—Standing behind or to the side of the student, place your hands lightly on the outside of the hips and gently move the hips so they are aligned over the ankle joints, with the legs perpendicular to the floor.

neck—Gently touch the back of the student's head, or just remind the student verbally to relax the neck.

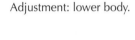
Adjustment: lower body.

MODIFICATIONS

tight hamstrings—Instruct the student to bend the knees slightly.

rounded back—Instruct the student to take a wider stance with the feet or to bend the knees.

pregnancy; stiff back, hips, or hamstrings—Suggest that the student use a wall or chair for support to relieve some of the physical work involved in the posture, promoting an easier release of the spine and hamstrings.

weakness—Student can be seated on a chair with the spine pressed against the chair back (or an exercise ball) and the feet placed comfortably apart. From there, the student folds as far forward as is comfortable.

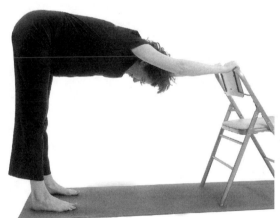
Modification: pregnancy; stiff back, hips, or hamstrings.

KINEMATICS

The most common mistake students make in practicing this posture is to bend forward from the lumbar or thoracic spine instead of the hip joint. If the knees bend, the hips usually move out of alignment. However, it is more important to protect the low back by bending the knees than it is to have the hips aligned over the knees. The legs will eventually lengthen, and the bend will initiate from the appropriate area in the hips.

Uttanasana

Body segment	Kinematics	Muscles active	Muscles released
Foot and toes	Toe abduction, foot stability	Dorsal interossei, abductor digiti minimi brevis, abductor hallucis (C, I)	
	Toe flexion (pressure into ground)	Flexor digitorum longus and brevis, flexor hallucis longus (C, I)	
Lower leg	Stability to counter body sway (muscles relax and contract as necessary to maintain balance)	Gastrocnemius, anterior and posterior tibialis, flexor digitorum longus and flexor hallucis longus (C, E, I)	Gastrocnemius
	Slight external rotation of lower leg	Peroneus longus, brevis, and tertius (C, I)	
Thigh	Knee extension	Quadriceps (C, I)	Hamstrings
Hip and pelvis	Hip flexion, stability	Hamstrings (E, I), iliopsoas (C, I)	Gluteus medius and minimus, deep external rotators*
	Hip stability	Adductors (I)	
Torso	Spine extension	Thoracic erector spinae (C, I)	Lumbar erector spinae, quadratus lumborum
	Rib and chest elevation	Pectoralis minor (C, I)	
Shoulder	Scapular abduction	(Gravity induced)	Latissimus dorsi, rhomboids, trapezius
	Humeral flexion	(Gravity induced)	Deltoids
Upper arm	Elbow extension	(Gravity induced)	Triceps brachii, biceps brachii, brachialis, brachioradialis
Lower arm	Wrist extension or hyperextension	(Gravity or ground induced)	Extensor carpi radialis, brevis and longus, extensor carpi ulnaris
Hand and fingers	Finger extension	(Gravity or ground induced)	
Neck	Extension	None	Sternocleidomastoid, splenius capitus and cervicis, cervical erector spinae

*Obturator externus and internus, gemellus superior and inferior, quadratus femoris, and piriformis.

C = concentric contraction, E = eccentric contraction, I = isometric contraction.

Extended-Leg Forward Bend

[pruh-SAAH-ree-tuh paah-doht-taahn-AAH-suh-nuh]

Prasarita means to expand or spread. This asana is a variation of a forward bend with the legs extended.

DESCRIPTION

Although Prasarita Padottanasana has a number of variations, four are traditionally practiced in the warm-up of the Ashtanga yoga series. All four of the variations described here begin

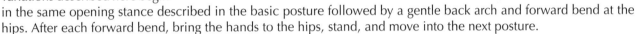

in the same opening stance described in the basic posture followed by a gentle back arch and forward bend at the hips. After each forward bend, bring the hands to the hips, stand, and move into the next posture.

BENEFITS

- Stretches the hamstrings and low back
- Builds stability in the feet and legs
- Stretches the shoulder joint throughout the range of motion
- Cools and recharges the mind and body

CAUTIONS

shoulder injuries—Students with shoulder problems should proceed cautiously with variation 3.

back problems—Anyone with low back problems should be extremely mindful of bending at the hips only as far as is comfortable.

VERBAL CUES

Variation 1

- From Tadasana (Mountain Pose), spread your legs as wide as is comfortable.
- Position your body so your knees, feet, hips, and chest point forward.
- Bring your hands to your hips, and roll your shoulders back and down toward your hips. Press your feet firmly against the ground, and feel your spine lengthen.
- Inhale and look up as you arch your back slightly. Lift your chest and press your pelvis forward. Try to lift your chest higher than your shoulders, and squeeze your shoulder blades toward each other behind your back.
- Reach your hands to the floor and place them shoulder-width apart between your feet.
- Inhale as you straighten your arms and look in the direction of your toes as you arch your back slightly.
- Exhale and bend the elbows as you lower the crown of your head toward the floor. Keep the elbows pulled in toward each other and roll the shoulders away from the ears.

- Adjust your body weight so that the hip joints are placed directly over your ankles and rolling more toward your toes. Doing so will straighten your knees slightly, giving you a deeper stretch in the hamstrings.
- If your head touches the floor, put as much weight on the crown of your head as feels comfortable to you.
- As you exhale, press through your legs and fold forward from the hips. Maintain the length in your upper back.
- To exit, place your hands on your hips and press firmly through your feet. Keep your elbows pointing away from you behind your back. Inhale as you lift yourself upright. Step or jump your feet together in Tadasana.

Variation 2

- From Tadasana, spread your legs as wide as is comfortable.
- Position your body so your knees, feet, hips, and chest point forward.
- Bring your hands to your hips, and roll your shoulders back and down toward your hips. Press your feet firmly against the ground, and feel your spine lengthen.
- Inhale and look up as you arch your back slightly. Lift your chest and press your pelvis forward. Try to lift your chest higher than your shoulders, and squeeze your shoulder blades toward each other behind your back.
- Breathe in deeply, and arch your back slightly while lifting the chest. Exhale and fold forward from your hips. Lower the crown of your head comfortably to the floor, keeping your hands on your hips.
- Allow your hips to press forward toward your toes and bring as much weight as you can comfortably to the top of your head.
- As you exhale, press through your legs and fold forward from the hips. Maintain the length in your upper back.
- To exit, place your hands on your hips and press firmly through your feet. Keep your elbows pointing away from you behind your back. Inhale as you lift yourself upright. Step or jump your feet together in Tadasana.

Variation 3

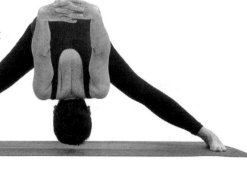

- From Tadasana, spread your legs as wide as is comfortable.
- Position your body so your knees, feet, hips, and chest point forward.
- Bring your hands to your hips, and roll your shoulders back and down toward your hips. Press your feet firmly against the ground, and feel your spine lengthen.
- Inhale and look up as you arch your back slightly. Lift your chest and press your pelvis forward. Try to lift your chest higher than your shoulders, and squeeze your shoulder blades toward each other behind your back.
- Clasp your hands behind your back. Press your hips forward, lifting out of the low spine. Lift the chest, and open the shoulders as you arch back as far as you can comfortably.
- Exhale as you bend at your hips, folding forward. Bring your head toward the floor as far as you can.
- Allow your arms to lift away from your back as you move your hands over your head toward the floor. With each exhalation feel your arms drop closer toward the floor, opening your chest and the front of your shoulders.
- Continue to focus on your breath.
- To exit from this variation, squeeze your elbows together, feeling the front of your arms and chest open even more deeply. Inhale as you press through the feet and pull yourself upright with your arms, lifting through the chest. Exhale and release the arms to your sides.

Variation 4

- From Tadasana, spread your legs as wide as is comfortable.
- Position your body so your knees, feet, hips, and chest point forward.
- Bring your hands to your hips, and roll your shoulders back and down toward your hips. Press your feet firmly against the ground, and feel your spine lengthen.
- Inhale and look up as you arch your back slightly. Lift your chest and press your pelvis forward. Try to lift your chest higher than your shoulders, and squeeze your shoulder blades toward each other behind your back.
- Exhale and fold forward as you reach your right hand toward your right big toe and your left hand toward your left big toe.
- Inhale and look up as you arch back as far as you can comfortably.
- As you exhale, bend your elbows and pull the crown of your head down toward the floor. Work to bring your hips into alignment over your ankles and find the edge of your balance.
- Keep your arms working to bring your chest closer to your thighs. Relax your neck.
- Continue to focus on your breath.
- To come out of the posture, bring your hands to your hips with your elbows squeezing together behind your back. Inhale and press through your feet as you lift up through your chest and head.

ADJUSTMENTS

balance—Stand behind a student with poor balance, and place the side of your hip against the back of the student's thigh to block the student from placing the weight too far back on the heels. You can also stand to the front of the student, place your hand to the hip, and slowly and gently bring the body weight more onto their toes to provide better alignment.

hands—When the hands are on the ground, they should be in line with the feet. Instruct the student to move the hands back if they are too far forward of the toes. Have the student accommodate moving the hands back by spreading the feet wider apart.

neck—If the student has hyperextended the neck, gently touch the back of the head to cue the student to relax.

elbows—If the student's elbows are not parallel, gently place your hands to the outside of each elbow and move them slowly together. Stand behind the student and place your hands on the upper arms and roll the arms toward each other. This adjustment also helps to further open the chest. To further stabilize and build strength in the chest and shoulders in variation 1, place a block between the student's elbows and instruct them to squeeze into it while keeping length in the spine.

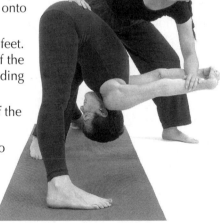

Adjustment: arms in variation 3.

arms in variation 3—Stand to the side of the student and place your thigh against the front of the student's thigh to support the student's balance. Place one hand on the low back, and hold the student's wrists with your other hand. Gently press the student's hands closer to the floor as the student exhales. Ask the student for constant feedback so that the adjustment is acceptable.

MODIFICATIONS

tight hamstrings or back—Instruct the student to bend the knees slightly to help lengthen the spine. Place the student's palms against a wall to keep from straining the back while gently and slowly stretching the hamstrings. Remind the student to focus on the length and straightness of the spine.

tight groin—If the student is unable to abduct the legs far enough to place the head on the floor, place a block under the head for support. Make certain that the block is on a secure surface so that it will not slip.

weakness—Place the student at the edge of a chair or on a fitness ball. Have the student bend forward from the hips and practice the variations of the arm positions.

KINEMATICS

As in Uttanasana, if the quadriceps contract concentrically, the hamstrings will relax more readily. Unlike Uttanasana, Prasarita Padottanasana stretches both the hip adductor group (inner thigh) and the peroneal group (outer calf) at the lateral ankle joint. Note: Although four variations of the asana are discussed, only variation 1 is described in the kinematic table.

Prasarita Padottanasana (Variation 1)

Body segment	Kinematics	Muscles active	Muscles released
Foot and toes	Toe abduction, foot stability	Dorsal interossei, abductor digiti minimi brevis, abductor hallucis (C, I)	
Lower leg	Stability to counter body sway (muscles relax and contract as necessary to maintain balance)	Gastrocnemius, anterior and posterior tibialis, flexor digitorum longus, flexor hallucis longus (C, E, I)	Gastrocnemius, soleus, peroneals
Thigh	Leg extension	Quadriceps (C, I)	Hamstrings, adductors
Hip and pelvis	Hip flexion	Hamstrings (E, I)	Deep external rotators*
	Thigh abduction, stability	Tensor fascia lata (C, I)	
Torso	Spine extension	Thoracic erector spinae (C, I)	Lumbar erector spinae
	Rib and chest elevation	Pectoralis minor (C, I)	
Shoulder	Scapular abduction	(Gravity induced)	Latissimus dorsi, rhomboids, mid trapezius
	Overhead extension	(Gravity induced)	
Upper arm	Humeral flexion	(Gravity induced)	Deltoids, triceps brachii, biceps brachii, brachialis, brachioradialis
Lower arm	Elbow flexion	(Gravity induced)	
	Wrist extension or hyperextension	(Gravity or ground induced)	Extensor carpi radialis brevis and longus, extensor carpi ulnaris
Hand and fingers	Finger extension	Extensor digitorum, indicis, and digiti minimi; lumbricales manus, interossei dorsales (I)	
Neck	Extension	None	Sternocleidomastoid, splenius capitus and cervicis, cervical erector spinae

*Obturator externus and internus, gemellus superior and inferior, quadratus femoris, and piriformis.

C = concentric contraction, E = eccentric contraction, I = isometric contraction.

Garudasana

Eagle Pose

[guh-rood-AAH-suh-nuh]

Garuda is the king of birds, an eagle. This word is also representative of the focus needed to remain steady in this position.

DESCRIPTION

This one-legged balancing posture involves crossing the nonweight-bearing leg over the standing leg. The thighs and hips are engaged by the slight crouch. The mid back and shoulders are stretched as the arms are crossed in front of the chest. Like an eagle focused and poised for action, practicing this pose helps one develop stillness and concentration.

BENEFITS

- Helps develop focus and concentration
- Provides a deep stretch in the hips, along the posterior shoulders, and between the shoulder blades
- Stretches and strengthens standing calf

CAUTION

hip replacements—For students with hip replacements, the crossing over of the legs is generally contraindicated. (See modifications.)

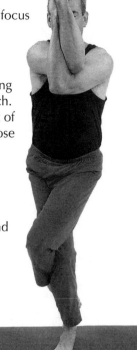

VERBAL CUES

- From Tadasana (Mountain Pose) find a focus point (*drishti*) somewhere in front of you. Keep your gaze fixed on this spot throughout the posture.
- Shift your weight to the right leg. Step the left leg out (abduct) to the left side approximately two feet (about one-half meter), and keep your toes on the ground. Inhale to create space in the spine and keep the pelvis square.
- Bring your hands to your hips, and roll your shoulders open as you exhale and bend both knees. Be sure that your body weight falls straight down from the spine and that your knees do not extend out beyond your feet. Flex your hips as if you were going to sit in a chair.
- Lift your left foot off the ground, and cross your left knee over your right leg above the right knee, keeping both knees bent. If possible, hook your left foot behind your right calf. Keep your tailbone extended toward the floor and your ribcage and chest lifted and open. With every breath in, reach the crown of the head upward.
- Maintain length in the entire spine from the low back to the neck. Keep your body weight balanced with your hips reaching back and your spine perpendicular to the floor.
- Inhale and stretch your arms apart out to your sides. Exhale and cross your arms in front of your chest by moving your right arm over your left arm above the elbows. Then bend your elbows so the backs of your hands come together in front of your face. If you can comfortably, press your palms together, essentially wrapping your arms. Bring your hands in line with your gaze.
- Continue to focus on your breath—the smoother and steadier the breath, the steadier the balance.
- Breathe into the space between your shoulder blades, feeling your shoulder blades move away from each other with each inhalation. Be sure to drop your shoulders away from your ears.
- To exit the posture, inhale and slowly unwind your arms. Uncross the left leg and place the foot on the floor. Inhale and straighten the right leg. Prepare to reverse the order for the other side.

ADJUSTMENTS

balance—First, have the student spread the toes for better balance. Stand behind the student, and place your hands on either side of the hips. While the student exhales, draw the hips back and down. At the same time encourage the student to lift and open the ribcage and chest. You can use your shoulder to press against the student's mid back to lift the shoulders.

knee of standing leg—If the knee of a student's standing leg extends too far forward, square the hips by standing to one side and slightly behind the person to support some of the body weight. Holding onto the hips, gently move the student's body weight back over the heels.

shoulders—Lightly touch the tops of students' shoulders to encourage them to relax the shoulders away from the ears.

elbows—If the student's arms are crossed below the elbow on the forearm, stand in front and grasp the opposite upper arm with each of your hands. Gently move each arm across the student's chest, toward the opposite shoulder.

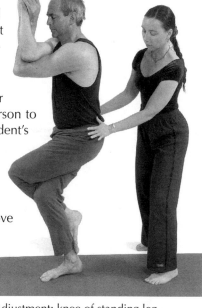

MODIFICATIONS

trouble balancing—Place the student with the back against a wall if available or, if no wall is available, instruct the student to keep the toes of the front foot lightly touching the ground.

Adjustment: knee of standing leg.

knee problems—Encourage the student to keep the toes of the nonweight-bearing leg on the floor to help balance. This placement also keeps the supporting leg from taking all the body weight. Another option, which is also helpful to those with balance difficulty, is to have the student sit at the edge of a chair or fitness ball or lean against a wall to keep the hips aligned and use the wall as a training wheel.

hip replacements or extremely tight hips—Have students cross the legs at the ankle joint, and keep the nonweight-bearing knee external to the line of the thigh.

KINEMATICS

To avoid placing undue stress on the weight-bearing leg, the knee joint should be aligned with or posterior to the foot. If a student's upper body is heavy, they will have difficulty wrapping the arms. In this case, instruct the students to "give themselves a hug" by reaching their hands toward the opposite shoulders. This allows for a stretch in the posterior musculature.

Garudasana (Standing on Right Leg)

Body segment	Kinematics	Muscles active	Muscles released
Foot and toes (R)	Toe abduction, foot stability	Dorsal interossei, abductor digiti minimi brevis, abductor hallucis (C, I)	
	Toe flexion (pressure into ground)	Flexor digitorum longus and brevis, flexor hallucis longus (C, I)	
Foot and toes (L)	Toe hyperextension	Extensor digitorum longus, extensor hallucis longus (C, I)	
Lower leg (R)	Ankle dorsiflexion	Gastrocnemius, soleus (E, I)	
	Ankle stability	Anterior and posterior tibialis, flexor digitorum longus, flexor hallucis longus, peroneals (C, E, I)	

Body segment	Kinematics	Muscles active	Muscles released
Lower leg (L)	Ankle dorsiflexion	Anterior tibialis (C, I)	Gastrocnemius, soleus
	Ankle eversion	Peroneals, extensor digitorum longus (C, I)	
Thigh (R)	Knee flexion	Quadriceps (E, I)	
	Knee stability	Adductors (I)	
Thigh (L)	Knee flexion	Hamstrings (C, I)	
Hip and pelvis (R)	Hip flexion, stability	Hamstrings, gluteus maximus (E, I)	
	Hip stability	Gluteus medius and minimus, adductors (I)	
Hip and pelvis (L)	Hip flexion	Iliopsoas, rectus femoris (C, I)	Gluteus medius, minimus; deep external rotators*
	Thigh adduction	Adductors, gracilis, pectineus (C, I)	
Torso	Trunk stability	Rectus abdominis, internal and external obliques, transverse abdominis, erector spinae, quadratus lumborum (I)	
	Postural support and downward pull of scapulae	Lower trapezius (C, I)	
Shoulder	Horizontal flexion of humerus	Pectoralis major, anterior deltoid, coracobrachialis (C, I)	Rhomboids, upper and mid trapezius, posterior deltoid
	Stability and external rotation of humerus	Infraspinatus, teres minor (I)	
	Scapular depression	Pectoralis minor, subclavius (C, I)	
	Scapular stability	Serratus anterior (C, I)	
Upper arm	Elbow flexion	Biceps brachii, brachialis, brachioradialis (C, I)	Triceps brachii
Lower arm	Pronation of lower arm	Pronator teres, pronator quadratus (C, I)	
Hand and fingers	Wrist extension	Extensor carpi radialis brevis and longus, extensor carpi ulnaris (C, I)	
	Wrist stability	Flexor carpi radialis and ulnaris, palmaris longus (I)	
	Finger extension	Extensor digitorum, extensor digiti minimi brevis (C, I)	
	Finger adduction	Flexor and extensor pollicis longus, adductor pollicis (C, I)	
Neck	Neck extension, stability	Splenius capitus and cervicis, suboccipitals, semispinalis (I)	

*Obturator externus and internus, gemellus superior and inferior, quadratus femoris, and piriformis.

C = concentric contraction, E = eccentric contraction, I = isometric contraction.

Utthita Parshvakonasana

Extended Side-Angle Stretch

[oot-T-HEE-tuh paarsh-vuh-kohn-AAH-suh-nuh]

Parshva is side or flank, and *kon* is angle. *Utthita* means extended. So Utthita Parshvakonasana is an extended side (or flank) angle stretch.

DESCRIPTION

This posture is a side-stretching lunge where one hand is placed on the ground of the lunging side and the other arm is extended overhead.

BENEFITS

- Stretches the side of the body
- Helps relieve sciatica
- Relieves hip, thigh, and low back pain caused by arthritis or imbalance
- Opens the groin
- Stabilizes the hip and knee joints
- Opens and stabilizes the chest and shoulders
- Increases circulation to structures around the heart and lungs
- Tones the abdominal muscles

CAUTION

knee problems—Those with knee injuries should be extra careful not to allow the bent knee to roll inward.

VERBAL CUES

- From Tadasana (Mountain Pose), extend your arms out to your sides with your palms facing downward.
- Continue to focus on your breath.
- Extend your legs apart; try to bring your feet as far apart as your outstretched hands.
- Rotate the left leg out 90 degrees, and then turn the right foot in slightly toward the left approximately 45 degrees.
- Bend the left knee and bring the top of the left thigh as parallel to the ground as possible, making sure not to extend the knee beyond the toes. Inhale and open and expand from the front center of the spine. Feel your hips and shoulders opening and your spine extending and lengthening.
- Exhale, keeping the foundation of the body open, and reach through your left arm. Continue to press through the right foot. Lengthen the left side of the torso as long as possible.
- Bring your left hand either in front of or behind the left foot on the ground. If you put the left arm in front of the knee it is easier to press back with the upper arm and keep the knee from rolling inward. If you place the hand behind the left foot it makes it easier to roll the right side of the body open as you extend outward. Place your hand where you feel your body needs the most support.
- Take your right hand to the hip as you roll both shoulders open to reestablish the space expanding through the torso.

- On the next inhalation, bring the right arm out in front of your body with the right palm facing the floor. Keep your shoulders moving down away from the ears, and extend the right arm over your head. Turn to look up at the right palm. Keep the space in your neck. Rotate your navel up toward the sky. Continue to press through the right foot while continuing to open your left hip. Visualize your thighs rolling away from each other, opening your pelvis more with each breath.
- Remain focused on your breathing.
- Keep the legs active. Feel the space on the right side expand with each breath. Imagine your right fingers moving farther away from your right foot.
- To exit the position, press firmly through both feet and inhale while extending the left knee and sweeping the right arm out to the right side of the body. Imagine that you are being pulled up by that right hand.

ADJUSTMENTS

bent knee—Ask students to check that the bent knee is at an angle where the thigh is nearing parallel with the floor. If the knee is not bent enough, the hips will remain too high and it will not be Parshvakonasana! Adjust the distance of the feet to correct the angle of the knee.

hips—Instruct the student to roll the top hip back so it is in the frontal plane with the shoulders. Stand behind the student and brace your knee against the back of the pelvis. Use your closest hand to roll the upper shoulder toward you as you use your other hand to stabilize the top hip.

hand placement—Help the student decide where to place the down arm—in front of or behind the foot—depending on the student's stability, flexibility, and openness in the hips.

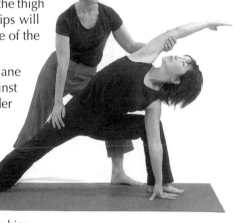

Adjustment: hips.

MODIFICATIONS

stiff hips—If the student cannot reach the ground without compromising the alignment, have the student bend the elbow of the downward facing arm and place the forearm on the bent thigh just above the knee. The student can also use a block for leverage. Caution: Students tend to sink into the shoulder in this modification. It is harder for them to press and lift out of the low back and neck.

balance issues—Place students with balance problems with their backs against the wall to help maintain balance.

stiff neck and shoulders—Instruct students to look forward instead of up toward the upper arm if the neck fatigues or is extremely stiff.

KINEMATICS

Many times students new to the posture will practice it in the modified position, where the lower arm rests on the thigh of the bent leg. Over time, as the student increases strength and flexibility in the hips and shoulders, the student will develop the ability to bring the hand to the floor. Generally, when you see a student's lower shoulder pressed up near the ear, presuming the student is not "resting" in the posture, you can suggest the student try to bring the hand to the floor.

Modification: stiff hips.

Parshvakonasana (Flexing to the Right)

Body segment	Kinematics	Muscles active	Muscles released
Foot and toes	Toe abduction, foot stability	Dorsal interossei, abductor digiti minimi brevis, abductor hallucis (C, I)	
	Toe flexion (pressure into ground)	Flexor digitorum longus and brevis, flexor hallucis longus (C, I)	
Lower leg (R)	Stability to counter body sway (muscles relax and contract as necessary to maintain balance)	Peroneals, anterior and posterior tibialis, gastrocnemius, soleus, flexor digitorum longus, flexor hallucis longus (C, E, I)	
Lower leg (L)	Ankle inversion, stability	Anterior tibialis, flexor hallucis longus (C, I)	Gastrocnemius, soleus, peroneals
	Ankle stability	Peroneals (E, I)	
Thigh (R)	Knee flexion, stability	Quadriceps (E, I)	
	Knee stability	Hamstrings, popliteus (I)	
Thigh (L)	Knee extension	Quadriceps (C, I)	
	External rotation of femur	Deep external rotators (C, I)*	
Hip and pelvis (R)	Hip flexion, stability	Hamstrings, gluteus maximus (E, I)	Adductors
	Hip flexion, abduction, and stability	Tensor fascia lata (E, I)	
	Pelvic stability	Rectus abdominis (C, I)	
	External rotation of femur, stability	Deep external rotators (C, I)*	
Hip and pelvis (L)	Hip extension and stability	Gluteus maximus, hamstrings (C, I)	Iliopsoas, adductors
	Abduction	Tensor fascia lata	
	Pelvic stability	Rectus abdominis (C, I)	
Torso	Torso stability	Erector spinae, rectus abdominis, internal and external obliques, rectus abdominis, transverse abdominis, quadratus lumborum (I)	
	Rib and chest elevation	Pectoralis minor (C, I)	
Shoulder (R and L)	External rotation	Infraspinatus, teres minor (C, I)	
	Scapular adduction	Rhomboids major and minor, mid trapezius (C, I)	
Shoulder (R)	Humerus abduction and shoulder stability	Deltoids, infraspinatus, teres minor (C, I)	
Shoulder (L)	Humerus flexion	Anterior deltoids, pectoralis major, biceps brachii (C, I)	Latissimus dorsi, pectoralis major

Body segment	Kinematics	Muscles active	Muscles released
Upper arm	Elbow extension	Triceps brachii (C, I)	Biceps brachii, brachialis, brachioradialis
Lower arm	Elbow	Anconeus (C, I)	
	Forearm supination	Supinator (C, I)	
Hand and fingers (R)	Wrist hyperextension, stability, and finger extension	Extensor carpi radialis brevis and longus; extensor carpi ulnaris; extensor digitorum, indicis, and digiti minimi; lumbricales manus; interossei dorsales (C, I)	Flexor carpi radialis and ulnaris, digitorum superficialis, palmaris longus
	Finger abduction, stability	Abductor pollicis longus, extensor pollicis brevis, interossei dorsales manus, abductor digiti minimi, abductor pollicis brevis, opponens pollicis (C, I)	
Hand and fingers (L)	Wrist extension	Extensor carpi radialis brevis and longus, extensor carpi ulnaris, extensor digitorum (C, I)	
	Finger extension	Extensor digitorum, indicis, and digiti minimi; lumbricales manus; interossei dorsales (C, I)	
	Finger adduction	Interossei palmaris, adductor pollicis (C, I)	
Neck (R)	Head rotation to left	Sternocleidomastoid (C, I)	
Neck (L)	Head rotation, neck stability against gravity	Splenius capitus and cervicis, occipitals, cervical erector spinae, scalenes, sternocleidomastoid (C, I)	

*Obturator externus and internus, gemellus superior and inferior, quadratus femoris, and piriformis.

C = concentric contraction, E = eccentric contraction, I = isometric contraction.

Half-Moon Pose

[AR-dhuh chuhn-DRAAH-suh-nuh]

Ardha is Sanskrit for half, and *chandra* is one of the Sanskrit words for moon.

DESCRIPTION

This posture is named more for the pattern the body follows when entering the posture than for what the body looks like once in the posture. From Utthita Trikonasana (Extended Triangle), the body weight is balanced on the forward leg as the trailing leg lifts up off the ground in an arcing motion. Visualize the moon as a big circle; the arc the nonweight-bearing leg moves through resembles the curve of the half-moon. As an extension of Utthita Trikonasana, Ardha Chandrasana provides similar benefits, most notably in that it opens the chest, hips, and pelvis.

BENEFITS

- Strengthens the leg musculature on the balancing leg as well as the hip and torso on the extended side
- Opens the chest and shoulders
- Builds concentration and focus
- Strengthens hip abductors

CAUTIONS

pregnancy—After the first trimester, this pose should be practiced with modifications.

weakness or balance problems—Those with extreme weakness or balance difficulties should use modifications.

VERBAL CUES

- Begin in Utthita Trikonasana extending to the right side, but with the feet a slightly shorter distance apart, such as 4 to 6 inches (10 to 15 centimeters).
- While extending the upper body over the right leg, bend the right knee and bring your right hand down to the floor in front of your toes. Turn your head to look at your right foot and watch that you keep the right knee aligned with the right foot. Do not let the knee roll inward.
- Breathe deeply in this position for a few breaths and focus on the balance in your right foot. Keep the space open in the low back, chest, and hips.
- Bring your top hand down to your left hip. Check that the right ankle is rotating externally and not inward to make sure your knee is in proper alignment.
- Continue to focus on your breath.
- While keeping your right knee bent, extend your fingertips 4 to 8 inches (10 to 20 centimeters) in front of your right toes. Inhale and slowly straighten your right leg as you lift your left leg until it is parallel to floor. Focus on the balance in your right leg.

- Concentrate on keeping the right leg externally rotated with your knee and toes in alignment. Roll your left hip back; imagine you are pressing your back and hips against a wall behind you. With each inhalation, expand the space from the front center of the spine. Remember: The steadier your breath is, the steadier your balance will be.
- Turn to look forward, keeping the length and space in the neck, shoulders, and chest. Raise your left hand in the air and keep both arms reaching out from the center of the spine.
- Continue to focus on rolling your left hip back; then press through the ball of the left foot to keep the action and energy moving through the leg.
- To exit from this posture, slowly bend the right knee and lower your left leg back to the ground. Inhale as you extend the right knee and bring yourself back into standing. Prepare to repeat on the other side.

ADJUSTMENTS

standing leg—Make sure the knee of the standing leg is aligned over the ankle and externally rotated by 90 degrees. It is usually best to have students come out of the posture and move back into it with any necessary modifications, or with you helping to guide them.

hip—Stand behind the student, facing toward the head, and position your hip against the student's top leg, hip, or low back for stability. Place your nearest hand on the student's top hip, and gently roll the hip toward you.

extended leg—Brace your nearest hip against the student's low back, and place one hand lightly under the student's knee joint to move the leg parallel to the floor.

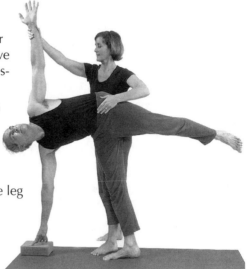

Adjustment: hip.

MODIFICATIONS

balance training—Place students with their backs against the wall for alignment as well as balance support. Instruct them to press the top hip and shoulder against the wall.

weakness in hip abductors—Position the student so the lifted foot is placed against a wall. The pressure helps with balance and lift of the leg. If no wall is available, you can stand facing the sole of the foot and instruct them to press the foot into your hand.

difficulty reaching hands to floor due to tight groin—Place a block under the student's lower hand to aid in balance and maintain proper alignment.

extremes in weakness and imbalance or pregnancy—Have the student kneel and place one hand laterally on the floor or block and lift the opposite leg off the ground.

KINEMATICS

Because the way to enter this position is from Utthita Trikonasana—first flexing then extending the balancing leg—the quadriceps are greatly utilized. With the spine and nonweight-bearing leg parallel to the ground, the pull of gravity challenges the neck, hips, and spine as the student works to maintain balance and alignment.

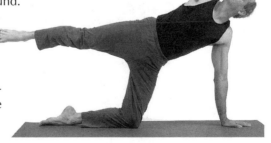

Modification: extremes in weakness and imbalance or pregnancy.

Ardha Chandrasana (Standing on Right Leg)

Body segment	Kinematics	Muscles active	Muscles released
Foot and toes (R)	Toe abduction, foot stability	Dorsal interossei, abductor digiti minimi brevis, abductor hallucis (C, I)	
	Toe flexion (pressure into ground)	Flexor digitorum longus and brevis, flexor hallucis longus (C, I)	
Foot and toes (L)	Toe extension	Extensor digitorum longus, anterior tibialis, extensor hallicus longus (C, I)	
Lower leg (R)	Stability to counter body sway (muscles relax and contract as necessary to maintain balance)	Peroneals, anterior and posterior tibialis, gastrocnemius, soleus, flexor digitorum longus, flexor hallucis longus (C, E, I)	
Lower leg (L)	Ankle dorsiflexion	Anterior tibialis, extensor digitorum longus, peroneus tertius (C, I)	Gastrocnemius, soleus
Thigh (R)	Knee flexion then extension and patellar elevation	Quadriceps (C, E, I)	Adductors, gracilis
	External rotation of femur, stability	Gluteus maximus, deep external rotators (C, I)*	
Thigh (L)	Knee extension and patellar elevation	Quadriceps (C, I)	
Hip and pelvis (R)	Hip flexion, stability	Hamstrings, gluteus maximus (E, I)	
	Hip stability	Gluteus medius and minimus, adductors (C,I)	
Hip and pelvis (L)	Hip extension	Hamstrings, gluteus maximus (C, I)	
	Hip stability (against gravity)	Tensor fascia lata, gluteus maximus, deep external rotators* (C, I)	
Torso	Trunk stability	Internal and external obliques, rectus abdominis, transverse abdominis, quadratus lumborum, erector spinae (I)	
	Rib and chest elevation	Pectoralis minor (C, I)	
Shoulder	Humerus abduction and shoulder stability	Deltoids, supraspinatus, (C, I)	Pectoralis major
	Humerus depression and stability	Subscapularis, infraspinatus, teres minor (C, I)	
	Scapular adduction	Rhomboids, mid trapezius (C, I)	
	Postural support in mid back and downward pull on scapulae	Lower trapezius (C, I)	
	External rotation of humerus	Infraspinatus and teres minor with some posterior deltoid (C, I)	

Body segment	Kinematics	Muscles active	Muscles released
Upper arm	Elbow extension	Triceps brachii (C, I)	
Lower arm	Forearm supination	Supinator (C, I)	
	Elbow extension	Anconeus (C, I)	
	Wrist hyperextension	Extensor carpi radialis brevis and longus, extensor carpi ulnaris, extensor digitorum (C, I)	Flexor carpi radialis and ulnaris, digitorum superficialis, palmaris longus
Hand and fingers	Finger extension	Extensor digitorum, indicis, and digiti minimi; lumbricales manus; interossei dorsales (C, I)	
	Finger adduction	Interossei palmaris, adductor pollicis (C, I)	
Neck (R)	Head rotation (to left)	Sternocleidomastoid (C, I)	
Neck (L)	Head rotation, neck stability	Splenius capitus and cervicis, occipitals, cervical erector spinae (C, I)	Sternocleidomastoid

*Obturator externus and internus, gemellus superior and inferior, quadratus femoris, and piriformis.

C = concentric contraction, E = eccentric contraction, I = isometric contraction.

Revolving Extended Side-Angle Stretch

[par-ee-VRT-tuh paarsh-vuh-kohn-AAH-suh-nuh]

Parshva means side or flank, and *kon* means angle. *Parivrtta* means the other side. This term is often translated as meaning to revolve or revolving. This posture is a twisted or revolving flank stretch.

DESCRIPTION

Starting from Utthita Parshvakonasana (Extended Side-Angle Stretch), the body twists or revolves around the upper torso. The trunk ends up in a position where the chest is pointing away from the hips. It is a challenge to keep the back foot on the ground, and the lower extremities are worked in a manner that connects the energy of the body while maintaining balance. The two

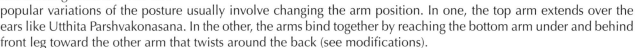

popular variations of the posture usually involve changing the arm position. In one, the top arm extends over the ears like Utthita Parshvakonasana. In the other, the arms bind together by reaching the bottom arm under and behind front leg toward the other arm that twists around the back (see modifications).

BENEFITS

- Combines the benefits of Utthita Parshvakonasana with a spinal twist
- Improves digestion
- Stimulates circulation
- Builds balance and focus
- Provides deep stretch in hips and shoulders and upward-facing flank

CAUTIONS

back problems—As with other twists, those with back injuries should be extra cautious.

pregnancy—It is not advised to practice this posture during pregnancy due to extreme rotation in the torso.

VERBAL CUES

- Starting from Utthita Parshvakonasana with the right leg forward and the right hand to the outside of the right foot, bring your left hand from over your head to your left hip. You may need to adjust the left leg by turning your hip toward the floor and lifting the heel off the ground so that you can square the hips and rotate the spine.
- Rotate the chest toward the right knee as you exhale and reach your left hand to the outside of the right leg.
- On each inhalation lengthen the spine and open the chest. On each exhalation, twist slightly more to the right. Stay mindful not to go past the edge of what is comfortable but challenging.
- Extend the right arm and reach the right hand over the head with your upper arm near your right ear. Look up at the palm.
- Continue to focus on your breath.
- To exit from this position, exhale and slowly lower your right hand back to the floor as you release the rotation in your torso. Inhale and lift your left hand off the floor, and imagine being pulled up out of the lunge with that hand as you also straighten your right knee, coming back into a standing position. Prepare for your next posture.

- Another option for exiting this position is to place both hands on the floor under the shoulders and step the right leg back into a plank to move on to other positions.

ADJUSTMENTS

balance—Enable the student to stay in position with greater stability by offering a block on which to place the lower hand.

bent back leg—Check the student's feet, making sure the bent knee is not turned inward. If it is, then guide the knee into deeper external rotation by gently pressing your hands against the inside of the student's knee.

shoulders—Instruct students that their shoulders should be as far away from their ears as possible. Gently touch the tops of their shoulders as a reminder.

spine—If the student is rounding the spine, touch the spine gently as a reminder. Cue the student to visualize the spine as a long straight line, with the crown of the head moving away from the back foot.

extended arm—The arm extended over the ear must be rotated externally to open the chest and shoulders. Be sure the student's palm is facing down toward the floor. Stand behind the student, and hold the upper arm and gently roll the elbow more toward the floor. Use the side of your body to stabilize the student if needed.

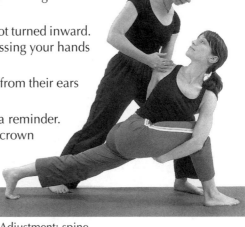

Adjustment: spine.

MODIFICATIONS

difficulty rotating and balancing—Have the student lower the back knee onto the floor, square the hips, and bring the lower arm to the outside of the opposite leg; they can then twist and open the body. From there the student can lift the back knee off the floor.

back knee pain—If the back knee is on the ground, you may have to provide the student with extra padding.

tight shoulders—The hands can be in prayer position (anjali mudra) so the bottom elbow is used to press against the outside bent knee to create more leverage to rotate the shoulders open.

deepening the posture—Binding the arms gives a deeper stretch in the chest and shoulders. Instruct the student as follows: Bend the arm that is placed to the outside of the bent knee, and then bring the elbow underneath the thigh. Rotate the arm inward and

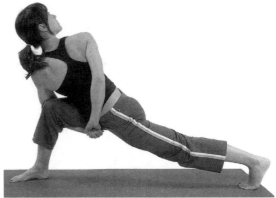

Modification: difficulty rotating and balancing.

reach the hand toward the outside of the same-side hip or onto the low back. Next, bend the opposite elbow and lift the shoulder toward the sky (hyperextending that arm). Bring the back of that hand against the spine, reaching toward the opposite hand. If the student cannot quite clasp the opposite hands together, she can hold onto a strap and work the hands toward each other.

This positioning stretches the chest and front of the shoulders more intensely. You can move students deeper in the position if they are stable by moving the hip of the bent knee toward their foot creating more space in the torso.

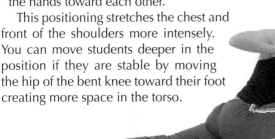

Modification: tight shoulders.

Modification: deepening the posture.

KINEMATICS

This posture utilizes a considerable amount of energy due to the stability required to maintain both balance and alignment.

Parivrtta Parshvakonasana (Flexing and Rotating to the Right)

Body segment	Kinematics	Muscles active	Muscles released
Foot and toes	Toe abduction, foot stability	Dorsal interossei, abductor digiti minimi brevis, abductor hallucis (C, I)	
	Toe flexion (pressure into ground)	Flexor digitorum longus and brevis, flexor hallucis longus (C, I)	
Lower leg (R)	Stability to counter body sway (muscles relax and contract as necessary to maintain balance)	Peroneals, anterior and posterior tibialis, gastrocnemius, soleus, flexor digitorum longus, flexor hallucis longus (C, E, I)	
Lower leg (L)	Ankle inversion, stability	Anterior tibialis, flexor hallucis longus (C, I)	Gastrocnemius, soleus, peroneals
Thigh (R)	Knee flexion	Quadriceps (E, I)	Hip adductors
Thigh (L)	Knee extension	Quadriceps (C, I)	
Hip and pelvis (R)	Hip flexion, stability	Hamstrings, gluteus maximus (E, I)	
	Hip flexion, abduction, stability	Tensor fascia lata (E, I)	
	External rotation of femur, stability	Deep external rotators,* gluteus maximus (C, I)	
Hip and pelvis (L)	External rotation of femur, stability	Deep external rotators,* gluteus maximus (C, I)	Iliopsoas, hip adductors
	Hip extension, stability	Hamstrings, gluteus maximus (C, I)	
Torso (R and L)	Trunk stability	Erector spinae, internal and external obliques, rectus abdominis, transverse abdominis, quadratus lumborum (I)	
	Rib and chest elevation	Pectoralis minor (C, I)	
Torso (R)	Rotation to right	Internal obliques, quadratus lumborum (C, I)	External obliques
Torso (L)	Rotation to right	External obliques (C, I)	Internal obliques, quadratus lumborum
Shoulder (R and L)	Scapular adduction	Rhomboids, mid trapezius (C, I)	
Shoulder (R)	Humerus flexion	Anterior deltoids, pectoralis major, biceps brachii (C, I)	Posterior deltoids, serratus anterior
	External rotation	Infraspinatus, teres minor (C, I)	
Shoulder (L)	Humerus abduction and shoulder stability	Deltoids, infraspinatus, teres minor, posterior deltoid (C, I)	
	External rotation	Infraspinatus, teres minor, posterior deltoid (C, I)	
	Slight hyperextension of humerus, stability	Posterior deltoid, teres major, latissimus dorsi (C, I)	

Body segment	Kinematics	Muscles active	Muscles released
Upper arm	Elbow extension	Triceps brachii (C, I)	Biceps brachii, brachialis, brachioradialis
Lower arm	Elbow extension	Anconeus (C, I)	
	Forearm supination	Supinator (C, I)	
Hand and fingers (R)	Finger extension	Extensor digitorum, indicis, and digiti minimi; lumbricales manus; interossei dorsales (C, I)	
	Finger adduction	Interossei palmaris, adductor pollicis (C, I)	
Hand and fingers (L)	Wrist hyperextension	Extensor carpi radialis brevis and longus, extensor carpi ulnaris, extensor digitorum (C, I)	Flexor carpi radialis and ulnaris, digitorum superficialis, palmaris longus
	Finger extension	Extensor digitorum, indicis, and digiti minimi; lumbricales manus; interossei dorsales (C, I)	
	Finger adduction	Interossei palmaris, adductor pollicis (C, I)	
Neck (R)	Head rotation (to left)	Sternocleidomastoid (C, I)	
Neck (L)	Head rotation, neck stability	Splenius capitus and cervicis, occipitals, cervical erector spinae (C, I)	Sternocleidomastoid

*Obturator externus and internus, gemellus superior and inferior, quadratus femoris, and piriformis.

C = concentric contraction, E = eccentric contraction, I = isometric contraction.

Parivrtta Ardha Chandrasana

Revolving Half-Moon Pose

[par-ee-VRT-tuh AR-dhuh chuhn-DRAAH-suh-nuh]

Parivrtta means the other side. It is often translated to mean to revolve or revolving. *Ardha* is Sanskrit for half, and *chandra* is one of the Sanskrit words for moon.

DESCRIPTION

Parivrtta Ardha Chandrasana is basically the half-moon posture with the upper torso revolving to the opposite side. One can enter this posture either from Ardha Chandrasana (Half-Moon Pose) or Parivrtta Trikonasana (Revolving Triangle Pose). This asana is much more challenging than Half-Moon because of the twist, which requires greater strength for balance and greater flexibility to twist and stay open. Many forces are working on the body in this posture. This asana is not generally practiced on a regular basis, but it is an excellent posture nonetheless. Students should be able to balance for at least 2-3 breaths in the other standing balance postures before attempting this one.

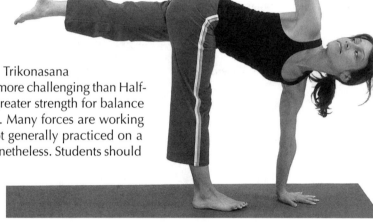

BENEFITS

- Improves flexibility and strength in the hips and torso
- Builds balance and focus
- Increases stamina
- Tones abdominal muscles

CAUTIONS

weakness or dizziness—If a student is feeling weak or dizzy, it is a good idea to have the student skip this posture.

pregnancy—It is inadvisable to attempt this posture during pregnancy due to extreme rotation in torso.

VERBAL CUES

- From Utthita Trikonasana (Extended Triangle), extend to the right side, pull the crease of the right hip back toward the left heel, and slowly rotate the left hip toward the right foot. Press firmly through the left foot.
- Bend the right knee, taking care not to let it turn inward. Place your left fingertips on the floor approximately 4 to 6 inches (10 to 15 centimeters) in front of the right foot.
- Place the right hand on your right hip and begin to transfer the weight of the left leg forward over the right foot and left hand. When you feel balanced, lift the left foot off the ground.
- Look down at the floor as you straighten the right leg. Maintain the length in your spine. When you find your balance and alignment in the hips, continue reaching out of the extended back leg. Lift your chest and roll the right side of the torso toward the sky.
- Roll the right shoulder back and down toward your hips. Lift the right arm up, and keeping the length in the neck, slowly turn your head to look up at your right hand.
- Continue to focus on your breath.
- To exit this position, inhale and slowly bend your left knee and set your right foot back on the floor. Take another breath, and on the next inhalation straighten your left leg and lift the torso. Exhale and bring your arms to your sides. Prepare for the next posture.

ADJUSTMENTS

support foot—Instruct students to spread the toes and to keep the supporting knee aligned with the foot. Remind them to press through the back lifted foot and leg.

balance—To help the student maintain balance, stand on the side of the elevated leg and use your hip or ribs to help provide support. Place the hand closest to the student's legs on the top hip, gently rotating it back. Use your other hand to lift or gently guide the lower shoulder forward for greater rotation.

hips—Create alignment in the hips by encouraging the student to point the lower hip toward the standing leg as much as possible. Brush your fingertips on the crease of the right hip.

exiting the posture—To come out of this posture, students really need to focus on moving slowly and being mindful of their body positioning. Focusing on their breath enables them to exit the posture as gracefully and as purposefully as possible. To physically assist students, stand to the side of the weight-bearing leg with your hip blocking the student's hip. Place your closest hand on the student's upper shoulder and your other hand on the opposite hip and gently guide the person to untwist and come upright.

Adjustment: balance; hips.

MODIFICATIONS

difficulty reaching ground with hand—Provide a block for the hand on the ground if lowering to the ground is difficult while maintaining balance.

balance—You can help your students establish and maintain balance in a number of ways. One way is to instruct them to place the upward rotating hand on the hip instead of extending the hand toward the sky. They can place the extended foot against a wall for stability. Also, you can have them place their hands against a wall for support.

building strength and balance, weakness or pregnancy—Instruct students to start with a "baby" Revolving Half-Moon to build strength, flexibility, and balance. Students begin by placing the right knee on the ground with the left hand on the floor to the outside of the right knee. Instruct them to rotate the torso to the right and extend the right hand in the air as they lift and extend the left leg back.

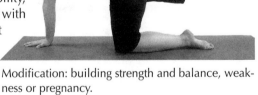
Modification: building strength and balance, weakness or pregnancy.

KINEMATICS

Because the lifted leg has nothing to press against, more effort is required to keep the spine lengthened and to open the chest. This posture requires the deeper stabilizing musculature of the pelvis and spine to achieve and maintain alignment and balance.

Parivrtta Ardha Chandrasana (Standing on Right Leg)

Body segment	Kinematics	Muscles active	Muscles released
Foot and toes (R)	Toe abduction, foot stability	Dorsal interossei, abductor digiti minimi brevis, abductor hallucis (C, I)	
	Toe flexion (pressure into ground)	Flexor digitorum longus and brevis, flexor hallucis longus (C, I)	
Foot and toes (L)	Toe extension	Extensor digitorum longus, anterior tibialis (I)	
Lower leg (R)	Stability to counter body sway and contract and relax as needed	Gastrocnemius, soleus, peroneals, posterior tibialis, flexor digitorum longus and flexor hallucis longus (C, E, I)	
Lower leg (L)	Ankle plantarflexion	Gastrocnemius, soleus (C, I)	Anterior tibialis, extensor digitorum longus
Thigh (R)	Knee extension, patellar elevation, stability	Quadriceps (C, I)	Adductors, gracilis
Thigh (L)	Knee extension, patellar elevation	Quadriceps (C, I)	
Hip and pelvis (R)	Flexion, stability	Hamstrings, adductors (E, I)	Hamstrings
	Hip stability	Gluteus medius and minimus (C, I)	
	External rotation of femur	Gluteus maximus, deep external rotators* (C, I)	
Hip and pelvis (L)	Hip extension	Hamstrings, gluteus maximus (C, I)	
Torso (R and L)	Trunk stability	Internal and external obliques, rectus abdominis, transverse abdominis, quadratus lumborum, erector spinae (I)	
	Rib and chest elevation	Pectoralis minor (C, I)	
Torso (R)	Trunk rotation to right	Internal obliques, quadratus lumborum (C, I)	Erector spinae, external obliques
Torso (L)	Trunk rotation to right	External obliques (C, I)	Quadratus lumborum, erector spinae, internal obliques
Shoulder	Humerus abduction and shoulder stability	Deltoids, infraspinatus, teres minor (C, I)	Pectoralis major
	Scapular adduction	Rhomboids major and minor, mid trapezius (C, I)	
	Supporting posture in mid back and downward pull of scapulae	Lower trapezius (C, I)	
	External rotation of humerus	Infraspinatus and teres minor with some posterior deltoid (C, I)	

Body segment	Kinematics	Muscles active	Muscles released
Upper arm	Elbow extension	Triceps brachii (C, I)	Biceps brachii, brachialis, brachioradialis
Lower arm (R)	Forearm supination	Supinator (C, I)	
	Elbow extension	Anconeus (C, I)	
Hand and fingers (R)	Finger extension	Extensor digitorum, indicis, and digiti minimi; lumbricales manus; interossei dorsales (C, I)	
	Finger adduction	Interossei palmaris, adductor pollicis (C, I)	
Hand and fingers (L)	Wrist hyperextension, stability, and finger extension	Extensor carpi radialis longus and brevis, extensor carpi ulnaris; extensor digitorum, indicis, and digiti minimi; lumbricales manus; interossei dorsales (C, I)	Flexor carpi radialis and ulnaris, digitorum superficialis, palmaris longus
Neck (R)	Head rotation to the right, neck stability	Splenius capitus and cervicis, occipitals, cervical erector spinae (C, I)	Sternocleidomastoid
Neck (L)	Head rotation to the right, stability	Sternocleidomastoid (C, I)	Splenius capitus and cervicis, occipitals, cervical erector spinae

*Obturator externus and internus, gemellus superior and inferior, quadratus femoris, and piriformis.

C = concentric contraction, E = eccentric contraction, I = isometric contraction.

Utkatasana

Fierce Pose, or Chair Pose

[OOT-kuht-AAH-suh-nuh]

This pose is fierce (*utkata* in Sanskrit) because draws significant energy from and builds strength in the thighs and hips. In Indian mythology, warriors drew much of their power and virility from these muscles. Utkatasana is a very symbolic pose.

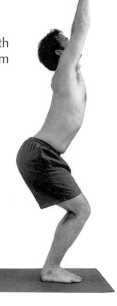

DESCRIPTION
Although the positioning appears as if one is sitting in an uncomfortable chair, it is actually considered a semistanding squat with the arms lifted overhead. This posture is part of Surya Namaskara B.

BENEFITS
- Builds strength and endurance in hips and thighs
- Strengthens balance
- Opens and tones the chest and shoulders

CAUTION
knee injuries—Those with knee pain or injury should avoiding bending the knees too deeply.

VERBAL CUES
- Begin from Tadasana (Mountain Pose) with the feet and legs together and parallel. Inhale and raise your hands overhead. Feel your ribcage expand. Press your palms together, although you may also keep your hands shoulder-width apart if that is more comfortable for you.
- Draw your shoulders down, keeping your chest lifted. Continue to stretch your tailbone down.
- On the next exhalation, bend your hips and knees. Try to keep your hips aligned behind your heels and your knees back behind your toes.
- Stretch your tailbone down and feel the extension out of the low spine. You can look up at your thumbs as you draw them back. Take time to breathe deeply, opening the chest. Keep your shoulders moving away from the ears.
- Be sure the neck is comfortable so there is space in the back of the neck. If you are uncomfortable at all, continue to look straight ahead. Otherwise, take the focus up toward your hands.
- Feel the inside of the knees pressing together and keep the knees aligned back of the toes. Notice that your hips feel as if they are being pulled backward and down, while during each inhalation your chest feels like it is lifting higher toward the sky.
- Find yourself in the space where you are the most comfortably challenged, and continue to focus on your breath.
- To exit this posture, inhale deeply as you straighten your hips and legs. Exhale as you bring your arms back down to your sides in Tadasana.
- A nice counterposture is Uttanasana (Intense Forward Bend).

ADJUSTMENTS
feet—Instruct student to position the feet so that they point directly forward. If the student's knees are not aligned in the same direction as the feet, gently press against the outside of the student's knees. Occasionally, a student will attempt to flex at the knees and hips too deeply, causing the knees to rotate externally to compensate. To regain alignment, instruct the student to straighten up slightly.

lower extremity—Often students align the hips and knees too far forward. Stand behind and to one side of the student and place your hands on the student's hips. Gently and slowly guide the hips backward. Because the student's balance will shift as you move the hips, you must move the person very slowly and with care. Remind the student to stretch the tailbone toward the floor to keep length in the low spine.

spine—If the student is standing with an accentuated swayback (lordosis), remind the student to stretch the tailbone toward the floor and to keep length in the low spine. You can place your hands lightly at the low spine, above the pelvis, as a reminder to lengthen the area.

chest—If the student's chest is "collapsing" inward, help the student rotate the arms externally to keep the shoulders open. Standing in front of the student, place your hands above the student's elbows and rotate the elbows closer toward each other. Also, you can gently guide the student's thumbs toward the back of the body to open the shoulders even more.

MODIFICATIONS

weakness or knee pain—Do not have students squat down as far. Focus on the alignment and lengthening the spine. Have them bend farther once they gain strength and endurance in the muscles over time.

balance difficulty and leg weakness—Place students with their backs against the wall for support in both balance and in gradually gaining strength in the thighs and hips.

Adjustment: lower extremity.

standing instability—Suggest that students place their feet wider apart for better stability. Remind them, however, to be sure the knees do not turn in.

strength building—Have students place a towel or small ball between the knees and a block between the hands to help target the knee and shoulder alignment. By pressing against the props, strength is increased at the point of proper alignment.

KINEMATICS

The body positioning of this asana is similar to that of a traditional squat without the weights. And although no additional load is placed on the body, the alignment in the sagittal plane in this asana is important in building and maintaining joint stability.

Utkatasana

Body segment	Kinematics	Muscles active	Muscles released
Foot and toes	Toe abduction, foot stability	Dorsal interossei, abductor digiti minimi brevis, abductor hallucis (C, I)	
Lower leg	Ankle dorsiflexion, stability	Gastrocnemius, soleus (E, I)	Gastrocnemius, soleus
	Stability to counter body sway (muscles relax and contract as necessary to maintain balance)	Peroneals, anterior and posterior tibialis, gastrocnemius, soleus, flexor digitorum longus, flexor hallucis longus (C, E, I)	
Thigh	Knee flexion, stability	Quadriceps (E, I)	
	Knee stability	Hamstrings, popliteus (I)	

(continued)

Utkatasana *continued*

Body segment	Kinematics	Muscles active	Muscles released
Hip and pelvis	Hip flexion	Hamstrings, gluteus maximus (E, I)	
	Pelvic stability	Rectus abdominis, quadratus lumborum, hamstrings (I)	
	Hip stability	Adductors, gluteus maximus (I)	
Torso	Spinal extension and stability	Erector spinae (C, I)	
	Rib and chest elevation	Pectoralis minor (C, I)	
	Trunk stability	Internal and external obliques, rectus abdominis, transverse abdominis, quadratus lumborum, erector spinae (I)	
Shoulder	Humeral flexion (90 to 180 degrees)	Anterior deltoids, pectoralis major, biceps brachii (C, I)	Latissimus dorsi, serratus anterior
	External rotation	Infraspinatus, teres minor, posterior deltoid (C, I)	
	Scapular adduction	Rhomboids major and minor, mid trapezius (C, I)	
Upper arm	Elbow extension	Triceps brachii (C, I)	Biceps brachii, brachialis, brachioradialis
Lower arm	Forearm supination	Supinator (C, I)	
	Elbow extension	Anconeus (C, I)	
Hand and fingers	Finger extension	Extensor digitorum, indicis, and digiti minimi; lumbricales manus; interossei dorsales (C, I)	
	Finger adduction	Interossei palmaris, adductor pollicis (C, I)	
Neck	Neck extension and stability	Splenius capitus and cervicis; suboccipitals, semispinals, and upper trapezius (I)	

C = concentric contraction, E = eccentric contraction, I = isometric contraction.

Virabhadrasana I

Warrior I

[veer-uhb-huh-DRAAH-suh-nuh, kuh]

In the Western hemisphere this pose is known as Warrior I. In India, they traditionally use letters of the alphabet rather than numerals. The first consonant letter of the Sanskrit alphabet is pronounced "kuh." *Virabhadra* is actually the name of a great and powerful mythological warrior. Legend says that he was so great, a hair of his dropped to the earth and a great army arose.

DESCRIPTION

Warrior poses are quite physical and symbolic of warrior energy in that they require considerable strength in the muscles of the legs, which symbolize virility and power. And yet, at the same time, all three warrior postures demand that the chest and heart area remain open. The arms and legs are active, while the heart center, when open, banishes the fear of death. The Warrior 1 variation is a standing forward lunge. Hips face forward with the legs in the sagittal plane; one leg is placed forward and the other one back instead of both legs out to the sides (frontal plane) like in Utthita Trikonasana (Extended Triangle) and Vrkshasana (Tree Pose). Virabhadrasana I works deep into the hip muscles. In many Vinyasa classes or Ashtanga classes, a common way to enter this posture is from Adho Mukha Shvanasana (Downward-Facing Dog).

BENEFITS

- Strengthens the lower extremities, particularly the thighs
- Stabilizes the hips and knees
- Builds strength and endurance
- Improves flexibility and stamina in the spine

CAUTION

knee injuries—Those with knee pain or injuries should be extra careful to flex the knee less than 90 degrees and not allow the knee to turn inward.

VERBAL CUES

- From Adho Mukha Shvanasana, inhale and take a giant step forward with the right leg so that the foot is between the hands. Rotate the left foot out approximately 45 degrees pressing the back heel on the ground. Lift the torso so it is perpendicular with the floor and your hips are level with the front knee. Keep your right knee bent at 90 degrees, so that your right thigh remains parallel to the floor.
- Inhale as you raise your arms overhead, palms pressed together or shoulder-width apart. Look up at your thumbs and press them back.
- Keep the hips square with the right knee opening toward the right pinky toe.
- Stretch the tailbone toward the floor as you feel your ribcage lifting and bending back slightly.
- With each exhalation drop your hips a little lower. With each inhalation lift your chest a little higher.
- Keep your left heel on the ground, pressing through the outer edge of the foot. This helps move the left hip forward, keeping the pelvis squared.
- Maintain smooth, steady breaths as you feel the strength in the energy of your body.
- To exit this position, press through the right leg by extending the knee, and step the left leg forward. Or, you can bend at the hips, place your hands to the floor, and step or jump back (vinyasa), flowing into another posture.

ADJUSTMENTS

back foot—To help keep the back foot pressing down, walk to the student's side and use your toes to brush against the outer edge of the heel to encourage the student to press the foot into the floor. Do not push too hard!

front knee—Lightly touch the medial side (inside) or top of the student's knee and guide the leg into external rotation, which keeps the knee from rolling inward. Instruct the student to lift the arch slightly, keeping better balance on the foot.

hips—To align a student's hips directly under the shoulders, place your fingers at the outer edge of the crease of the flexed hip and gently guide the hip back. At the same time, press the back hip forward.

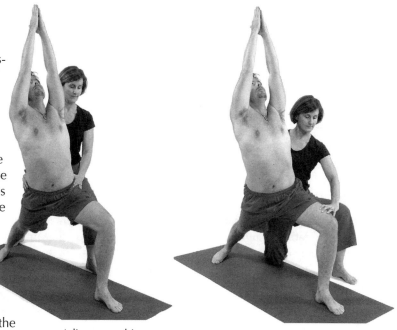

Adjustment: hips.

Adjustment: knee.

spine—Remind the student to stretch the tailbone down. Brush your hand on the low spine, encouraging the low spine to lengthen.

upper torso—Stand behind the student and place your hands on the upper arms with your thumbs to the inside and your fingers to the outside of the arm near the shoulders. Rotate the student's arms externally.

shoulders—Instruct students to draw their shoulders down. Encourage them to relax the shoulders away from the ears. Place your hands gently on top of their shoulders and press gently downward.

chest—Remind students to keep their chests lifted. Place your fingertips or the palm of your hand on the student's mid spine. Ask them to lift their backs off of your hand.

MODIFICATIONS

weakness, tiredness, pregnancy—Students can place a chair, stool, or fitness ball under their hips to take some of their body weight off the front leg. The props increase stabilization and balance because less energy is required. This also allows students to focus on balance and the rest of their body alignment. Using chairs with backs, turn the chair sideways so that the back of the chair is nearest to their forward leg. Here, the student can use the closest hand to hold onto the chair back for support.

weak shoulders—The arm position can be modified. Place a block between students' hands and instruct them to press against the block while lifting it up and back. This action activates the shoulders more specifically. If students have an acute shoulder condition with limited range of movement, then have them raise the arms up as high as they can lift them. Arms can be flexed forward with the palms facing each other at shoulder height and the thumbs pointed up to keep external shoulder rotation. Direct students to squeeze the shoulder blades together to open the chests, or have them bend their arms to 90 degrees in front and roll their shoulders open and down, pressing the shoulders back. The thumbs should be touching.

knee problems—The lunge in this asana is beneficial in strengthening the quadriceps and aligning the knee caps. However, instruct those with knee pain to avoid flexing the front knee too deeply, so the hips remain higher than the knees. Keeping the front lower leg perpendicular to the floor helps protect the knee joint. Another modification can be considered "baby" warrior, where the back knee rests on the floor instead of straight and lifted. This lunge is similar to that practiced in classical Sun Salutations.

Modification: weakness, tiredness, pregnancy.

KINEMATICS

Many times students will not realize that their hips are not aligned and that the hip of the back leg is rotated backward because they are so focused on the front knee. The more firmly they press through the back foot the more the hip flexors stretch to allow the pelvis to rotate freely forward.

Virabhadrasana I (Right Leg Forward)

Body segment	Kinematics	Muscles active	Muscles released
Foot and toes	Toe abduction, foot stability	Dorsal interossei, abductor digiti minimi brevis, abductor hallucis (C, I)	
Lower leg (R)	Slight ankle dorsiflexion, stability	Gastrocnemius, soleus (E, I)	Gastrocnemius, soleus
	Ankle stability	Peroneals, anterior and posterior tibialis, flexor digitorum longus, flexor hallucis longus (C, E, I)	
Lower leg (L)	Ankle inversion, stability	Anterior tibialis, flexor hallucis longus (C, I)	Peroneals, gastrocnemius, soleus
Thigh (R)	Knee flexion, stability	Quadriceps (E, I)	
	Knee stability	Hamstrings, popliteus (I)	
Thigh (L)	Knee extension	Quadriceps (C, I)	
Hip and pelvis (R)	Pelvic stability	Rectus abdominis (I)	
	Hip flexion	Hamstrings, gluteus maximus (E, I)	
	Hip stability, hyperextension	Adductors, gluteus maximus, hamstrings (C, I)	
Hip and pelvis (L)	Pelvic stability	Rectus abdominis, hamstrings (I)	Rectus femoris, iliopsoas
	External rotation	Gluteus maximus, deep external rotators* (C, I)	
Torso	Rib and chest elevation	Pectoralis minor (C, I)	
	Slight spinal hyperextension and stability	Iliopsoas, rectus abdominis (E, I)	
	Trunk stability	Internal and external obliques, transverse abdominis, quadratus lumborum, erector spinae (I)	Rectus abdominis
Shoulder	Humeral flexion, stability	Deltoids, pectoralis major, biceps brachii (C, I)	Latissimus dorsi, serratus anterior
	External rotation	Infraspinatus, teres minor, posterior deltoids (C, I)	
	Scapular adduction	Rhomboids major and minor, mid trapezius (C, I)	
Upper arm	Elbow extension	Triceps brachii (C, I)	Biceps brachii, brachialis, brachioradialis

(continued)

Virabhadrasana I (Right Leg Forward) *continued*

Body segment	Kinematics	Muscles active	Muscles released
Lower arm	Forearm supination	Supinator (C, I)	
Head and fingers	Elbow extension	Anconeus (C, I)	
	Finger extension	Extensor digitorum, indicis, and digiti minimi; lumbricales manus; interossei dorsales (C, I)	
	Finger adduction	Interossei palmaris, adductor pollicis (C, I)	
Neck	Slight neck hyperextension and stability	Sternocleidomastoid (E, I)	
	Neck stability	Splenius capitus and cervicis, suboccipitals (I)	Sternocleidomastoid

*Obturator externus and internus, gemellus superior and inferior, quadratus femoris, and piriformis.

C = concentric contraction, E = eccentric contraction, I = isometric contraction.

Virabhadrasana II

Warrior II

[veer-uhb-huh-DRAAH-suh-nuh, k-huh]

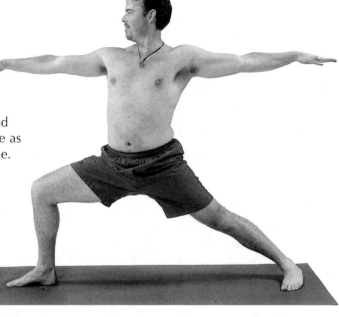

In the Western hemisphere this pose is known as Warrior II. It is the second asana named after the warrior Virabhadra. The second consonant in Sanskrit is pronounced "k-huh" and is similar to that in Warrior I, but the sound is aspirated. For proper pronunciation, it takes twice as much breath to say "k-huh" rather than "kuh" for one.

DESCRIPTION

This posture, as a lunge, is similar to Virabhadrasana I, but instead of the body lunging forward in the sagittal plane, the lunge occurs in the frontal plane. The bent knee is externally rotated, directly out to the side and the arms are abducted and parallel to the floor. The spine is perpendicular to the ground without arching the back.

BENEFITS

- Opens and strengthens the musculature of the hips
- Tones the lower extremities
- Continues to work on subtle alignments of the upper body and opening and strengthening of the shoulder joint
- Builds muscular endurance
- Tones the abdominal muscles

CAUTIONS

knee problems—Those with knee injuries or weakness should practice with modification.

pregnancy—After the first trimester, pregnant women should proceed with caution.

VERBAL CUES

- From Tadasana (Mountain Pose), inhale and reach your hands over your head. Exhale and lower your arms out to your sides until they are parallel to the floor. Now step your right leg out to the side.
- Place your feet wider than your outstretched hands, if comfortable. Turn your left foot toward the right heel and the right leg out 90 degrees so that the heel of your right foot, if you drew a line, would bisect through the left arch.
- Keep your arms outstretched and your hips and shoulders squared in the frontal plane.
- Point your tailbone down to lengthen the low back, and picture both legs rolling open from the center away from each other.
- Feel your chest lifting up, the crown of your head extending upward and away from the tailbone, and your ears back and aligned over the shoulders.
- Exhale and bend the right knee until your hips and right knee are bent approximately 90 degrees, making your right thigh parallel to the ground.

- Keep extending through the left leg and left hand. Feel your left hip and ribcage press back to keep the torso from rotating out of the frontal plane.
- Turn your head to look over your right hand so your gaze is past the right fingertips. Align your chin with your right shoulder.
- Continue to focus on your breath.
- Keep your right knee opening out to the right. Continue to press your left hip, ribcage, and shoulders back and aligned as if you had a wall behind you and you were pressing your shoulder blades and hips against it.
- On each exhalation, drop the hips lower toward the floor as you bring the top of your right thigh parallel to the floor.
- Inhale and lift the chest higher than before. Feel the lower ribs lifting away from your hips.
- To exit the posture, inhale and straighten the right leg. Rotate the toes forward and bring your arms to your side. Prepare for the next posture.

ADJUSTMENTS

bent knee—Remind students to roll the front thigh outward by brushing your hand against the outside of the knee, or simply point to the knee and remind students verbally. You can also use both of your hands to slowly roll a student's thigh more open.

hips and knees—If the student has difficulty keeping the bent knee and opposite hip apart, place the student's back against a wall so less energy is expended on balancing and more can be used to open the front of the body. Sit on the floor in front of the student with your hands behind your hips for support. Place one foot on the middle of the student's bent-leg thigh and your other foot on the hip of the student's straight leg. Press the student's hips and thigh back against the wall. Always ask for feedback. This adjustment takes significant energy on the part of the teacher, so continue to remind the student to try to take on some of the effort by pressing the pelvis against the wall.

Adjustment: hips; knee.

hips—If the student's bent knee is rolling to the outside, there will be a tendency for the student to roll the opposite hip inward. Stand behind the student and step your closest leg over the student's bent thigh, pressing your heel into the leg, just above the knee joint. Use your foot to guide the student to rotate the thigh externally. At the same time, use your opposite hand to pull the other hip back toward you. Instruct the student to feel the hips and shoulders opening up.

hip height—Stand behind the student and place your hands lightly on the student's hips and guide the hips lower. Be sure the student is both strong and balanced enough to handle this adjustment. You may need to suggest that the student take the legs farther apart to avoid placing excessive stress on the bent knee while working to engage the hips and legs more fully.

shoulders—Instruct students to draw their shoulders down. Encourage them to relax the shoulders away from their ears. Place your hands softly on the tops of their shoulders and press gently downward.

spine—If the student's spine is leaning out over the leg such that the spine is no longer perpendicular to the floor, stand behind the student with your hands on either shoulder and lightly guide the torso back to center by gently moving the shoulders upright.

MODIFICATION

pregnancy, weakness, or rehabilitating students—Instruct students to bend their front knees less than 90 degrees. This modification requires less muscular energy and endurance. Students may also use a chair or fitness ball for support.

Modification: pregnancy, weakness, or rehabilitating students

KINEMATICS

Usually it is best to instruct students to place their feet slightly wider than the distance of their outstretched hands. If they do not, the feet will tend to be too close together when they move into the lunge and the bent knee will extend past the foot causing a loss of stability and alignment. Feet too close together make it harder to open the hip and easier to roll the bent knee inward, so the body weight will be off center. This lack of stability could harm the bent knee rather than strengthening the supporting structures to protect it.

Virabhadrasana II (Right Knee Bent)

Body segment	Kinematics	Muscles active	Muscles released
Foot and toes	Toe abduction, foot stability	Dorsal interossei, abductor digiti minimi brevis, abductor hallucis (C, I)	
	Toe flexion (pressure into ground)	Flexor digitorum longus and brevis, flexor hallucis longus (C, I)	
Lower leg (R)	Ankle dorsiflexion, stability	Gastrocnemius, soleus (E, I)	Gastrocnemius, soleus
	Stability to counter body sway (muscles relax and contract as necessary to maintain balance)	Peroneals, anterior and posterior tibialis, gastrocnemius, soleus, flexor digitorum longus, flexor hallucis longus (C, E, I)	
Lower leg (L)	Ankle inversion, stability	Anterior tibialis, flexor hallucis longus (C, I)	Gastrocnemius, soleus, peroneals
Thigh (R)	Knee flexion, stability	Quadriceps (E, I)	
Thigh (L)	Knee extension	Quadriceps (C, I)	
Hip and pelvis (R)	Hip flexion	Hamstrings, gluteus maximus (E, I)	Adductors
	External rotation, stability	Gluteus medius and minimus (C, I)	
	Abduction, stability	Tensor fascia lata (E, I)	
	Hip flexion, abduction, stability	Tensor fascia lata (E, I)	
Hip and pelvis (L)	Hip extension and stability	Gluteus maximus, hamstrings (C, I)	Iliopsoas, adductors
	External rotation, stability	Gluteus maximus, deep external rotators* (C, I)	
	Abduction, stability	Tensor fascia lata, gluteus medius, minimus (I)	
	Pelvic stability	Hamstrings, rectus abdominis (I)	
Torso	Torso stability	Erector spinae, internal and external obliques (I)	
	Rib and chest elevation	Pectoralis minor (C, I)	

(continued)

Virabhadrasana II (Right Knee Bent) *continued*

Body segment	Kinematics	Muscles active	Muscles released
Shoulder	Humerus abduction and shoulder stability	Deltoids, infraspinatus, teres minor, supraspinatus, pectoralis major (C, I)	
	Scapular adduction	Rhomboids, mid trapezius (C, I)	
	Scapular rotation	Serratus anterior, mid and lower trapezius (C, I)	
	Supporting posture in mid back and downward pull of scapulae	Lower trapezius, subscapularis (C, I)	
	External rotation of humerus	Infraspinatus and teres minor with some posterior deltoid (C, I)	
Upper arm	Elbow extension	Triceps brachii, brachioradialis (C, I)	
Lower arm	Forearm pronation	Pronator teres, pronator quadratus (C, I)	
	Elbow extension	Anconeus (C, I)	
Hand and fingers	Finger extension	Extensor digitorum, indicis, and digiti minimi; lumbricales manus; interossei dorsales (C, I)	
	Finger adduction	Interossei palmaris, adductor pollicis (C, I)	
Neck (R)	Head rotation to right, stability	Splenius capitus and cervicis, cervical erector spinae, occipitals (C, I)	Sternocleido-mastoid
Neck (L)	Head rotation to right	Sternocleidomastoid (C, I)	

*Obturator externus and internus, gemellus superior and inferior, quadratus femoris, and piriformis.

C = concentric contraction, E = eccentric contraction, I = isometric contraction.

Virabhadrasana III

Warrior III

[veer-uhb-huh-
DRAAH-suh-nuh,
guh]

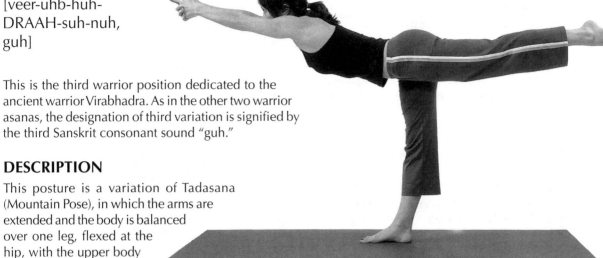

This is the third warrior position dedicated to the ancient warrior Virabhadra. As in the other two warrior asanas, the designation of third variation is signified by the third Sanskrit consonant sound "guh."

DESCRIPTION

This posture is a variation of Tadasana (Mountain Pose), in which the arms are extended and the body is balanced over one leg, flexed at the hip, with the upper body and opposite leg parallel to the ground. Deeper hip muscles in the standing leg are worked considerably to create stability. Fatigue occurs faster in these postures. Also, the length of the person's leg and the force of gravity working against both the extended upper body and leg create the need for considerable strength and endurance building. Be sure to counterstretch the low back after performing this posture.

BENEFITS

- Strengthens the spine and posterior shoulder muscles
- Builds stamina and endurance
- Opens chest
- Promotes awareness of proper hip alignment
- Builds abdominal strength

CAUTION

balance or vertigo—Those with extreme balance difficulties or vertigo should practice with support.

VERBAL CUES

- Begin from Tadasana or from Virabhadrasana I.
- From Virahabhadrasana I,
    - With right foot forward, keep the hips square, pulling back through the crease in the hip of the bent leg. Continue to press forward with the left hip. The arms remain overhead.
    - Fold forward at your hips and straighten the bent right leg as you begin to lift the left leg straight up off the ground. Balance here for a breath or two.
    - Inhale as you move your body weight completely onto the front leg, bringing your torso, arms, and lifted leg parallel to the floor.
    - Gaze straight ahead and look at your hands, pulling your shoulders down away from your ears.
- From Tadasana,
    - Inhale and raise the arms above your head. Drop the shoulders down from the ears. Transfer the weight of your body onto your right leg and then step your left leg straight behind you so the toes are barely touching the floor. Remain balanced for a couple of breaths. Stay mindful of keeping your hips squared and level.

- Inhale and lengthen the spine. Exhale as you slowly begin to fold forward from the right hip, lifting your left leg off the ground and lowering your torso until both are parallel to the ground.
- With each breath in, continue to extend and lengthen through the arms, torso, and the extended back leg. On each exhalation, square the hip of the lifted left leg toward the floor.
- Gaze straight ahead and look at your hands, pulling your shoulders down away from your ears.
- To exit the posture, inhale and begin to slowly drop the left leg down to the ground as you lift your chest and torso upright. Use the strength of the legs and hips, and keep lifting through the low back to keep those muscles from straining as you lower the leg. Drop your hands to your sides and prepare for the other side.

ADJUSTMENTS

standing leg bent—Many times students will bend the support leg slightly to compensate for balance. Instruct them to spread the toes and straighten the supporting knee. By spreading the toes they create a slightly wider base of support, which helps their balance. Also, remind students to focus on evenly distributing their body weight on the foot.

hips—If the hip of the student's lifted leg is higher than the hip of the supported leg, stand to the supporting-leg side and gently hold the student's hips. Lower the elevated side of the pelvis so the hips are aligned in the frontal plane with the rest of the torso. Make certain to move slowly and gently so the student does not lose balance. You also can press your hip against the student's hip to keep the student from falling.

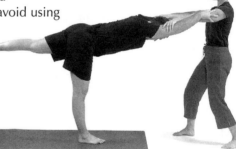

Adjustment: hips.

balance—Place your outstretched arms under the student's arms and let the student lean into your arms until balanced. Be sure to remove your arms away slowly and only when the student is balanced. You should be at the student's side in a relaxed stance with knees slightly bent; avoid using your own shoulder or back to hold them up.

arms—To help students straighten their arms and lift or press their thumbs higher, hold on to their upper arms and gently rotate their shoulders externally. Also, you may simply brush your hands on the outside of their arms to cue them to relax their shoulders away from their ears.

MODIFICATIONS

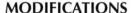

Adjustment: balance.

shoulder or neck tightness or pain—Instruct students to hold their arms at their sides, hands by the hips. This also makes it easier to balance and keep the torso straight.

balance difficulty—Place the student's hands on a ballet bar, against a wall, or even on the back of a chair to help provide lift in the upper body and aid in balance. Also, students can place the foot of their lifted leg against a wall for balance.

weakness—Do not keep anyone in the posture for too long if it is the first time a student has practiced it or if the student is experiencing significant weakness, as might be the case for those recovering from illness.

KINEMATICS

This posture requires a great deal of low back and hip-extensor strength for the lifted leg to remain parallel to the floor. Follow this posture with a resting forward bend, such as Uttanasana, as an appropriate counterposture.

Virabhadrasana III (Standing on Right Leg)

Body segment	Kinematics	Muscles active	Muscles released
Foot and toes (R)	Toe abduction, foot stability	Dorsal interossei, abductor digiti minimi brevis, abductor hallucis (C, I)	
	Toe flexion (pressure into ground)	Flexor digitorum longus and brevis, flexor hallucis longus (C, I)	
Foot and toes (L)	Toe flexion	Flexor digitorum and hallucis longus (C, I)	
Lower leg (R)	Stability to counter body sway (muscles relax and contract as necessary to maintain balance)	Peroneals, anterior and posterior tibialis, gastrocnemius, soleus, flexor digitorum longus, flexor hallucis longus (C, E, I)	
Lower leg (L)	Plantar flexion	Gastrocnemius, soleus (C, I)	Anterior tibialis
Thigh (R)	Knee extension, patellar elevation	Quadriceps (C, I)	
	Stability and adduction (magnus also helps extend knee)	Adductors (C, I)	
Thigh (L)	Knee extension	Quadriceps (C, I)	
Hip and pelvis (R)	Hip flexion and stability	Hamstrings, gluteus maximus (E, I)	
	Hip stability	Gluteus medius and minimus, adductors (C, I)	
Hip and pelvis (L)	Hip extension	Hamstrings, gluteus maximus (C, I)	Iliopsoas
	Pelvic stability	Rectus abdominis, quadratus lumborum, hamstrings (I)	
Torso	Spinal extension and stability	Erector spinae, quadratus lumborum (C, I)	
	Rib and chest elevation	Pectoralis minor (C, I)	
	Trunk stability	Internal and external obliques, rectus abdominis, transverse abdominis, quadratus lumborum, erector spinae (I)	
Shoulder	Humeral flexion, stability	Anterior deltoids, pectoralis major, biceps brachii (C, I)	Latissimus dorsi, serratus anterior
	Maintaining humeral flexion against gravity	Deltoids, rhomboids, trapezius (C, I)	
	External rotation, stability	Infraspinatus, teres minor (C, I)	
	Scapular adduction, stability	Rhomboids major and minor, mid trapezius (C, I)	
	Stability	Subscapularis (C, I)	

(continued)

Virabhadrasana III (Standing on Right Leg) *continued*

Body segment	Kinematics	Muscles active	Muscles released
Upper arm	Elbow extension	Triceps brachii (C, I)	Biceps brachii, brachialis, bracioradialis
Lower arm	Forearm supination	Supinator (C, I)	
	Elbow extension	Anconeus (C, I)	
Hand and fingers	Finger extension	Extensor digitorum, indicis, and digiti minimi; lumbricales manus; interossei dorsales (C, I)	
	Finger adduction	Interossei palmaris, adductor pollicis (C, I)	
Neck	Neck extension and stability	Splenius capitus and cervicis, cervical erector spinae, suboccipitals, (C, I)	

C = concentric contraction, E = eccentric contraction, I = isometric contraction.

Parshvottanasana

Intense Side Stretch

[paarsh-voht-taahn-AHH-suh-nuh]

Parshva is side or flank, and *ottana* is intense extension or stretch. *Parshvottanasana* means an intense stretch in the side.

DESCRIPTION

Parshvottanasana is similar to Uttanasana (Intense Forward Bend), but one leg is forward and one leg is back. This placement of the legs requires more balance and creates a deeper stretch through the hips and side. The arms are in anjali mudra, or prayer pose, behind the back. The stretch extends from the backs of the heels all the way up into the neck, releasing tension throughout the entire back of the body.

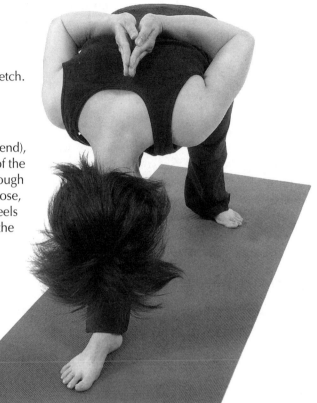

BENEFITS

- Relieves neck, shoulder, elbow, and wrist stiffness
- Opens chest
- Provides deep stretch for the legs and hips
- Relieves arthritis in the neck and spine

CAUTIONS

glaucoma—In general, students with glaucoma should not place the head below the heart.

shoulder injuries—Anyone with shoulder injuries should practice a modified version.

VERBAL CUES

- From Tadasana (Mountain Pose), step the legs three to four feet (about one meter) apart. Turn to the right so that your right leg is forward and your left leg is back. Adjust the width of your feet so that you can keep the left heel on the ground. Square the hips to the front.
- Press the palms of your hands together behind your back with the fingertips pointed up. Draw the tips of your fingers up the spine as you roll the wrists down away from your head. Only go as far as you feel comfortably challenged; never force or strain! Keep your shoulders rolling open.
- Continue to focus on your breath.
- Press your left hip forward as you move your right hip backward. Extend the tailbone down to begin as you breathe in deeply. Focus up as you gently arch back, lifting the front of the chest. Draw your shoulders down and keep the space in the neck as you look up as much as feels comfortable to you.
- Exhale, pull the right hip back, and take your time as you maintain length in the spine and begin to fold forward until the spine is parallel with the floor. Keep the hips squared and ribs parallel to the ground. With the next exhalation, release your torso down over the right leg as much as you can without rounding the back. Feel the left side of your ribcage move down toward your right thigh a little more.
- Relax your neck and soften your abdomen as you breathe deeply into the back. Feel the balance in your feet from front to back and press through the back heel.
- Create as much space in the low spine as you can by reaching through the crown of your head and stretching your tailbone toward the sky. Continue moving the right hip back. You should feel the right hip and hamstring lengthening deeply.

- To come out of this position press down firmly through both feet and extend up through the crown of the head. Press the ribcage and chest forward as you inhale and lift your body upright.

ADJUSTMENTS

front hip—Standing either behind or to the side of the student, use your fingertips to guide the front hip back and square the hips forward in the sagittal plane.

ribcage—Stand behind the student to the side of the back leg. Place your closest hand on the opposite side of the student's ribcage and your other hand on the side of the ribcage nearest you. With a light touch, slightly rotate the far side toward you and the near side more toward the student's front leg.

shoulders—Gently place your hands on top of the student's shoulders and guide the shoulders down away from the ears.

neck—Lightly touch the back of the student's head as a reminder to release the tension in the neck.

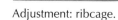
Adjustment: ribcage.

MODIFICATIONS

tight shoulders—If students cannot place their palms together behind their backs, instruct them to fold their arms behind their waists, clasping opposite elbows. Or, have them clasp their hands behind them with their elbows straight. As they fold forward they can lift their arms up to help stretch the fronts of the shoulders and chests.

increase shoulder stretch—If students can press their palms together, instruct them to point their elbows up toward the sky.

tight hamstrings—If the hamstring stretch is too intense for a student, have the student bend the front leg slightly, taking care not to let the knee turn inward if it is bent.

rounded back—Do not have the student go down toward the thigh all the way. Instruct the student to keep the back parallel to the floor. Also, the student can have the legs in position, but instead of the arms behind the back place the hands against a chair or wall.

KINEMATICS

As in Virabhadrasana I, the more firmly the student presses through the back foot, the more the hip flexors stretch to allow the pelvis to rotate forward. This action also helps create better balance as the student folds forward and deepens the stretch in the hip extensors. The arm kinematics shown in the chart reflect arms in prayer position.

Modification: tight shoulders.

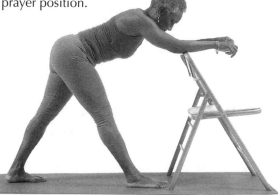
Modification: rounded back; tight hamstrings.

Parshvottanasana (Right Leg Forward)

Body segment	Kinematics	Muscles active	Muscles released
Foot and toes	Toe abduction, foot stability	Dorsal interossei, abductor digiti minimi brevis, abductor hallucis (C, I)	
	Toe flexion (pressure into ground)	Flexor digitorum longus and brevis, flexor hallucis longus (C, I)	
Lower leg (R)	Stability to counter body sway (muscles relax and contract as necessary to maintain balance)	Peroneals, anterior and posterior tibialis, gastrocnemius, soleus, flexor digitorum longus, flexor hallucis longus (C, E, I)	Anterior tibialis
Lower leg (L)	Ankle dorsiflexion, stability	Gastrocnemius, soleus, peroneals (E, I)	Gastrocnemius, soleus, peroneals
Thigh (R and L)	Knee extension, patellar elevation	Quadriceps (C, I)	
Hip and pelvis (R)	Flexion, stability	Hamstrings, gluteus maximus (E, I)	Hamstrings, gluteus maximus
	Pelvic stability	Rectus abdominis, quadratus lumborum, hamstrings (I)	
Hip and pelvis (L)	Hip extension	Hamstrings, gluteus maximus (C, I)	Iliopsoas
	Slight external rotation and stability	Deep external rotators,* gluteus maximus (C, I)	
Torso	Spinal extension and stability	Erector spinae, quadratus lumborum (C, I)	
	Trunk stability	Internal and external obliques, rectus abdominis, transverse abdominis, quadratus lumborum, erector spinae (I)	
	Rib and chest elevation	Pectoralis minor (C, I)	
Shoulder	Scapular adduction	Rhomboids major and minor and mid trapezius (C, I)	Pectoralis major, anterior deltoid, coracobrachialis
	Postural support in mid back and downward pull of scapulae	Lower trapezius (C, I)	
	External rotation	Infraspinatus, teres minor, posterior deltoid (C, I)	
Upper arm	Hyperextension of humerus	Posterior deltoid, latissimus dorsi, teres major (C, I)	
Lower arm	Elbow flexion	Biceps brachii, brachialis, brachioradialis (C, I)	
	Forearm pronation	Pronator teres and quadratus (C, I)	

(continued)

Parshvottanasana (Right Leg Forward) *continued*

Body segment	Kinematics	Muscles active	Muscles released
Hand and fingers	Wrist hyperextension	Extensor carpi radialis longus and brevis, extensor carpi ulnaris, extensor digitorum (C, I)	Flexor carpi radialis and ulnaris, palmaris longus
	Finger extension	Extensor digitorum, indicis, and digiti minimi; lumbricales manus and interossei dorsales manus (C, I)	
Neck	Extension and stability	Splenius capitis and cervicis, cervical erector spinae, upper trapezius (C, I)	

*Obturator externus and internus, gemellus superior and inferior, quadratus femoris, and piriformis.

C = concentric contraction, E = eccentric contraction, I = isometric contraction.

Utthita Hasta Padangusthasana

Extended Hand-to-Toe Pose

[oot-T-HEE-tuh HAAS-tuh paah-daahng-oost-AHH-suh-nuh]

In this pose, *utthita* means extended, *hasta* refers to hand, *pada* is the entire leg or foot, and *gusth* means big toe. The name of this asana refers to a number of different positions, but in the standing position it usually refers to standing on one leg while the other leg is extended parallel to the floor while you hold on to the big toe of the lifted foot.

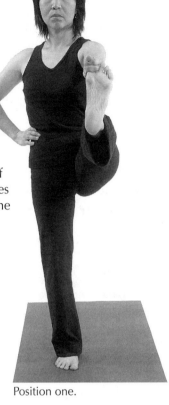

DESCRIPTION

This asana utilizes strength in the quadriceps of both the standing and, especially, the extended legs. Once you are balanced on one leg and holding onto the big toe of your extended leg with either your fingers or a strap, then you can go through the series of extending the leg to the side, then back to the center, then bending forward from the hips, and finally allowing the leg to slowly lower to the ground.

BENEFITS

- Increases concentration
- Builds stability and strength
- Balances stability and symmetry in the pelvis and spine
- Tones the abdominal muscles

VERBAL CUES

Position one.

- Starting from Tadasana (Mountain Pose), bring your weight onto the right leg. Place your hands to your hips for stability and roll the shoulders open. Exhale and bend the left knee, and then draw it up toward your chest. Keep your right hand on your right hip, and reach down with the first two fingers of your left hand to hook your big toe. Keep the spine straight and lifted. Take your time as you maintain your alignment and balance. Begin to straighten the left leg out in front of you so it is parallel to the floor.

- Inhale and lengthen the spine and roll the shoulders back to open the chest. Keep your shoulders and hips squ+ared. Stack your shoulders over your hips.

- Pull the left hip back and down to maintain balance in the pelvis. Press firmly through your right leg. (See position one.)

- Stay here for a few breaths, maintaining your focal point. Keep your breathing steady.

- Act like you have blinders on when you practice. Focus somewhere out in front of your body so that noticing anything in your peripheral vision does not cause you to lose your balance.

- You can remain here or externally rotate the left leg out to the left side, grounding your balance through the right heel. Look over your right shoulder. You can extend your right arm out to the right side, parallel to the floor, to maintain balance. Stretch your chin out over the right shoulder to keep the openness in the chest and shoulders. (See position two.)

Position two.

- Exhale as you slowly bring the left leg and head forward again. Keep the shoulders down and chest lifted. Bend the left arm slightly, and pull your leg up toward your chest as far as you feel comfortable. On the exhalation, fold from your hips as much as possible as you drop your head toward your left knee. You can hold on to the left foot with both hands if it is more comfortable. (See position three.)
- Inhale and lift your chest and shoulders up away from your hips. Exhale as you bring your hands back to your hips; keeping your left leg extended in front for a couple more breaths before gently lowering it to the floor. (See position four.)

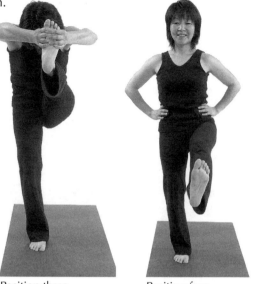

Position three.   Position four.

ADJUSTMENTS

standing foot—If the supporting foot is not pointed directly forward they will have difficulty keeping balance. Remind the student to keep the toes and knees pointed forward.

legs—Stand in front of the student and provide gentle support to the lifted leg. Hold the leg lightly at the heel. You can help the student to rotate the leg slowly to the side as you aid with the balance.

hips—To help the student maintain hip alignment and to keep the top of the pelvis parallel to the floor, stand behind the person and lightly place your hands on the student's hips as you make the necessary adjustment.

shoulders—Be sure the student's shoulders do not roll forward. Stand behind the person and place one hand between the shoulder blades. Instruct the student to squeeze the shoulder blades toward your hand. This opens the shoulders and lifts the chest.

MODIFICATIONS

lack of hamstring or hip flexibility—Give the student a strap to wrap around the foot as an extension of the arms. This allows the student to keep the spine straight and aids significantly in balance. If no straps are available, you can instruct students to keep their knees bent slightly. Doing so helps alleviate strain in the low back.

increase strength and flexibility—Students can use a wall or ballet bar to rest the lifted foot against as they focus on spinal alignment while building strength and flexibility in the legs.

weakness—Students can sit in a chair or on a fitness ball to work on balance and flexibility.

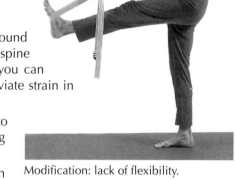

Modification: lack of flexibility.

KINEMATICS

An added benefit of this posture is the subtle strengthening and stretching of the posterior shoulder in the arm reaching for the extended foot.

Utthita Hasta Padangusthasana (Standing on Right Leg)

Body segment	Kinematics	Muscles active	Muscles released
Foot and toes (R)	Toe abduction, foot stability	Dorsal interossei, abductor digiti minimi brevis, abductor hallucis (C, I)	
	Toe flexion (pressure into ground)	Flexor digitorum longus and brevis, flexor hallucis longus (C, I)	
Foot and toes (L)	Toe extension	Extensor digitorum longus, anterior tibialis (C, I)	
Lower leg (R)	Stability to counter body sway (muscles relax and contract as necessary to maintain balance)	Peroneals, anterior and posterior tibialis, gastrocnemius, soleus, flexor digitorum longus, flexor hallucis longus (C, E, I)	
Lower leg (L)	Ankle dorsiflexion	Anterior tibialis, extensor digitorum longus (C, I)	Gastrocnemius, soleus
Thigh (R)	Knee extension, patellar elevation	Quadriceps (C, I)	
	Stability, adduction (adductor magnus helps extend knee)	Adductors (C, I)	
Thigh (L)	Knee extension	Quadriceps (C, I)	Hamstrings
Hip and pelvis (R)	Hip extension, stability	Hamstrings, gluteus maximus (C, I)	
	Hip stability	Gluteus maximus and medius, adductors, deep external rotators (I)*	
Hip and pelvis (L)	Hip flexion	Iliopsoas, rectus femoris, pectineus, tensor fascia lata (C, I)	Hamstrings, gluteus maximus, deep external rotators*
Torso	Pelvic stability	Rectus abdominis, quadratus lumborum, hamstrings (I)	
	Spinal extension and stability	Erector spinae, quadratus lumborum (I)	
	Rib and chest elevation	Pectoralis minor (C, I)	
	Trunk stability	Internal and external obliques, rectus abdominis, transverse abdominis, quadratus lumborum (C, I)	
Shoulder (R)	Humerus abduction	Deltoids, supraspinatus (C, I)	Pectoralis major
	External humeral rotation	Infraspinatus, teres minor, posterior deltoid (C, I)	
	Scapular adduction	Rhomboids, trapezius (C, I)	

(continued)

Utthita Hasta Padangusthasana (Standing on Right Leg) *continued*

Body segment	Kinematics	Muscles active	Muscles released
Shoulder (L)	Shoulder flexion	Anterior deltoid, pectoralis major, biceps brachii(C, I)	Posterior deltoid, rhomboids
	External humeral rotation	Infraspinatus, teres minor (C, I)	
	Stability	Latissimus dorsi (C, I)	
	Scapular stability	Serratus anterior, pectoralis minor (I)	
Upper arm (R)	Elbow flexion	Biceps brachii, brachioradialis, brachialis (C, I)	
Upper arm (L)	Elbow extension	Triceps brachii, brachialis, brachioradialis (C, I)	
Lower arm (R)	Forearm supination	Supinator (C, I)	
Lower arm (L)	Elbow extension	Anconeus (C, I)	
	Forearm pronation	Pronator teres, pronator quadratus (C, I)	
Hand and fingers (R)	Wrist extension	Extensor carpi radialis brevis and longus, extensor carpi ulnaris (C, I)	
	Finger adduction	Interossei palmaris, adductor pollicis (C, I)	
Hand and fingers (L)	Finger flexion	Flexor digitorum, superficialis and profundus; lumbricales manus, interossei palmaris (C, I)	
	Finger adduction	Interossei palmaris, adductor pollicis (C, I)	
Neck	Neck extension and stability	Splenius capitus and cervicis, cervical erector spinae (C, I)	

*Obturator externus and internus, gemellus superior and inferior, quadratus femoris, and piriformis.

C = concentric contraction, E = eccentric contraction, I = isometric contraction.

King Dancer

[nut-tuh-raahj-AHH-suh-nuh]

Nata means dancer, and *raja* is royal, so this posture translates to King Dancer. This is one of the many forms of Shiva (a Hindu god) as the "Lord of the Dance."

DESCRIPTION

Natarajasana is a one-legged balance posture with a back bend and is rather regal looking with the "puffed-out" chest. The nonweight-bearing leg is drawn behind the back with the arms reaching overhead to the foot of the lifted leg.

This posture has many variations. Most people cannot achieve the back arch and shoulder opening of the original posture, so a modified version is generally taught. This posture is described in three separate phases, building from least demanding to most.

BENEFITS

- Stretches chest and shoulders deeply
- Enhances balance and concentration
- Lengthens and strengthens the front of the torso and spine
- Stretches the quadriceps and iliopsoas (deep hip flexors) in the nonweight-bearing leg

CAUTIONS

acute back pain—Students with acute low back injuries should refrain from the back-arching phase of this posture.

pregnancy—Pregnant students should practice phase one.

weakness—Students who may feel weak should practice phase one of the pose.

VERBAL CUES

From Tadasana (Mountain Pose), shift your weight to the left foot. Find your drishti (gazing point) and remain focused.

Phase One

- Bend your right knee and bring your right foot toward your bottom. Reach back and hold on to your right foot or ankle with your right hand. Hold wherever you can comfortably with your hands or a strap.
- Firmly press the tailbone down toward the ground and begin to point your right knee backward while keeping your hips squared. Your thighs should remain close together so that your bent knee does not rotate.
- Continue to focus on your breath.

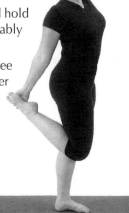

Phase Two

- Inhale and lift your left arm overhead. As you exhale, keep the pelvis level and the chest lifted as you bend slowly forward from your hip joint.
- Create a slight back bend as you strive to stretch your hips and ribcage away from each other. Keep the front of your shoulders rolled open by drawing your shoulder blades together.
- Look up toward your left fingertips. Imagine your tailbone and the crown of your head stretching away from each other.
- Continue to focus on your breath.

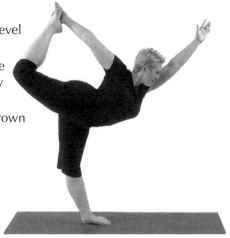

Phase Three

- If you have good balance and substantial flexibility in the shoulders and spine, stand up straight instead of folded forward at the hips. Reach both hands back and hold the right foot or ankle. You can use a strap to hold the foot for greater comfort.
- Maintain the upright position of the spine and continue to reach the spine out of the low back area. With every inhalation, lift higher and feel your chest puff open. Maintain your grip on the foot, lifting it as high as you comfortably can.
- To exit this posture, slowly release the foot and bring the arms back to your sides. Slowly lower the leg to the ground and prepare to practice on the other side.

ADJUSTMENTS

balance—Stand in front of the student and hold on to the top hand with one or both of your hands. Extend the student's arm overhead, lifting slowly. You may need to place your hand on the hip of the student's support leg for stability.

nonweight-bearing leg—Stand behind or to the side of the student and gently tap the front of the thigh, cuing them to lift the thigh higher. You can also place your hand gently under the student's heel to aid in balance while helping the person lift the leg higher.

low back—Many times students will arch the low back to reach the foot behind them. Stand to the side of the student and place one hand on the student's hip and the other on the shoulder. Guide the hip down and the ribcage forward and help the student draw the shoulders down away from the ears.

shoulders—Stand behind the student, and place your hands on the student's upper arms and rotate the shoulders externally.

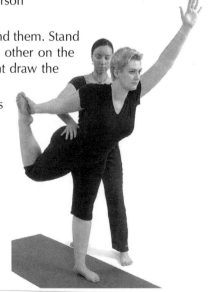

Adjustment: low back.

MODIFICATIONS

building flexibility—Modify the position by wrapping a strap around the student's lifted ankle or foot. For those with sufficient flexibility, they can use a strap in phase three and walk the hands down the strap closer to the foot.

tight shoulders—Make sure students' arms are rotated externally by keeping their elbows parallel to each other. If the elbows point away from the body, then the arms are not externally rotated and it will be difficult or impossible for them to reach the hands closer to the foot.

pregnancy, weakness, or acute low back issues—Have students stay in phase one of the posture. For increased balance, place a chair in front of them so they can place a hand on the chair for balance.

KINEMATICS

People with sufficient flexibility in the shoulders, hips, and spine can arch the back so that they touch the head to the lifted foot.

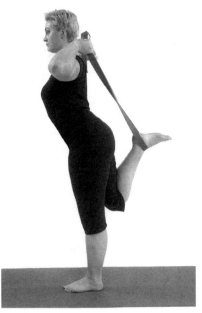

Modification: building flexibility.

Natarajasana, Phase Three (Standing on Left Leg)

Body segment	Kinematics	Muscles active	Muscles released
Foot and toes (R)	Toe extension	Extensor digitorum (C)	
Foot and toes (L)	Toe abduction, foot stability	Dorsal interossei, abductor digiti minimi brevis, abductor hallucis (C, I)	
	Toe flexion (pressure into ground)	Flexor digitorum longus and brevis, flexor hallucis longus (C, I)	
Lower leg (R)	Ankle dorsiflexion, ankle plantarflexion	Gastrocnemius, soleus (C, I)	Anterior tibialis extensor digitorum longus
Lower leg (L)	Stability to counter body sway (muscles relax and contract as necessary to maintain balance)	Peroneals, anterior and posterior tibialis, gastrocnemius, soleus, flexor digitorum longus, flexor hallucis longus (C, E, I)	
Thigh (R)	Knee flexion	Hamstrings (C, I)	Quadriceps
	Thigh adduction, stability	Adductors (C, I)	
Thigh (L)	Knee extension, patellar elevation	Quadriceps, gracilis (C, I)	
	Stability, adduction (adductor magnus helps extend knee)	Adductors (C, I)	
Hip and pelvis (R)	Hip hyperextension, stability	Hamstrings, gluteus maximus (C, I)	Iliopsoas
Hip and pelvis (L)	Hip stability	Gluteus maximus and medius, hamstrings, adductors, deep external rotators* (C, I)	
	Pelvic stability	Rectus abdominis, quadratus lumborum, hamstrings (I)	

(continued)

Natarajasana, Phase Three (Standing on Left Leg) *continued*

Body segment	Kinematics	Muscles active	Muscles released
Torso	Rib and chest elevation	Pectoralis minor (C, I)	
	Trunk stability	Internal and external obliques, rectus abdominis, transverse abdominis, quadratus lumborum (C, I)	
Shoulder	Hyperflexion, humerus adduction	Anterior deltoid, pectoralis major, biceps brachii (C, I)	Posterior deltoid
	Scapular adduction	Rhomboids, mid trapezius, (C, I)	
	External rotation	Infraspinatus, teres minor (C, I)	
	Scapular stability	Serratus anterior (C, I)	
Upper arm	Elbow flexion, stability	Triceps brachii, biceps brachii (C, I)	
Lower arm	Forearm supination	Supinator (C, I)	
Hand and fingers	Finger flexion	Flexor digiti minimi brevis, interossei palmaris, flexor pollicis brevis (C, I)	
Neck	Neck stability	Splenius capitus and cervicis, occipitals, cervical erector spinae (I)	

*Obturator externus and internus, gemellus superior and inferior, quadratus femoris, and piriformis.

C = concentric contraction, E = eccentric contraction, I = isometric contraction.

chapter 8

Seated Postures

This chapter describes 21 seated asanas. These are postures in which the hips are placed on the floor. The one exception is Malasana (Seated Squat), where the hips hover slightly above the ground. Seated postures can include forward bends, side bends, twists, or cross-legged poses. The Sanskrit word *asana* can be translated as "a way of being" or "a way of being seated."

Padmasana (Lotus pose) often comes to the minds of students and would-be yogis when they think about asanas and meditation. Seated poses might appear easier because they require less energy and strength in the legs. It is the support of the legs pushing against the ground and channeling gravity to lift the back, however, that allow the back

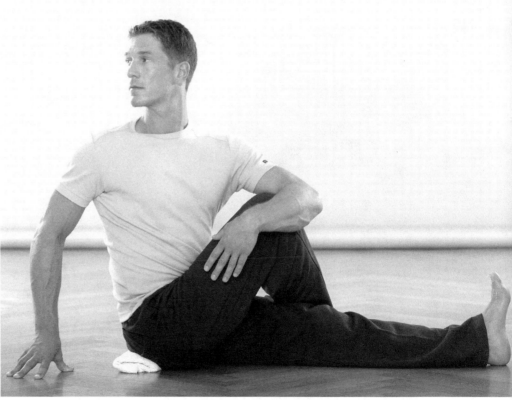

© Jumpfoto

to work less hard to maintain good posture. And if a student has not developed good postural muscles, seated asanas may feel very uncomfortable. Most people cannot tolerate sitting with a straight spine for more than a few moments because the back muscles are weak and lack endurance. In order for the back to be free to lift, the hips also need to be relaxed and flexible. When a student is able to sit comfortably with a straight spine, then the shoulders and chest can open more completely, warding off degeneration of the neck, wrists, and the whol1e body. Whether students are seeking to strengthen and release the upper body after long hours in front of the computer or to develop the strength to sit comfortably for long periods of meditation, seated poses can empower students by deepening the opening of the hips, relaxing the shoulders and neck, and improving the muscular endurance of the spine and abdominals.

The standing postures often warm up the body and circulate blood out to the limbs. Once seated, the blood has a chance to go back into the internal organs, lymph nodes, and joints more substantially.

With residual warmth and more concentrated circulation, deeper stretches and detoxification can occur. One gains greater hip and shoulder stability from practicing standing poses, whereas flexibility and spinal endurance improve with seated poses, which allow one to develop the ability to sit comfortably at length. Although most people believe seated postures are more elementary because they appear easier to do, they actually are more demanding on the spine and can be considered "more advanced." Perspective and experience, however, are what make any pose more or less "advanced."

The asanas in this chapter are sequenced in a way that lends itself to flow in a class as movements and positions progress from the first few poses to those that follow. The order is for your reference and planning. The easiest-to-teach and the most popular poses are presented first. Poses toward the end of the chapter are not necessarily more difficult for students, but these poses do tend to be more sophisticated to teach and to arrange for easy flow into and out of other asanas.

Malasana

Basic Squat Pose

[maahl-AAH-suh-nuh]

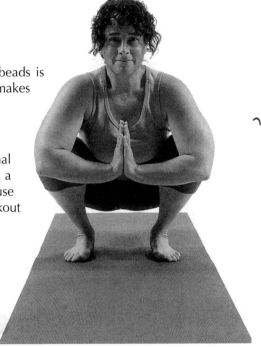

In Sanskrit, *mala* means bead. In yoga tradition, a string of prayer beads is called a *mala*. It is thought that the squatting position of this posture makes a person look curled up like a bead.

DESCRIPTION

Malasana can be considered a seated posture. It is a good transitional posture when moving from a standing to a seated posture or in a Vinyasa practice when moving from one posture to the next. Because of the restorative nature of Malasana, it can be incorporated in a workout at any time.

BENEFITS

- Stretches the back muscles
- Opens the pelvic area by as much as 30 percent
- Massages the internal organs
- Stabilizes and builds strength in the ankles and feet

CAUTION

knee problems—Students with knee injuries should practice with modifications.

VERBAL CUES

- From Tadasana (Mountain Pose), place your feet hip-width apart with toes straight ahead and parallel. Be sure that your feet are not pointed inward or your knees will roll in as you lower to the floor. This strains the joint.
- As you begin to bend at the hips, knees, and ankles, sink your hips and knees back behind your heels as if you are going to sit in a chair just beyond your reach.
- Keep your ribcage floating up and your chest and shoulders open. Gently squeeze your shoulder blades together to keep your shoulders from rolling forward.
- As you exhale, lower your hips down farther. Keep your knees apart in the center. If you need to, you can reach your arms out in front of you to keep yourself balanced as you lower down toward the floor.
- Move slowly and breathe deeply as you lower down to where you are most comfortably challenged. When you find your balance, adjust your position accordingly.
- Keep your knees from rolling toward each other, and do the best you can to sink your heels all the way to the ground.
- Stay in this position for a few breaths. Interlace your fingers, resting your forehead on your thumbs, or bring your hands together in anjali mudra (prayer position). Soften your abdomen, and relax your shoulders as you focus your breath into your back.
- To exit this position, lower your bottom onto the floor as slowly and gracefully as possible.

ADJUSTMENTS

heels—Many students have tight calf muscles, which requires lifting the heels off the floor. The ideal solution is to place a towel or blanket under the heels for support and comfort. You also can simply roll up the student's mat. This is the most common adjustment needed for this posture.

knees—Many times the student's knees will roll in toward each other. Place the student's arms between the knees as a wedge to hold the knees out. Have the student check to be sure the knees are pointed in the same direction as the toes.

balance—Squat in front of the student. Each of you should hold on to the other's wrists. Take on some of the student's weight until well balanced. Gently pull forward so the student does not sink back too far back on the heels.

MODIFICATIONS

knee problems—Use a bar, such as a ballet bar, if available, so students can hold onto it as they squat down, thus taking the body weight off the knees. You also can place pillows under students' heels so they can lower themselves down. The use of pillows should cause no stress to the knees because it allows more of the effort to be taken on by the person's thighs and hips, with the body weight back behind the line of the knees. You also can have students sit on the floor with bent knees pulled into the chest and shoulders so that the feet and pelvis are on the floor.

Adjustment: heels.

foot injury, very stiff ankles, weak knees, or hip replacement—Students can lie on their back with the knees pulled into the chest. The knees should be held apart wider than the shoulders for a restorative posture.

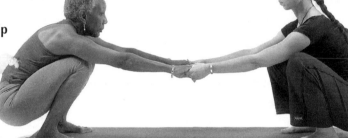

KINEMATICS

Although this posture might seem completely contraindicated for those with knee injuries because of the deep squat, it can be beneficial

Adjustment: balance.

to some because of the stretching in both the thighs and calves. By gently stretching overly tight calf muscles it may be possible to help alleviate some of the causes of knee hyperextensions.

This is a particularly beneficial posture for pregnant students as the squat opens and stretches the pelvis and perineum.

Malasana

Body segment	Kinematics	Muscles active	Muscles released
Foot and toes	Toe abduction, stability	Dorsal interossei, abductor digiti minimi brevis, abductor hallucis (C, I)	
	Toe flexion (pressure into ground)	Flexor digitorum longus and brevis, flexor hallucis longus (C, I)	
Lower leg	Ankle dorsiflexion, stability	Gastrocnemius, soleus (E, I)	Gastrocnemius, soleus
	Ankle stability	Anterior tibialis, extensor digitorum longus, peroneals (I)	
Thigh	Knee flexion	Quadriceps (E, I)	Quadriceps
Hip and pelvis	Hip flexion	Hamstrings, gluteus maximus (E, I)	Gluteus maximus, deep external rotators*
	Stability	Adductors, deep external rotators* (I)	
Torso	Trunk stability	Internal and external obliques, rectus abdominis, transverse abdominis, quadratus lumborum, erector spinae (I)	Quadratus lumborum, erector spinae
Shoulder	Internal rotation	Latissimus dorsi, anterior deltoid, pectoralis major (C, I)	Rhomboids, trapezius
Upper arm	Elbow flexion	Biceps brachii, brachioradialis, brachialis (C, I)	Triceps brachii
Lower arm	Forearm supination	Supinator (C, I)	
Hand and fingers	Finger extension	Extensor digitorum, indicis, and digiti minimi; lumbricales manus; interossei dorsales (C, I)	
	Finger adduction	Interossei palmaris, adductor pollicis (C, I)	
	Thumb abduction	Abductor pollicis longus and brevis, extensor pollicus brevis (C, I)	
Neck	Neck flexion	Splenius capitus and cervicis, levator scapulae, cervical erector spinae, upper trapezius (E, R)	Splenius capitus and cervicis, levator scapulae, cervical erector spinae, upper trapezius

*Obturator externus and internus, gemellus superior and inferior, quadratus femoris, and piriformis.

C = concentric contraction, E = eccentric contraction, I = isometric contraction, R = relaxed.

Dandasana

Staff Pose

[duhnd-AAH-suh-nuh]

Danda is Sanskrit for staff, or walking stick. Dandasana describes the straightness and strength of the upper torso and back.

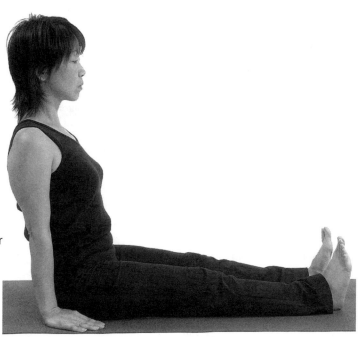

DESCRIPTION

In Dandasana, the spine and the lower body are straight and strong with the hips bent to 90 degrees. It is an active posture with the upper spine, lower abdominal muscles, and thighs all working to keep length in both the upper and lower body. This posture is generally the point from which many other seated postures build.

BENEFITS

- Massages internal organs
- Strengthens upper back
- Strengthens abdominal muscles, lower back, and thighs
- Can soothe heartburn
- Helps build postural awareness

CAUTION

back pain—Students with acute back pain should practice with modifications.

VERBAL CUES

- Sit on the ground, and stretch your legs out in front of you. Keep your legs and feet together with your sits bones level on the floor. Place your hands on the floor to either side of your hips with your fingers pointed forward toward the toes.
- Breathe in deeply as you lengthen the spine, lifting the ribcage up from the pelvis. Pull your shoulder blades together, and drop your shoulders toward your hips.
- Roll your upper thighs toward each other slightly, but keep your toes pointed upward. Lift your kneecaps toward your hips. Do not allow your heels to lift off the floor.
- Press down through your hands and sits bones to lift the spine higher. Feel your shoulders drop away from your ears, and the front of the shoulders rolling open.
- With each exhalation, feel your ears align over your shoulders and your shoulders align over your hips. With each inhalation, feel the crown of your head stretching up.
- Focus on the breath.

ADJUSTMENTS

legs—Remind the students to keep the feet pointed upward. Gently brush the outsides of the feet to cue student to press the feet together.

spine and shoulders—Most students will not realize that the upper back is rounded. Stand or kneel behind the student (watch your mechanics), and place your hands to the sides of the student's ribs and gently cue the student to lift the ribcage upward. You also can press your knee gently against the student's back to encourage more length in the spine. At the same time, place your hands to the front of the student's shoulders and gradually roll the arms back to open the chest.

head—Observe students to see if the chins are jutting forward. Place your hands lightly to the sides of the student's head, and move the head back to align the ears directly over the shoulders. You can also place your hand lightly on top of a student's head and ask the student to push against your hand to lengthen the neck and spine.

MODIFICATIONS

tight hamstrings or weak upper spine—The most common adjustment for Dandasana is to place a folded blanket or towel under the student's pelvis. It is also acceptable to allow the student to keep the knees flexed slightly as the student works, over time, to stretch the hamstrings. Another modification is to place students with the hips and back against a wall, stick, or other sturdy linear object, and instruct the student to press against the wall or stick and align the spine. To focus on keeping the spine straight and folding from the hips, students can wrap a strap around the straight leg foot and slowly walk the hands down the strap toward the toes, bringing the upper bands closer to the legs.

tight shoulders—Allow the student to point the fingers backward instead of forward to open the shoulders more completely.

KINEMATICS

The common modification of placing a blanket or towels under the student's hips helps alleviate strain in the low back by repositioning the front of the pelvis slightly more forward. By allowing more flexion at the hip joint, the

Modification: tight hamstrings or weak upper spine.

student works the upper spine muscles more to align the shoulders over the hips. This modification is beneficial to practicing the other seated postures because it trains the spinal muscles properly so that they are not compromised in the other positions.

Dandasana

Body segment	Kinematics	Muscles active	Muscles released
Foot and toes	Toe extension	Extensor digitorum longus (C, I)	
Lower leg	Ankle dorsiflexion	Anterior tibialis, extensor digitorum longus (C, I)	Gastrocnemius, soleus
Thigh	Knee extension	Quadriceps (C, I)	Hamstrings
Hip and pelvis	Hip flexion, stability	Iliopsoas, rectus femoris (C, I)	
	Pelvic stability	Rectus abdominis, quadratus lumborum, hamstrings (I)	
Torso	Rib and chest elevation	Pectoralis minor (C, I)	
	Trunk extension and stability	Internal and external obliques, rectus abdominis, transverse abdominis, quadratus lumborum, erector spinae, latissimus dorsi (I)	

(continued)

Dandasana *continued*

Body segment	Kinematics	Muscles active	Muscles released
Shoulder	Scapular adduction, stability	Rhomboids, mid trapezius (C, I)	Pectoralis major
	Postural support in mid back and downward pull of scapulae	Lower trapezius (C, I)	
	External rotation of humerus	Infraspinatus and teres minor with some posterior deltoid (C, I)	
Upper arm	Elbow extension	Triceps brachii (C, I)	Biceps brachii, brachialis, brachioradialis
Lower arm	Elbow extension	Anconeus (C, I)	Flexor carpi radialis and ulnaris, palmaris longus
	Wrist hyperextension	Extensor carpi ulnaris, radialis longus and brevis, extensor digitorum (C, I)	
Hand and fingers	Finger extension	Extensor digitorum, indicis, and digiti minimi; lumbricales manus; interossei dorsales (C, I)	
Neck	Neck extension and stability	Splenius capitus and cervicis, cervical erector spinae, upper trapezius (I)	

C = concentric contraction, E = eccentric contraction, I = isometric contraction.

Janu Shirshasana

Head-to-Knee Pose

[JAAH-noo sheer-SHAAH-suh-nuh]

Janu is Sanskrit for knee and *shirsha* is head; so this Sanskrit term translates to Head-to-Knee pose.

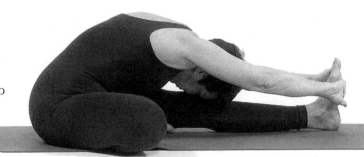

DESCRIPTION

In this seated forward bend one leg is extended forward and the knee of the opposite leg is flexed and lowered laterally to the floor. This posture is broken down into two separate parts. The first part concentrates on the lengthening of both the upper and lower halves of the body. In the second, or resting, phase of this posture the head rests close to the knee. There are several variations of Janu Shirshasana. In some of the variations the foot of the bent knee is flexed and rotated with the toes pointing toward the floor. In other variations, the student sits on the foot or the leg is in Ardha Padmasana (Half-Lotus).

BENEFITS

- Stretches and strengthens the spine
- Stretches the hamstrings and groin
- Calms the nervous system
- Helps relieve mild depression
- Improves digestion
- May alleviate symptoms of menstrual discomfort or menopause
- Can reduce anxiety, fatigue, and headache
- Relieves symptoms of high blood pressure, insomnia, and sinusitis

CAUTION

acute knee or back pain—Practice with modifications.

VERBAL CUES

Phase One

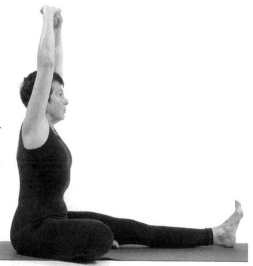

- From Dandasana (Staff Pose), bend your right knee toward your chest and point your sits bones toward the back edge of your mat. Keep your hips as squared as possible as you roll your right leg out, dropping the knee toward the floor.
- As your right thigh lowers to the floor, picture the top of that thigh as a bottle top opening; as the right thigh rotates out (externally), the twisting action opens the hips by creating more space and releasing tension. The more the hips open, the less stress you place on your knee.
- Interlace your fingers in front of you. As you inhale, raise your arms overhead. Press up through your palms with your arms as straight as possible. Press your thumbs toward the sky and point your pinky fingers toward the ground behind you. This action helps the posterior shoulder and upper back muscles to engage more fully. Move your shoulders down away from your ears, creating more space between your ears and shoulders.
- Exhale and turn your torso slightly toward the left so that you line up your spine to the straight left leg.
- Inhale and lengthen the spine as much as possible. Feel the ribcage lift out of the low back.

- Exhale and bend from the hips like a hinge. Go only as far as you can without rounding the spine, and then place your hands on the floor. Square your torso to your left leg. Align your navel toward the outside of your left knee.
- Maintain all the length and extension in your spine, and reach your hands toward your left foot. Hold on wherever you can reach comfortably with your hands or using a strap.
- With each inhalation, lift the front of your ribcage forward and up. Press your collarbones back while you press the back of your lower ribs forward. Reach your tailbone and the crown of the head away from each other.
- Continue to focus on your breath.

Phase Two

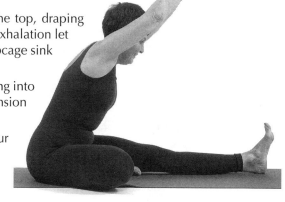

- On the next inhalation, arch your back slightly; lift your chest, and imagine your navel reaching toward the ceiling.
- Exhale and fold your torso forward from the bottom to the top, draping your upper body over the front of your left leg. With each exhalation let your head drop closer to your knee. Really let your right ribcage sink forward.
- Soften your abdomen. Feel and visualize your breath moving into your back, and focus your breath on any place you feel tension or resistance.
- To exit the posture, bring your hands to the floor beside your hips. Inhale and press through your arms to raise your torso. Exhale and stretch your right leg out, and prepare for the opposite side.

ADJUSTMENTS

feet—If the student's bent-leg ankle feels uncomfortable, adjust by either increasing the angle of the knee or placing some light padding under the ankle.

knee—If the student's bent knee is off the floor, you can offer support with a folded blanket or adjust for hip and back tightness (explained next).

hips—If the student's hips are not square toward the outstretched leg, you can start to move the hips toward proper alignment. Use your hand to gently pull the hips back, or cue the student to move the hips in a manner such that the hip of the straight leg pulls back a little. You also can press the other hip (of the bent knee) more forward at the same time. Note: The forward bend should come from the hips; otherwise the back will have a tendency to round, especially the low spine. Many teachers instruct students to move the fleshy tissue away from the sits bones while entering into seated forward bends.

torso—The back should be square toward the extended foot. Kneel beside the student, and, using your hands on the student's ribcage, turn the ribs toward the outstretched leg. At the same time, encourage the student to lift the ribcage out of the low spine as much as possible. Kneel behind or beside the student as you place one of your hands at the bottom of the ribcage in back and your other hand on the student's shoulder in a way to help pull the shoulders down and open. As you press the student's back forward and up, you can also guide the shoulders down. These two actions together should begin to lift the back and open the chest.

head—In the resting phase of this posture the neck and head relax. If the student's neck is holding any tension, brush your fingers against or lightly tap the neck or head to release.

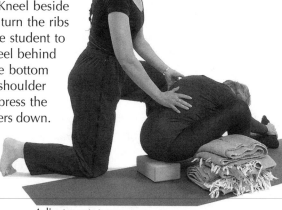

Adjustment: torso.

arms—The arm and hand positioning for this pose can be held in many ways. Once everything else in the pose is in good order, you can begin to address the hands. As long as the student keeps the shoulders relaxed and away from the ears, various options of hand positioning can be explored without detracting from the general benefits of the pose. If a student has enough flexibility to reach the hands to the foot, then the arms can be active or passive. If the student is flexible enough to reach beyond the foot, then the student may apply a grip with one hand holding the other wrist.

MODIFICATIONS

raised bent knee, rounded back and shoulders—Place a pillow or folded blanket and maybe even a block under the student's hips. This helps to open the hips and takes effort off the low back allowing for more relaxation in the posture. It also allows for a straighter upper spine.

tight hips or hamstrings—Provide a strap wrapped around the outstretched foot if the student cannot reach without rounding the spine.

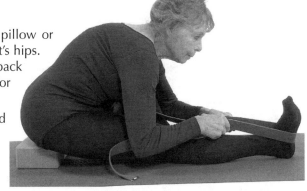

Modification: raised bent knee, rounded back and shoulders; tight hips or hamstrings.

KINEMATICS

This posture uses the concentric contraction of the quadriceps to help release the hamstrings and hip rotators as the torso lengthens over the outstretched leg. As the student continues to reach the torso out over the straight leg, the adductors of the bent leg are stretched. In the torso, the scapulae (shoulder blades) are drawn slightly together and toward the hips by the concentric contraction of the rhomboids and trapezius (muscles between the scapulae), which aid in keeping the torso long throughout the posture.

The torso should be elongated as much as possible, especially during the first phase of this pose. If a student's upper back is rounded, then it is important to help the student lift the ribs and open the chest.

Janu Shirshasana (Left Leg Extended)

Body segment	Kinematics	Muscles active	Muscles released
Foot and toes	Toe extension	Extensor digitorum and hallucis longus, tibialis anterior (C, I)	
Lower leg	Ankle dorsiflexion	Anterior tibialis, extensor digitorum longus (C, I)	Gastrocnemius, soleus
Thigh (R)	Knee flexion	Hamstrings, sartorius (C, I)	Adductors, gracilis
Thigh (L)	Knee extension	Quadriceps (C, I)	Hamstrings, adductors
Hip and pelvis (R)	Hip flexion	Iliopsoas, rectus femoris (C, I)	Adductors
	Initial hip external rotation	Adductors (E, R)	
	Hip abduction and external rotation	Gluteus medius and minimus, deep external rotators*	
Hip and pelvis (L)	Initial hip flexion (forward bend)	Hamstrings (E)	Hamstrings, gluteus maximus, deep external rotators
	Hip flexion over 120 degrees	Iliopsoas, rectus femoris (C, I)	

(continued)

Janu Shirshasana (Left Leg Extended) *continued*

Body segment	Kinematics	Muscles active	Muscles released
Torso	Spinal extension with forward flexion	Erector spinae (C, E, I)	Quadratus lumborum, latissimus dorsi
	Trunk stability	Internal and external obliques, rectus abdominis, transverse abdominis (I)	
Shoulder	Humeral flexion	Anterior deltoids, biceps brachii, coracobrachialis, pectoralis major (C, I)	
	Scapular adduction, stability	Rhomboids major and minor, mid trapezius (C, I)	
	Scapular stability	Serratus anterior (I)	
	Postural support in mid back and downward pull of scapulae	Lower trapezius (C, I)	
	External rotation	Infraspinatus and teres minor with some posterior deltoid (C, I)	
Upper arm	Elbow extension	Triceps brachii (C, I)	Biceps brachii, brachioradialis, brachialis
Lower arm	Forearm supination	Supinator (C, I)	
Hand and fingers	Finger flexion	Flexor digitorum profundus and superficialis, flexor digiti minimi, interossei palmaris (C, I)	
Neck	Neck extension, stability	Splenius capitus and cervicis, suboccipitals, semispinalis, cervical erector spinae, upper trapezius (C, I)	

*Obturator externus and internus, gemellus superior and inferior, quadratus femoris, and piriformis.

C = concentric contraction, E = eccentric contraction, I = isometric contraction, R = relaxed.

Ardha Matsyendrasana

Half Lord of the Fishes

[AR-dhuh muht-see-yen-DRAAH-suh-nuh]

Matsya is fish in Sanskrit, and *endra* is ruler. In one of the legends explaining the origin of the asanas, a fish overheard Shiva (a Hindu god) explaining the secrets of yoga and was fascinated with the knowledge. The fish began to twist its body in order to hear the words more clearly. Shiva noticed the fish and gave it the divine form of Matsyendra, who then spread the knowledge of yoga throughout the land. This twisting asana is the foundation of all the seated twists.

DESCRIPTION

Ardha Matsyendrasana is a seated twist where one leg is straight out in front of the body and the other leg is bent and usually crossed over the straight leg near the opposite hip. The upper torso is rotated in the direction of the bent leg.

BENEFITS

- Increases energy level
- Massages the internal organs
- Aligns the spine
- Builds the trunk muscles
- Opens the shoulders

CAUTIONS

migraines or cold symptoms—Students with severe cold symptoms or migraine headaches should substitute this posture with a gentle, restorative supine twist.

hip replacement—Those with hip replacements should not cross the foot of the bent knee over the straight leg.

pregnancy—Pregnant students should only rotate through the upper spine if they are beyond the first trimester.

VERBAL CUES

- From Dandasana (Staff Pose), inhale and lengthen the spine. Exhale and pull the right knee into the chest. Cross the right foot to the outside of the left leg.
- Press both hips into the ground as you rotate your right shoulder behind you and place the heel of your right hand on the floor against your spine. Point the fingers of your hand away from your body.
- Place your left arm wherever it feels most comfortable yet challenging—wrapped around your right knee or with the back of your elbow to the outside of your right thigh.
- Continue to focus on your breath.

- Inhale and lengthen the spine. As you exhale, turn your head to look over your right shoulder. Rotate your ribcage around as much as you can comfortably so that your right shoulder points as far back from the front of your body as possible.
- To exit this posture, slowly turn your head and chest forward and extend your legs out. Prepare for the next side.

ADJUSTMENTS

legs and hips—Make sure the student's outstretched leg is extended but comfortable and that the hip of the bent knee remains on the floor.

spine—Position yourself behind the student, and gently press against the middle spine with your hands or knee. Cue the student to lift the chest and lengthen the spine.

shoulders—Cue the student to relax the shoulders away from the ears by placing your hand gently on top of the shoulders. Also, remind the student to lengthen the crown of the head upward.

rotation—For students with a limited range in rotation or with shoulder problems, instruct them to keep the elbow of the front hand straight and to place the other hand wherever it is comfortably challenged. Stand or kneel behind the student, and place one hand on the shoulder closest to you and your other hand to the student's ribcage. Gently press the student's ribcage forward as you pull the shoulder around a little farther, creating more spinal rotation. As the student inhales, guide the ribcage forward and up and as the student exhales, lightly pull the shoulder down and back.

hand position—Encourage the student to keep the back arm as straight and as close to the spine as possible. Note that this position is dependent on the length of the student's arm and the width of the shoulders.

finger positioning—Instruct the student to rotate the back arm externally so that the fingers point away from the spine. Standing or kneeling behind the student, place one hand on

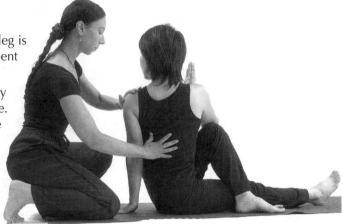

Adjustment: spine; shoulders.

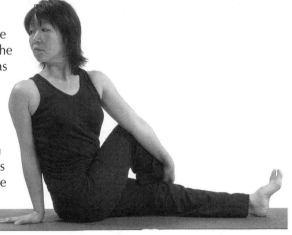

Adjustment: rotation.

the student's extended upper arm and rotate the shoulder externally. At the same time, place your other hand on the student's opposite shoulder to create length through the front of the chest.

MODIFICATIONS

low back weakness, hip or hamstring tightness—Place a folded blanket under the student's hips to help align the pelvis.

hip replacement—The student should not cross the bent knee over the opposite leg but instead keep it aligned with the same-side hip by placing the foot of the bent leg against the inside of the straight leg.

KINEMATICS

Ardha Matsyendrasana focuses on toning the abdominal and spinal muscles as well as creating a gentle stretch in the deep external hip rotators and the shoulders. Because both legs are grounded, this helps to create more length in the torso, as does the grounding of the arm that rotates behind the body. The twist is initiated in the lumbar-spine region and, depending on a person's spinal flexibility, continues up through the spine into the cervical spine (neck). The firmness of the abdominal muscles also helps to keep the torso lifted and stable.

Ardha Matsyendrasana (Rotating to the Right)

Body segment	Kinematics	Muscles active	Muscles released
Foot and toes	Toe extension	Extensor digitorum and hallucis longus (C, I)	
Lower leg	Ankle dorsiflexion	Anterior tibialis extensor digitorum longus (C, I)	Gastrocnemius, soleus
Thigh (R)	Knee flexion	Hamstrings, sartorius (C, I)	
	Thigh adduction	Adductors, gracilis, pectineus (C, I)	
Thigh (L)	Knee extension	Quadriceps (C, I)	
Hip and pelvis (R)	Hip flexion	Iliopsoas (C, I)	Tensor fascia lata, deep external rotators,* gluteus medius
Hip and pelvis (L)	Hip flexion	Iliopsoas, rectus femoris (C, I)	
Torso (R and L)	Trunk stability	Erector spinae, transverse abdominis, rectus abdominis (C, I)	
	Chest and rib elevation	Pectoralis minor (C, I)	
Torso (R)	Rotation to right	Internal obliques, latissimus dorsi (C, I)	Erector spinae (L), external obliques
Torso (L)	Rotation to right	External obliques (C, I)	Quadratus lumborum, serratus anterior, internal oblique
Shoulder (R and L)	External rotation	Posterior deltoid, teres minor, infraspinatus (C, I)	
Shoulder (R)	Humeral hyperextension, stability	Latissimus dorsi, posterior deltoid, teres major (C, I)	Anterior deltoid, pectoralis major
	Scapular adduction	Rhomboids, trapezius (C, I)	
Shoulder (L)	Humeral extension, leverage against right knee	Latissimus dorsi, posterior deltoid, teres major (C, I)	Latissimus dorsi, posterior deltoid, teres major, rhomboids, mid trapezius
Upper arm (R)	Forearm extension	Triceps brachii (C, I)	Biceps brachii, brachialis, brachioradialis
Upper arm (L)	Elbow flexion	Biceps brachii, brachialis, brachioradialis (C, I)	
Lower arm (R)	Elbow extension	Anconeus (C, I)	
	Forearm supination	Supinator (C, I)	
Lower arm (L)	Forearm pronation	Pronator teres and quadratus (C, I)	

(continued)

Ardha Matsyendrasana (Rotating to the Right) *continued*

Body segment	Kinematics	Muscles active	Muscles released
Hand and fingers (R)	Wrist hyper-extension	Extensor carpi radialis longus, brevis, extensor carpi ulnaris (C, I)	Flexor carpi radialis, ulnaris, digitorum superficialis, palmaris longus
Hand and fingers (L)	Wrist extension	Extensor carpi radialis longus and brevis, extensor carpi ulnaris (C, I)	
	Finger extension	Extensor digitorum, indicis, and digiti minimi; lumbricales manus; interossei dorsales (C, I)	
	Finger adduction	Interossei palmaris, adductor pollicis (C, I)	
Neck (R and L)	Neck extension, stability	Cervical erector spinae, splenius capitis and cervicis, semispinalis (C, I)	
Neck (R)	Head rotation to right	Splenius capitus and cervicis, occipitals (C, I)	Sternocleidomastoid
Neck (L)	Head rotation to right	Sternocleidomastoid (C, I)	Upper trapezius, splenius capitus and cervicis, occipitals

*Obturator externus and internus, gemellus superior and inferior, quadratus femoris, and piriformis.

C = concentric contraction, E = eccentric contraction, I = isometric contraction.

Marichyasana A

Marichi's Pose, Variation A

[mar-EE-chee-YAHH-suh-nuh, kuh]

Marichi is the name of a great sage in Hindu mythology and can be translated as "the way of light." The Marichyasana variations are symbolically and energetically powerful poses, as Marichi himself is said to be. This posture and its variations are named for him. This is the first of four poses.

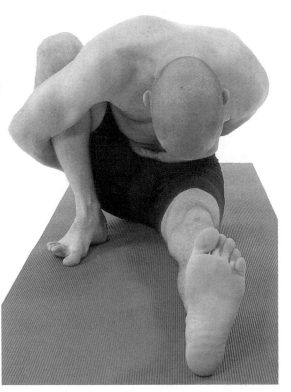

DESCRIPTION

Marichyasana and its variations are extensions of the spinal twist of Matsyendrasana. The main difference between the two postures is that in the Marichyasana variations the arms are bound around the body to create a deeper stretch into the joints. Marichyasana has four commonly practiced variations—A, B, C, and D. In variation A, the bent leg does not cross the opposite leg, and the arms wrap behind the back in a forward bend.

BENEFITS

- Increases energy level
- Massages the internal organs
- Bring the spine into alignment
- Builds strength in the trunk muscles
- Strengthens the hip and shoulder joints
- Increases circulation in the joints

CAUTIONS

pregnancy—After the first trimester, pregnant students should avoid doing this posture because of the compression into the abdomen.

shoulder injuries—Proceed with caution and modifications.

VERBAL CUES

- From Dandasana (Staff Pose), inhale to lengthen the spine. As you exhale, bend the right knee to your chest with your heel as close to your bottom as possible.
- Inhale and bring your extended right arm to the inside of your right knee.
- Exhale and imagine someone pulling your right hand forward so that your right shoulder is reaching beyond your right shin. Rotate your chest slightly to the left. Bend your right elbow and press against the shin as you lift your ribcage away from your hips.
- Rotate your right hand toward the floor then reach your hand around the outside of your right leg toward your spine.
- Bring your left arm behind your back, with the palm facing out and reach toward the right hand. Inhale and lengthen the spine, arching back slightly.
- Exhale and fold forward from the hips, reaching your chest toward your left knee. Relax your spine and neck. Release your muscles with each exhalation.

- Continue to focus on your breath.
- To exit this position, exhale and release the arms slowly. Bring the hands by your hips and inhale as you lift your chest upright. Straighten your right leg and prepare for the left side.

ADJUSTMENTS

extended leg—If the student's extended leg is rotated externally it generally means the student has relaxed the leg. Brush the outside of the foot to cue the student to activate the leg throughout the posture with the toes and knee pointing up.

bent leg—Sometimes a student will need to take the knee wider than hip-width apart to accommodate the ribcage rotation. However, instruct the student to align the knee with the hip to make it easier to wrap the arm around the leg. Gently press against the student's outer thigh to bring the leg into alignment.

shoulders—Kneel behind the student, and place your closest hand to the front of the shoulder the student is rotating toward you and gently guide the shoulder into greater external rotation. At the same time, place your opposite hand on the lower back ribs, near the kidneys, and gently press forward and up. This adjustment creates length as well as rotation in the torso.

hands—If the student's hands are almost touching, tell the person to relax and breathe deeply. Kneel behind the student, and grab each of the student's wrists in your hands. As the student exhales bring the fingertips closer together, if not touching. The student also can bend farther forward to help shorten the space between the thigh and ribcage. Only have the student stay in this position for a few breaths until more strength and flexibility are gained.

MODIFICATIONS

tight hips—If the hip of the bent leg is lifted off the ground, place a rolled-up blanket or towel under the student's opposite hip.

tight shoulders—Have the student hold the ends of a strap between both hands to allow the person to hold the arms in a static position to deepen the stretch.

KINEMATICS

Because of the deep shoulder stretch, students new to the pose may feel like their circulation is being cut off when binding the arms. After practice, the muscles lengthen and the students will have more range within the joint to allow the posture to be comfortable for longer periods of time.

Marichyasana A (Right Knee Bent)

Body segment	Kinematics	Muscles active	Muscles released
Foot and toes (R and L)	Toe extension	Extensor digitorum and hallucis longus (I)	
Lower leg (R)	Ankle dorsiflexion	Anterior tibialis (I)	
Lower leg (L)	Ankle dorsiflexion	Anterior tibialis (C, I)	Gastrocnemius, soleus
Thigh (R)	Knee flexion	Hamstrings (C, I)	
Thigh (L)	Knee extension	Quadriceps (C, I)	
Hip and pelvis	Hip flexion	Iliopsoas, sartorius, left rectus femoris (C, I)	
Torso	Spinal extension and stability	Erector spinae, quadratus lumborum (C, I)	
	Trunk stability	Internal and external obliques, rectus abdominis, transverse abdominis, quadratus lumborum (I)	
	Chest and rib elevation	Pectoralis minor (C, I)	
Shoulder (R and L)	Hyperextension, adduction of humerus	Latissimus dorsi, posterior deltoid (C, I)	Pectoralis major and minor, anterior deltoid
	Scapular adduction	Rhomboids, mid trapezius (C, I)	
Upper arm (R)	Elbow flexion	Biceps brachii, brachialis, brachioradialis (C, I)	
Upper arm (L)	Elbow flexion	Biceps brachii, brachialis, brachioradialis, triceps brachii (C, I)	
Lower arm (R and L)	Forearm pronation	Pronator teres and quadratus (C, I)	
	Wrist extension	Extensor carpi radialis brevis and longus, extensor carpi ulnaris, extensor digitorum (C, I)	
Hand and fingers (R and L)	Finger flexion	Flexor digiti minimi brevis, interossei dorsales manus and palmaris, opponens digiti minimi, flexor pollicis brevis (C, I)	
Neck	Head extension or slight hyperextension, stability	Splenius capitus and cervicis, occipitals, cervical erector spinae, semispinalis, upper trapezius (I)	Sternocleidomastoid

C = concentric contraction, E = eccentric contraction, I = isometric contraction.

Marichyasana B

Marichi's Pose, Variation B

[mar-EE-chee-YAHH-suh-nuh, k-huh]

This asana is the second of the four variations of Marichyasana.

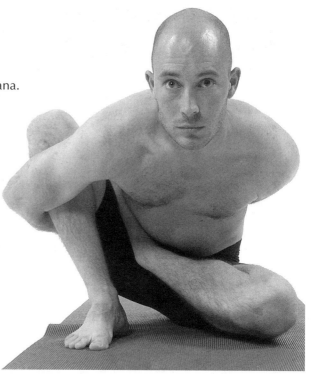

DESCRIPTION

This variation of Marichyasana is similar to variation A, except that where before the leg was extended in front of the body, the knee is now flexed and the ankle is placed in Ardha Padmasana (Half-Lotus).

BENEFITS

- Increases energy level
- Massages the internal organs
- Aligns the spine
- Builds strength in the trunk muscles
- Deeply strengthens the hip and shoulder joints
- Increases circulation in the joints
- Relieves stiffness in the hips, knees, and ankles
- Strengthens the low spine and abdominal muscles

CAUTIONS

knee injuries—Students should be extremely mindful of the knee in Ardha Padmasana whether they have a knee injury or not. If it is difficult to rotate the leg externally because the hips are tight, the knees will take on the strain to compensate.

pregnancy—Due to the compression into the abdomen, women in the second or third trimester of pregnancy should not practice this posture.

shoulder injuries—Those with shoulder injuries should proceed with caution and modifications.

VERBAL CUES

- From Dandasana (Staff Pose), inhale to lengthen the spine. On the next inhalation, bend your left knee and rotate it outward toward the floor. Exhale and bring your left ankle to the crease of your right hip into Ardha Padmasana. Please see modifications for Ardha Padmasana, page 195, for students who cannot accommodate this positioning comfortably.
- With your next exhalation, bend the right knee to the chest.
- Inhale and bring your extended right arm to the inside of your right knee.
- Exhale and imagine someone pulling your right hand forward so that your right shoulder is reaching beyond your right shin. Rotate your chest slightly to the left. Bend your right elbow and press against the shin as you lift your ribcage away from your hips.
- Rotate your right hand toward the floor and then reach your hand around the outside of your right leg toward your spine.
- Bring your left arm behind your back, with the palm facing out, and reach toward the right hand. Inhale and lengthen the spine, arching back slightly.
- Exhale and fold forward from the hips, reaching your chest toward your left knee. Relax your spine and neck with each exhalation.

- Continue to focus on your breath.
- To exit this position, exhale and release the arms slowly. Bring the hands by your hips and inhale as you lift your chest upright. Uncross your left leg and straighten both legs back into Dandasana. Prepare for the opposite side.

ADJUSTMENTS

positioning—Use Ardha Padmasana to help the student into the most appropriate positioning.

feet—The foot in Ardha Padmasana should not be overstretched on the outside of the ankle.

hips—If student's hips are not level, stand or kneel behind the student with your hand touching the hips lightly. Press down gently and pull back on the hip that is not in Ardha Padmasana.

extended leg—If the student's leg is rotated externally, it generally means the student has relaxed the leg. Brush the outside of the foot to cue the student to activate the leg throughout the posture with the toes and knee pointing up.

bent leg—Sometimes a student will need to take the knee wider than hip width to accommodate the ribcage rotation. Encourage the student to align the knee with the hip to make it easier to wrap the arm around the leg. Gently press against the student's outer thigh and bring the leg into alignment.

hands—If the hands are almost touching, remind the student to relax and breathe deeply. The student can bend farther forward to help shorten the space between the thigh and ribcage. Have the student stay in this position for only a few breaths until the student gains more strength and flexibility.

MODIFICATIONS

tight hip on Ardha Padmansana—If the student is unable to sit in Ardha Padmansana, instruct the student to keep the bent leg on the floor. Place a blanket under the bent knee to relax the leg in either position.

tight shoulders—Have the student hold the ends of a strap between both hands to allow the student to hold the arms in a static position to deepen the stretch in the shoulders.

KINEMATICS

Because of the deep shoulder stretch, students new to the pose may feel like their circulation is being cut off when binding the arms. After practice, the muscles lengthen and the students will have more range within the joint to allow the posture to be comfortable for longer periods of time. Since the foot of the leg in Ardha Padmasana is wedged against the opposite thigh and abdomen, it makes it somewhat easier to hold the leg in position for those working on the external rotation in Padmasana (Lotus Pose).

Marichyasana B (Right Knee Bent, Left Leg in Ardha Padmasana)

Body segment	Kinematics	Muscles active	Muscles released
Foot and toes (R and L)	Toe extension	Extensor digitorum and hallucis longus (I)	
Lower leg (R)	Ankle dorsiflexion	Anterior tibialis (I)	
Lower leg (L)	Ankle dorsiflexion	Anterior tibialis (R)	
Thigh (R and L)	Knee flexion	Hamstrings (R)	
Hip and pelvis (R)	Hip flexion	Iliopsoas (C, I)	

(continued)

Marichyasana B (Right Knee Bent, Left Leg in Ardha Padmasana) *continued*

Body segment	Kinematics	Muscles active	Muscles released
Hip and pelvis (L)	Hip flexion	Iliopsoas (C, I)	Adductors
	Hip external rotation	Adductors, sartorius (E, R)	
	External rotation, stability	Gluteus medius and minimus, deep external rotators* (C, I)	
Torso	Spinal extension and stability	Erector spinae, quadratus lumborum (C, I)	
	Trunk stability	Internal and external obliques, rectus abdominis, transverse abdominis, quadratus lumborum, erector spinae (I)	
	Chest and rib elevation	Pectoralis minor (C, I)	
Shoulder (R and L)	Hyperextension, adduction of humerus	Latissimus dorsi, posterior deltoid (C, I)	Pectoralis major and minor, anterior deltoid
	Scapular adduction	Rhomboids, mid trapezius (C, I)	
Upper arm (R)	Elbow flexion	Biceps brachii, brachialis, brachioradialis (C, I)	
Upper arm (L)	Elbow flexion	Triceps brachii (C, I)	
Lower arm (R and L)	Forearm pronation	Pronator teres and quadratus (C, I)	
	Wrist extension	Extensor carpi radialis brevis and longus, extensor carpi ulnaris, extensor digitorum (C, I)	
Hand and fingers (R and L)	Finger flexion	Flexor digiti minimi brevis, interossei dorsales manus and palmaris, opponens digiti minimi, flexor pollicis brevis (C, I)	
Neck	Head extension, stability	Splenius capitus and cervicis, occipitals, cervical erector spinae, semispinalis, upper trapezius (I)	Sternocleidomastoid

*Obturator externus and internus, gemellus superior and inferior, quadratus femoris, and piriformis.

C = concentric contraction, E = eccentric contraction, I = isometric contraction, R = relaxed.

Marichyasana C

Marichi's Pose, Variation C

[mar-EE-chee-YAHH-suh-nuh, guh]

This is the third of the four variations of Marichyasana.

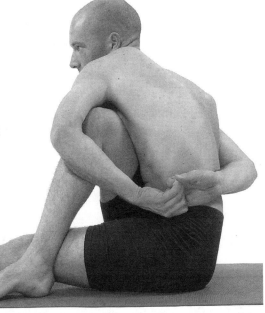

DESCRIPTION

This variation of Marichyasana is similar to variation A, except that the foot of the bent leg is crossed over the opposite thigh. The arms are bound behind the back, but the torso twists in the direction of the bent leg.

BENEFITS

- Increases energy level
- Massages the internal organs
- Aligns the spine
- Builds strength in the trunk muscles
- Deeply strengthens the hip and shoulder joints
- Increases circulation in the joints
- Increases focus

CAUTIONS

pregnancy—Due to the compression into the abdomen, women in the second or third trimester of pregnancy should not practice this posture.

shoulder injuries—Those with shoulder injuries should proceed with caution and modifications.

VERBAL CUES

- From Dandasana (Staff Pose), inhale to lengthen the spine. Exhale and bend the right knee to the chest.
- Inhale and roll your right shoulder back and turn to look over the shoulder.
- On your next breath, bring your left arm across your body to the outside of the right leg, and reach your left shoulder blade toward the outside of your right knee as you turn your torso to the right.
- Bend your left elbow and press the arm against the outside of the right knee as you lift your ribcage away from your hips.
- Reach your right arm behind your back toward your left hip. Rotate your left hand toward the floor, and then reach your hand around your right leg toward your spine.
- Inhale, lengthening the spine, and create as much space between the lower ribs and pelvis as possible.
- As you exhale, rotate your right shoulder and ribcage back as you press your left ribcage forward. Press the back of your left upper arm against the right thigh for leverage.
- Continue to focus on your breath.
- To exit this position, exhale and release the arms slowly. Rotate your chest forward and bring the hands by your hips. Uncross your left leg and straighten both legs back into Dandasana. Prepare for the opposite side.

ADJUSTMENTS

extended leg—If the student's leg is rotated externally it generally means the student has relaxed the leg. Brush the outside of the foot to cue the student to activate the leg throughout the posture with the toes and knee pointing up.

hips—If the student's hips are not level and touching the floor, stand or kneel behind the student with your hand lightly touching the student's hips. Press down gently and pull back on the hip that is not in Half-Lotus.

torso—Kneel behind the student, and place your same-side hand to the student's shoulder. Pull back gently as you use your other hand to press forward and up on the student's ribcage, creating more spinal rotation.

hands—If the student's hands are almost touching, encourage the student to relax and breathe deeply. The student can bend farther forward to help shorten the space between the thigh and the ribcage. Only have the student stay in this position for a few breaths until the student gains more strength and flexibility.

MODIFICATIONS

tight hips—If the hip of the bent leg is lifted off the ground, place a rolled-up blanket or towel under the opposite hip, or both hips, if necessary.

tight shoulders—Have the student hold the ends of a strap between both hands. This allows the student to hold the arms in a static position to deepen the stretch.

shoulder injury or extremely tight chest—Instead of asking the student to bind the arms behind the back, have the student place the back arm against the spine and wrap the opposite arm around the bent knee. You can also have student practice Matsyendrasana instead.

KINEMATICS

The pressure of the bent arm against the opposite thigh aids in giving leverage to rotate the torso more fully.

Modification: shoulder injury or extremely tight chest.

Marichyasana C (Right Knee Bent, Rotation to Right)

Body segment	Kinematics	Muscles active	Muscles released
Foot and toes (R and L)	Toe extension	Extensor digitorum and hallucis longus (I)	
Lower leg (R)	Ankle dorsiflexion	Anterior tibialis (I)	
Lower leg (L)	Ankle dorsiflexion	Anterior tibialis (C, I)	
Thigh (R)	Knee flexion	Hamstrings (C, I)	
Thigh (L)	Knee extension	Quadriceps (C, I)	
Hip and pelvis (R)	Hip flexion	Iliopsoas, sartorius (C, I)	Gluteus maximus
Hip and pelvis (L)	Hip flexion	Iliopsoas, rectus femoris, sartorius (C, I)	Hamstrings
Torso (R and L)	Spinal extension and stability	Erector spinae (C, I)	
	Trunk stability	Rectus abdominis, transverse abdominis, quadratus lumborum, erector spinae (I)	
Torso (R)	Rotation to right	Internal obliques, erector spinae, latissimus dorsi (C, I)	External oblique
Torso (L)	Rotation to right	External oblique (C, I)	Internal oblique, quadratus lumborum
Shoulder (R)	Humerus hyperextension and adduction	Latissimus dorsi, posterior deltoid (C, I)	Pectoralis major and minor, anterior deltoid
	External rotation	Posterior deltoid, infraspinatus, teres minor (C, I)	
	Scapular adduction	Rhomboids, mid trapezius (C, I)	
Shoulder (L)	Internal rotation	Pectoralis major, anterior deltoid (C, I)	
	Humerus hyperextension	Latissimus dorsi, teres major (C, I)	
	Scapular adduction	Rhomboids, mid trapezius (C, I)	
Upper arm (R and L)	Elbow flexion	Biceps brachii, brachialis, brachioradialis (C, I)	
Lower arm (R and L)	Forearm pronation	Pronator teres and quadratus (C, I)	
	Wrist extension	Extensor carpi radialis brevis and longus, extensor carpi ulnaris, extensor digitorum (C, I)	
Hand and fingers (R and L)	Finger flexion	Flexor digiti minimi brevis, interossei dorsales manus and palmaris, opponens digiti minimi, flexor pollicis brevis (C, I)	
Neck (R)	Head rotation to right, stability	Splenius capitus and cervicis, occipitals, cervical erector spinae (C, I)	Sternocleidomastoid
Neck (L)	Head rotation	Sternocleidomastoid (C, I)	

C = concentric contraction, E = eccentric contraction, I = isometric contraction.

Marichyasana D

Marichi's Pose, Variation D

[mar-EE-chee-YAHH-suh-nuh, g-huh]

This is the fourth of four variations of Marichyasana.

DESCRIPTION

This variation of Marichyasana is a combination of the Ardha Padmasana (Half-Lotus) element of variation B and the twisting direction of variation C. This is by far the most challenging variation of Marichyasana because it combines Ardha Padmasana, a spinal twist, and binding of the arms in one posture.

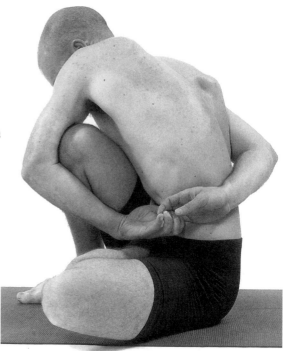

BENEFITS

- Increases energy level
- Massages the internal organs
- Bring the spine into alignment
- Builds strength in the trunk muscles
- Opens the shoulder joints
- Deeply strengthens the hip and shoulder joints
- Increases circulation in the joints
- Increases focus

CAUTIONS

knee injuries— Students should be extremely mindful of the knee in Ardha Padmasana whether they have a knee injury or not. If it is difficult to rotate the leg externally because the hips are tight, the knees will take on the strain to compensate.

pregnancy—Due to the compression into the abdomen, women in the second or third trimester of pregnancy should not practice this posture.

VERBAL CUES

- From Dandasana (Staff Pose), inhale to lengthen the spine, creating as much space between the ribs and hips as possible. Keep the hips level and on the ground.
- Inhale and bend your left knee and rotate it outward toward the floor. Exhale and bring your left ankle to the crease of your right hip into Ardha Padmasana. Please see modifications for Ardha Padmasana, page 195, for students who cannot accommodate this positioning comfortably.
- With your next exhalation bend the right knee to the chest with your heel as close to the right hip as comfortable.
- Breathing in, bring your right arm behind your spine for leverage. Then bring the back of your left arm across to the outside of your right knee. Reach as far as you can, using the energy of your right arm to lift the spine.
- Bend your left elbow and press the arm against the outside of the right knee as you lift your ribcage away from your hips.
- Reach your right arm behind your back toward your left hip. Rotate your left hand toward the floor, and then reach your hand around your right leg toward your spine.
- Bind your hands as best you can.
- Continue to focus on your breath.

- To exit this position, exhale and release the arms slowly. Bring your hands beside your hips and inhale as you lift your chest upright. Uncross your left leg and straighten both legs back into Dandasana. Prepare for the opposite side.

ADJUSTMENTS

Ardha Padmasana positioning—Please refer to page 195 to help the student into the most appropriate positioning. The foot in Ardha Padmasana should not be overstretched on the outside of the ankle.

hips—If the hips are not level, stand or kneel behind the student with your hand touching the student's hips lightly. Press down gently and pull back on the hip that is not in Ardha Padmasana.

extended leg—If the student's leg is rotated externally it generally means the student has relaxed the leg. Brush the outside of the foot to cue the student to activate the leg throughout the posture with the toes and knee pointing up.

bent leg—Sometimes a student will need to take the knee wider than hip-width apart to accommodate the ribcage rotation. However, instruct the student to align the knee with the hip to make it easier to wrap the arm around the leg. Gently press against the student's outer thigh and bring the leg into alignment.

hands—If the student's hands are almost touching, encourage the student to relax and breathe deeply. The student can bend farther forward to help shorten the space between the thigh and ribcage. Only have the student stay in this position for a few breaths until the student gains more strength and flexibility.

MODIFICATIONS

tight hip on Ardha Padmasana—If the student is unable to sit in Ardha Padmasana, suggest that the student keep the bent leg on the floor. Place a blanket under the bent knee to relax the leg in either position.

tight shoulders—Have the student hold the ends of a strap between both. This allows the person to hold the arms in a static position to deepen the stretch.

inability to bind arms—Suggest to the student that instead of binding with the initial balancing arm, the student can keep the hand on the floor behind the spine and place the outside of the opposite arm against the outside of the bent knee. You can also instruct the student to bind in the opposite direction.

balance issues—If the student has extreme difficulty attaining this posture without strain, or cannot maintain positioning and stay balanced, it is best to substitute another posture.

KINEMATICS

The Ardha Padmasana positioning of the leg in this posture will most likely require modification for a large number of students. As always, it is important that students refrain from forcing the legs into this position if they experience any discomfort.

Marichyasana D (Right Knee Flexed, Left Leg in Ardha Padmasana, Torso Rotated to Right)

Body segment	Kinematics	Muscles active	Muscles released
Foot and toes (R and L)	Toe extension	Extensor digitorum and hallucis longus (I)	
Lower leg (R)	Ankle dorsiflexion	Anterior tibialis (C)	
Lower leg (L)	Ankle dorsiflexion	Anterior tibialis (C, I)	
Thigh (R)	Knee flexion	Hamstrings (C, I)	
Thigh (L)	Knee flexion	Hamstrings (C, I)	

(continued)

Marichyasana D (Right Knee Flexed, Left Leg in Ardha Padmasana, Torso Rotated to Right) *continued*

Body segment	Kinematics	Muscles active	Muscles released
Hip and pelvis (R and L)	Pelvic stability	Rectus abdominis, quadratus lumborum, hamstrings (I)	
Hip and pelvis (R)	Hip flexion	Iliopsoas, sartorius (C, I)	
Hip and pelvis (L)	Hip flexion	Iliopsoas (C, I)	Adductors
	Hip external rotation	Adductors, sartorius (E)	
	External rotation, stability	Gluteus medius, deep external rotators (C, I)*	
Torso (R and L)	Spinal extension and stability	Erector spinae (C, I)	
	Trunk stability	Rectus abdominis, transverse abdominis, quadratus lumborum, erector spinae (I)	
Torso (R)	Rotation to right	Internal obliques, erector spinae, latissimus dorsi (C, I)	External obliques
Torso (L)	Rotation to right	External obliques, internal oblique, quadratus lumborum, erector spinae (C, I)	
Shoulder (R)	Humerus hyperextension and adduction	Latissimus dorsi, posterior deltoid (C, I)	Pectoralis major, anterior deltoid
	External rotation	Posterior deltoid, infraspinatus, teres minor (C, I)	
	Scapular adduction	Rhomboids, mid trapezius (C, I)	
Shoulder (L)	Internal rotation	Pectoralis major, anterior deltoid (C, I)	
	Humerus hyperextension	Latissimus dorsi (C, I)	
	Scapular adduction	Rhomboids, mid trapezius (C, I)	
Upper arm (R and L)	Elbow flexion	Biceps brachii, brachialis, brachioradialis (C, I)	
	Forearm pronation	Pronator teres and quadratus (C, I)	
Lower arm (R and L)	Wrist extension	Extensor carpi radialis brevis and longus, extensor carpi ulnaris, extensor digitorum (C, I)	
Hand and fingers (R and L)	Finger flexion	Flexor digiti minimi brevis, interossei dorsales manus and palmaris, opponens digiti minimi, flexor pollicis brevis (C, I)	
Neck (R)	Head rotation to right, stability	Splenius capitus and cervicis, occipitals, cervical erector spinae (C, I)	Sternocleidomastoid
Neck (L)	Head rotation	Sternocleidomastoid (C, I)	

*Obturator externus and internus, gemellus superior and inferior, quadratus femoris, and piriformis.

C = concentric contraction, E = eccentric contraction, I = isometric contraction.

Paschimottanasana

Seated Forward Bend

[puhsh-chee-moht-tuhn-AHH-suh-nuh]

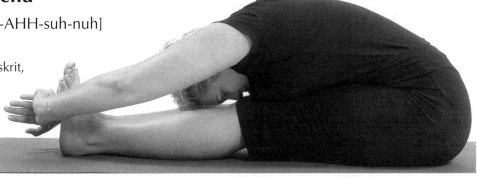

Paschima means west in Sanskrit, and *uttana* means intense stretch. Traditionally, it is ideal to face the east to meditate; therefore, the east direction is considered the front of the body and the west direction is the back of the body. *Paschimottanasana* is literally translated as "intense stretch of the west."

DESCRIPTION

This is a seated, full forward bend. The legs are outstretched in front of the body, and the torso is folded forward at the hips and laid on the front of the legs to the best of the student's ability.

BENEFITS

- Calms and soothes the nervous system
- Stretches the hamstrings as well as the entire back, both in the passive and the active practice variations
- Stimulates circulation to the liver, kidneys, ovaries, and uterus
- Improves digestion
- Can relieve some symptoms of menstrual discomfort and menopause
- May alleviate headaches, anxiety, and fatigue
- Can be therapeutic for high blood pressure, infertility, insomnia, and sinusitis

lungs-asthma

CAUTION

back injury—Perform this pose with the back straight and little or no forward bend. Until the student is strong enough to release the spine while sitting, the pose should be practiced with a modification or substitute a different pose.

VERBAL CUES

Active

- From Dandasana (Staff Pose), inhale and sit tall. Roll the upper legs toward each other slightly and reach your sits bones back.
- Expand the space between your hip bones and naval, and begin to bend at your hips, like a hinge, folding forward only as much as you can without rounding your back.
- Place your hands on the floor and use your arms to assist lengthening your spine.
- Gently reach your hands toward your feet and hold wherever you can while maintaining a straight back and relaxed legs.
- Inhale, lift, and open the chest. Roll your upper arms out, collarbones apart, and reexpand the length in the front of your torso. Lift your ribs forward and up, and press your shoulders down and back.
- Inhale and arch back slightly. Lift your chin, chest, and abdomen as high as you can.

Resting

- Exhale and roll down the spine from the bottom to the top, relaxing your torso over your legs.
- Soften the abdomen and find your breath moving in your back. Relax the shoulders far down from your ears. Feel your body sink into the earth.
- Imagine your breath moving into any place that is resistant or holding tension to release that area completely. Relax your neck.
- To exit this position, place your hands on the floor beside your hips. Inhale and press down through your hands as you slowly lift your torso and head up.

ADJUSTMENTS

feet—The student's feet are not of much concern in this pose; however, if the student can reach the hands beyond the feet, then you can help the person deepen the posture. Instruct the student to bring the feet together and pull the toes toward the head. You can assist by gently pushing up against the bottom of the toes.

legs—If the student's knees are bent, check for proper back alignment and support. It is better to have the student back off, focus on the legs, and sit more upright than to let the student struggle with tight hamstrings. Note: If the student has finished with the active phase of the posture and is resting, the student may bend the knees slightly as a modification as long as the body remains relaxed. Instruct the student to bring the legs as close together as possible.

hips—If the forward bend does not start in the hips because of tight hamstrings, modify with a strap (see modifications).

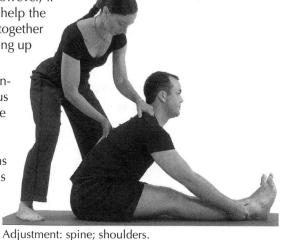

Adjustment: spine; shoulders.

spine—It is extremely common for students to have trouble getting and keeping the back straight. To help the student lengthen the spine, squat or kneel behind the student and place your hands at the bottom edge of the person's ribcage and gently press the lower ribcage up and slightly forward. Press, ever so lightly, as the student exhales. Another adjustment is to stand behind the student and instruct the student to reach the hands overhead and interlace the fingers. As you squat down, bending from your hips and knees, have the student reach back and hold the base of your neck. Place your arms on the student's upper arms and lift the student up. Step your feet to straddle the student's hips. Slowly walk yourself forward and take the student's hands from around your neck as you help the student lower, with length in the spine, to the ground.

IMPROPER

Improper Paschimottanasana form: spine and shoulders rounded.

shoulders—Usually, if the back is rounded the shoulders will be also. You can use your hands to roll the student's shoulders open. Kneel behind the student and place your hands on each of their shoulders with your fingers draped just in front of the junction of the arm, shoulder, and chest. Use your hands to gently pull the collarbones apart and the shoulders down. You can also simultaneously press your knee into the student's mid back, thus lifting the chest and opening the shoulders.

neck—The student's neck can be actively aligned with the spine in the active variation or it can be relaxed in the resting phase. The key is to keep space in the neck between the head and shoulders regardless of the phase.

MODIFICATIONS

spinal weakness—Props such as straps, pillows, or folded blankets are commonly needed in this pose. A blanket or pillow propped under the hips will take some of the pressure and work out of a weak or rounded back.

tight hamstrings or hips—When the student cannot reach the hands to the feet, the person can wrap a strap around the feet. The strap allows the student to get an extra stretch in the shoulders and lateral torso.

KINEMATICS

If a student is very close to bringing the chest down to the legs, you can assist in deepening the flexion. However, be sure that you move slowly and in a way that is mechanically appropriate. To begin, kneel behind the student and lightly place your palms flat against the student's pelvis with your fingers pointing toward the floor. Gently move your hands in a lifting and lengthening

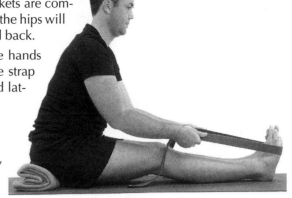

Modification: tight hamstrings or hips.

motion in the direction of the head. This movement actually helps the student flex at the hip joint, rather than allowing the low spine to round. When applying adjustments in this posture, be certain that your hand placement and the movement of the adjustment is mechanically sound. *Never* press down on the student's spine to deepen the forward bend! Doing so would put excessive strain on the spine. Also, make certain that you move according to the student's breath pattern; as the student exhales, begin to press your hands gently on the spine in an upward motion.

Paschimottanasana

Body segment	Kinematics	Muscles active	Muscles released
Foot and toes	Toe extension	Extensor digitorum and hallucis longus (C, I)	
Lower leg	Ankle dorsiflexion	Anterior tibialis, extensor digitorum longus (C, I)	Gastrocnemius, soleus
Thigh	Knee extension	Quadriceps (C, I)	Hamstrings
Hip and pelvis	Hip flexion	Iliopsoas, sartorius, rectus femoris (C, I)	Deep external rotators, hamstrings, gluteus maximus
	Hip flexion more than 120 degrees	Rectus abdominis (C, I)	
Torso	Spinal extension, stability	Erector spinae (E, I)	Quadratus lumborum, erector spinae
	Trunk stability	Internal and external obliques, rectus abdominis, transverse abdominis, quadratus lumborum, erector spinae (I)	
Shoulder	Scapular adduction	Rhomboids and mid trapezius (C, I)	Latissimus dorsi
	Scapular stability	Serratus anterior	
	Humeral flexion	Deltoids, pectoralis major, biceps brachii coracobrachialis, supraspinatus (C, I)	
	Postural support in mid back and downward pull of scapulae	Lower trapezius (C, I)	
	External rotation of humerus	Infraspinatus and teres minor with some posterior deltoid (C, I)	

(continued)

Paschimottanasana *continued*

Body segment	Kinematics	Muscles active	Muscles released
Upper arm	Elbow extension	Triceps brachii (C, I)	Biceps brachii, brachioradialis, brachialis
Lower arm	Elbow extension	Anconeus (C, I)	
	Forearm supination	Supinator (C, I)	
Hand and fingers	Finger flexion	Flexor digitorum profundus and superficialis, flexor digiti minimi interossei palmaris (C, I)	
Neck	Head extension, stability	Splenius capitus and cervicis, suboccipitals, semispinalis, upper trapezius (C, I)	

C = concentric contraction, E = eccentric contraction, I = isometric contraction.

Gomukhasana

Cow's Face Pose

[go-mook-AHH-suh-nuh]

Go in Sanskrit means cow. *Mukha* is the word for face. This pose is referred to as "Cow's Face." At first glance, this pose might not seem to resemble the face of the gentle and symbolically nurturing creature it is named after. You might see the pattern, however, if you look at your image in the mirror while practicing this pose. The arms are like a cow's ears, and the legs form the shape of a cow's mouth.

DESCRIPTION

In this seated posture, the legs are on the ground, stacked in front of the hips with the knees bent. One knee is folded on top of the other, aligned with the middle of the body. The spine is upright and the arms are bent with one elbow pointed up and the other pointed down and reaching behind the back. Note: Sometimes the upper-body portion of the pose is done on its own.

BENEFITS

- Opens the chest and shoulders
- Renews circulation of and stretches the arms and wrists
- Relieves discomfort for headache sufferers and postnatal women
- Relieves sciatica

CAUTIONS

hip replacements—Students with a hip replacement are advised not to cross the legs over. They may practice the arm portion of the posture and sit in any other comfortable cross-legged position.

shoulder injury—Have students with any shoulder injuries use caution. For students with rotator-cuff tears, the anterior shoulder of the bottom arm is usually sensitive and tight in this pose, making it hard to rotate the arm externally. Students with a history of shoulder dislocation might need to use a strap and not reach as far.

VERBAL CUES

- From Dandasana (Staff Pose), exhale and bend your right knee toward your chest. Cross your right leg over your left leg and place your right foot on the ground outside your left thigh.
- Rotate your left leg out and then bend your left knee. Place your left foot beside your right hip. Relax your right knee down on top of your left knee and place your right foot by your left hip.
- Feel your right hip sinking downward. With each exhalation relax your legs more.
- Inhale and reach your right arm up in the air alongside your ear. Press your thumb back as you look over your right shoulder.

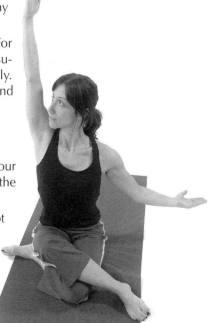

Extend your left arm out to the side with your palm facing up.

- Turn to look forward and bend your right elbow. Reach the palm of your right hand down your back to the lowest vertebra you can.
- Extend your left arm out to the side with your palm facing up (see photo). Keep your shoulder rolled open and place your left hand to the floor behind you. Bend your left elbow and reach the back of your left hand up toward your right hand.
- Inhale and lift your chest. Exhale and let your shoulders drop. Your right elbow points directly up and your left elbow directly down. Feel the space opening between your ears and shoulders, keeping your neck long.
- To exit this posture, inhale and release your fingers. Slowly bring both hands down to your sides. Exhale and straighten your legs and prepare for the next side.

ADJUSTMENTS

back—If the student's upper back is rounded, kneel behind the student and press the ribcage forward and up by placing the palms of your hands just below the scapulae.

arms—If the student's elbows are wider than shoulder-width apart, place your hand against the outside of the elbows and gently press the arms closer toward the student's head.

hands—If the student's hands do not touch, but they seem very close, you might be able to move the student's hands the extra little bit to enable the hands to meet. Carefully and slowly hold each wrist and draw the hands closer together.

MODIFICATIONS

hips—If the hips are not level on the ground, place a blanket under the lower hip. As an option, the student can sit on the foot of the bottom leg to raise the hips level.

hip replacement—Instruct the student to sit in any comfortable position where the thighs do not cross over each other.

tight shoulders—Have the student hold the ends of a strap between the hands if the student cannot reach the hands together without assistance.

KINEMATICS

Gomukhasana is an excellent stretch for the triceps. If a student is unable to touch the hands together, it is beneficial for the student to use a strap of some type between the hands. The resistance allows the student to hold the arm positioning much more easily.

Modification: tight shoulders.

Gomukhasana (Right Elbow Up, Left Elbow Down)

Body segment	Kinematics	Muscles active	Muscles released
Foot and toes	Toe extension	Extensor digitorum and hallucis longus (I)	
Lower leg	Ankle dorsiflexion	Anterior tibialis, extensor digitorum longus (C, I)	
Thigh	Knee flexion	Hamstrings (C, I)	
Hip and pelvis	Hip flexion	Iliopsoas (C, I)	Adductors, tensor fascia lata, gluteus medius and minimus
	Initial external rotation, adduction	Adductors, sartorius (E)	
	Initial external rotation	Gluteus medius, deep external rotators* (C, I, R)	
	Pelvic stability	Rectus abdominis, quadratus lumborum, hamstrings (I)	
Torso	Torso stability	Rectus abdominis, internal and external obliques, transverse abdominis (C, I)	
	Spinal extension and stability	Erector spinae, quadratus lumborum (C, I)	
	Sternoclavicular stability	Subclavius (I)	
Shoulder (R)	Horizontal flexion of humerus	Pectoralis major, coracobrachialis, anterior and middle deltoid (C, I)	Latissimus dorsi, trapezius, pectoralis major and minor
	Stability and external rotation of humerus	Infraspinatus, teres minor (C, I)	
	Supporting posture in mid back and downward pull of scapulae	Lower trapezius (C, I)	
	Scapular stability, lateral rotation	Serratus anterior (I)	
Shoulder (L)	Hyperextension and adduction of humerus	Latissimus dorsi, teres major (C, I)	Anterior deltoid, upper trapezius, levator scapulae, subscapularis
	Stability and external rotation of humerus	Infraspinatus, teres minor, posterior deltoid (C, I)	
Upper arm (R and L)	Elbow flexion	Biceps brachii (C, I)	Triceps brachii
Lower arm (R)	Forearm supination	Supinator (C, I)	
Lower arm (L)	Forearm pronation	Pronator teres and quadratus (C, I)	
Hand and fingers	Wrist extension	Extensor carpi radialis brevis and longus, extensor carpi ulnaris (C, I)	
	Finger extension	Extensor digitorum, extensor digiti minimi brevis, dorsal interossei (C, I)	
	Finger adduction	Interossei palmaris, adductor pollicis (C, I)	
Neck	Neck extension	Splenius capitus and cervicis, suboccipitals, semispinalis (I)	

*Obturator externus and internus, gemellus superior and inferior, quadratus femoris, and piriformis.

C = concentric contraction, E = eccentric contraction, I = isometric contraction, R = relaxed.

Boat Pose

[naah-VAAH-suh-nuh]

Nava is Sanskrit for ship or boat. The shape of the body in Navasana resembles a boat balanced in the water.

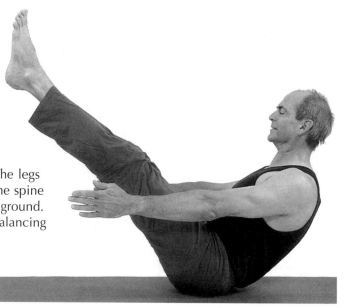

DESCRIPTION

Navasana is a seated jack-knife balancing position. The legs are together and straight with the toes at eye level. The spine is straight while the arms are extended parallel to the ground. When a student is strong in this pose, the student is balancing on the sits bones.

BENEFITS

- Strengthens the thighs, hips, abdominal muscles, and back; targets the core musculature
- Massages the internal organs
- Builds balance and concentration

CAUTION

pregnancy or injuries—Pregnant or injured students are advised to avoid this posture.

VERBAL CUES

- From Dandasana (Staff Pose), exhale and bend your knees to your chest. Bring your hands as close to your hips as possible, hugging your arms to your sides. Bend your elbows and begin to recline the torso back with the spine straight. Feel the balance starting in the hip joint. Keep your spine long and lifted.
- Engage your abdominal and thigh muscles and lift your feet off the floor. Balance here between your sits bones and your tailbone, making sure not to roll back on your pelvis.
- If this position feels challenging, stay here and focus on your breath.
- If you feel strong and comfortable, especially in the low back, then lift your hands off the floor and reach your arms out from your chest. Turn your palms so they are facing each other.
- Be sure to keep your chest lifted and your back lengthened.
- Continue to focus on your breath.
- To go further into the full Navasana, place your hands behind and underneath your knees. Use your arms to hold on to the legs to assist or relieve your low back and legs as you gradually straighten your legs bringing your toes to eye level.
- If and when you feel ready, release your hands so your arms are parallel to the ground. You are in full Navasana *if* you are breathing!
- To exit the position, exhale and slowly lower your feet back to the floor. To rest your thighs and abdominal muscles, lower your legs into Baddha Konasana (Bound Angle) and rest before the next posture.

ADJUSTMENTS

spine—Often it takes a little practice before a student has enough strength to keep the spine from rounding. If the torso is collapsing inward, you can modify the pose to take the load off the student's back and other muscles. Another option is to stand behind the student and lightly nudge the spine with your knee to create more length.

legs—If the student's legs are shaking, and the student has difficulty keeping the legs extended, kneel beside the student to support the legs briefly. Supporting the legs will enable the student to straighten the legs fully.

MODIFICATIONS

weakness or fatigue—Bending the knees will reduce the work for weak or tired students.

building strength—The student can use the arms for support by placing the hands on the floor behind the hips, elbows bent. The wall or an exercise ball are great props. Place the student facing the wall or ball with the legs extended. The student can then rest the feet on the wall or on top of the ball at eye level.

KINEMATICS

It is important that the balance point of the body fall between the ischial tuberosities (sits bones) and the tailbone. If the body is balanced above the tailbone, higher onto the pelvis, the likelihood of flexion in the lumbar spine increases, as does the possibility of injury.

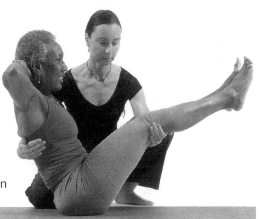

Adjustment: spine.

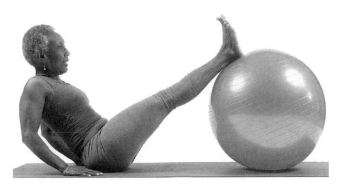

Adjustment: legs; spine.

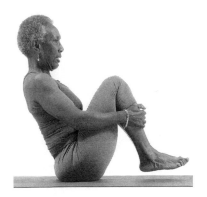

Modification: weakness or fatigue.

Modification: building strength.

Navasana

Body segment	Kinematics	Muscles active	Muscles released
Foot and toes	Toe extension	Extensor digitorum and hallucis longus (I)	
Lower leg	Plantar flexion	Gastrocnemius, soleus (C, I)	Anterior tibialis, extensor digitorum longus
Thigh	Knee extension	Quadriceps (C, I)	Hamstrings
	Thigh adduction	Adductors, gracilis (C, I)	
Hip and pelvis	Hip flexion	Iliopsoas, rectus femoris (C, I)	
Torso	Spinal extension, stability	Erector spinae, quadratus lumborum (C, I)	
	Trunk stability	Internal and external obliques, rectus abdominis, transverse abdominis, latissimus dorsi (C, I)	
Shoulder	Humerus flexion	Pectoralis major, anterior deltoid, coracobrachialis (C, I)	
	Joint stability	Trapezius, rhomboids, teres minor (I)	
Upper arm	Elbow extension, stability	Biceps brachii, brachialis, brachioradialis, triceps brachii (E, I)	
Lower arm	Forearm supination	Supinator (C, I)	
Hand and fingers	Wrist extension	Extensor carpi radialis brevis and longus, extensor carpi ulnaris, extensor digitorum (C, I)	
	Finger extension	Extensor digitorum, indicis, and digiti minimi; lumbricales manus; interossei dorsales (C, I)	
Neck	Neck extension against gravity	Sternocleidomastoid, scalenes (C, I)	

C = concentric contraction, E = eccentric contraction, I = isometric contraction.

Baddha Konasana

Bound Angle

[BUD-dhuh kohn-AAH-suh-nuh]

Baddha is Sanskrit for bound, and *kona* is angle. This posture is often called "Cobbler's Pose" because it is the traditional seated position for East Indian shoemakers. While working, the shoemakers use their feet to hold a shoe so that both of their hands are free.

DESCRIPTION

In this seated asana, the knees are bent and rotated out to the sides with the soles of the feet pressed together or held together with the hands to make a seal or lock. Variations to this posture involve making the space between the ankles and the groin more or less open.

BENEFITS

- Promotes healthy urinary and reproductive organs
- Increases general circulation by stretching the major arteries and lymph glands in the groin, legs, and thighs
- Stretches the adductor muscles of the thighs
- Can help alleviate pain from sciatica
- Relives discomfort for pregnant and menstruating women

CAUTION

knee, hip, or groin injuries—Students with these injuries should use modifications and props.

VERBAL CUES

- From Dandasana (Staff Pose), exhale and bring the knees into the chest. Inhale and let the knees slowly drop to the sides toward the floor.
- The hips should remain on the floor with the body weight even between both sides. Keep the spine lifted and strong, and reach your tailbone and sits bones toward the back of your mat.
- Bring your hands to the floor behind you and press the soles of your feet together. Feel your knees move closer to the floor. Use your arms to create more length through the spine without lifting the hips off the floor.
- Maintain the lift in the spine and place your hands on your ankles or clasp your fingers around your ankles.
- Continue to focus on your breath.
- Inhale deeply and as you exhale fold forward from your hips as you lower your chest toward the floor beyond your feet. Keep your hands around your ankles or around your shins for leverage. You can also place the hands on the floor wherever you are most comfortable.
- Try using your hands to roll the outer legs closer to the floor to open the groin more deeply. As always, when you inhale, lengthen your spine and extend the crown of your head beyond your feet.
- To exit this posture, bring your hands to the floor beside your hips. Press firmly through your arms and inhale as you lift slowly through the chest and the crown of the head. Exhale and stretch your legs out in front of you as you move back into Dandasana.

ADJUSTMENTS

feet—Instruct the student to press the inner edges of the soles together. Gently brush the feet with your hands as a reminder.

knees—If the student has difficulty pressing the knees to the floor, help the student roll the soles of the feet up by pressing the tops of the feet toward the floor. Instruct the student to open the soles of the feet like opening a book. This action rotates both legs externally.

spine—To help support the student's back, sit or kneel behind the student and place your hands to the mid thigh and gently rotate the legs externally. Press your shoulder against the student's spine and lift. This action encourages the length in the back.

MODIFICATIONS

groin or knee injuries—Place blankets under the student's knees and hips for support.

tight hips—Instruct the student to make the knee angle larger by moving the feet farther away from the body. The student may also keep the feet slightly apart for comfort.

weak spine or injury—Place the student on the back for spinal support, but open the angle between the legs to stretch the groin for the Supta Baddha Konasana (Reclining Bound Angle) version. If this positioning still creates a strain on the spine, instruct the student to lie on the floor with the legs against a wall and place the soles of the feet together as the student presses the knees toward the wall.

pregnancy—Place stacked bolsters, blankets, or a chair in front of the student and have the student rest the arms and forehead on the prop for support. This modification is also works well for all seated forward bends.

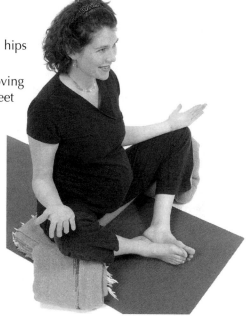

Modification: groin or knee injuries.

KINEMATICS

In this posture it is sometimes difficult for students to establish why their knees do not drop down to the floor. Common sense states that tight adductors are the culprits, and this is true in many cases. However, tight hip rotators are often involved as well.

For students with tight hips, the forward-bend portion of the posture is made possible by a coordinated effort between the hip flexors (iliopsoas), the spinal extensors (erector spinae), and sometimes the arms. The forward bend is initiated by an eccentric contraction of the spinal muscles. Then, to aid in the flexion, the hip flexors contract concentrically to help draw the torso down farther. Because of the external rotation of the femurs, the angle of contraction in the flexors may not allow a person to lower any farther without the arms pulling the torso down as well.

If the head touches the floor in the forward bend, the posterior neck muscles are relaxed. If, however, the torso is suspended over the floor, the posterior neck muscles, as well as the upper trapezius muscle, work to maintain extension in the neck.

Baddha Konasana

Body segment	Kinematics	Muscles active	Muscles released
Foot and toes	Toe extension	Extensor digitorum and hallucis longus (I)	
Lower leg	Ankle inversion	Anterior tibialis (C, I)	Peroneals
Thigh	Knee flexion	Hamstrings (C, I)	
Hip and pelvis	Hip flexion (aids)	Iliopsoas, quadriceps (C, I)	Iliopsoas, quadriceps (after external rotation), gracilis, sartorius
	Initiates external rotation	Adductors (E)	
	External rotation	Deep external rotators,* gluteus medius (C, I)	
	Flexion, external rotation	Sartorius (C, I)	
Torso	Spine extension, stability	Erector spinae, semispinalis, quadratus lumborum (C, I)	
	Rib and chest elevation	Pectoralis minor (C, I)	
	Trunk stability	Internal and external obliques, rectus abdominis, transverse abdominis (C, I)	
Shoulder	External rotation of humerus	Infraspinatus and teres minor, posterior deltoid (C, I)	
	Scapular adduction	Rhomboids major and minor, mid trapezius (C, I)	
	Postural support in mid back, downward pull of scapulae	Lower trapezius (C, I)	
Upper arm	Elbow flexion	Brachialis, biceps brachii, brachioradialis (C, I)	
Lower arm	Forearm supination	Supinator (C, I)	
Hand and fingers	Finger and thumb flexion	Flexor digiti minimi brevis, interossei dorsales manus and palmaris, opponens digiti minimi, flexor pollicis brevis (C, I)	
Neck	Neck extension and stability	Splenius capitus and cervicis, cervical erector spinae, semispinalis (I)	

*Obturator externus and internus, gemellus superior and inferior, quadratus femoris, and piriformis.

C = concentric contraction, E = eccentric contraction, I = isometric contraction.

Upavishtha Konasana

Wide-Angle Seated Forward Bend

[oo-puh-VISH-tuh kohn-
AAH-suh-nuh]

Upavishtha means seated, or sitting, in Sanskrit. *Kona* means angle.

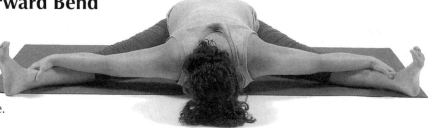

DESCRIPTION

Upavishtha Konasana is a seated straddle position. With the legs outstretched from the center, the torso folds forward toward the floor from the hips.

BENEFITS

- Opens the hips
- Stretches the groin and hamstrings
- In a complete forward bend, deeply stretches the hips and lengthens the torso

CAUTION

back pain or injury—Practice with modification or skip the pose.

VERBAL CUES

- From Dandasana (Staff Pose), inhale and move your feet apart as wide as you can comfortably. Point your tailbone and sits bones toward the back of your mat while tilting your pelvis slightly.
- Point your toes and knees up as much as possible by gently rolling your thighs back. Breathe deeply and slowly and lift the ribcage away from the hips.
- Inhale and reach your arms up and out to your sides as you expand your chest. Look up as you lift your chest.
- As you keep your chin and chest lifted, exhale and fold forward from your hips. Maintain length in the spine as you bring your chest closer to the floor. Do not allow your shoulders to roll forward.
- Lower your hands above or below your knees or to the floor in front of you. Use your hands to assist your back and ribcage as you fold forward more deeply.
- Continue to focus on your breath.
- When you get to the point where you feel you must release your back, stay there and breathe, allowing the breath to loosen the muscles.
- Then, allow your body to fold forward to completely relax. Make certain that your spine feels comfortable, and use your hands for support.
- To exit this posture, bring each hand above each knee and press down firmly. Inhale as you slowly lift through the chest and crown of the head to a seated position. Exhale and bring your legs together again in Dandasana.

ADJUSTMENTS

legs—If the student's knees and feet are rolling in, kneel behind the student and place your hands above the knees and rotate the student's legs externally.

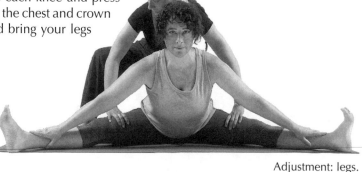

Adjustment: legs.

knees—If the student needs to have the knees bent slightly, sit the student on some folded blankets to help realign the hips and decrease stress on the hamstrings and low back.

spine—If the student is rounding the spine, have the student come upright slowly and aid the student in folding forward from the hips. Place your hand lightly on the student's back and encourage length by lifting the fingers up the spine toward the head or if you are standing, you can use your knee. Another adjustment is to stand behind the student and instruct the student to reach the hands overhead and interlace the fingers. As you squat down, bending from your hips and knees, have the student reach back and hold the base of your neck. Place your arms on the student's upper arms and lift the student up. Step your feet in front of both of the student's thighs so that you are straddling the student. Slowly walk yourself forward and take the student's hands from around your neck as you help the student lower, with length in the spine, to the ground. Make certain that you use proper mechanics by keeping your spine straight and bending from the hips and knees.

Adjustment: pregnancy.

MODIFICATIONS

tight back or hamstrings—Place a folded blanket under the student's hips to tilt the pelvis forward. You can also allow the student to keep the knees bent slightly.

pregnancy—Do not allow the student to round the back or to squash the abdomen. Place a chair in front of the student to rest the hands on. As the student flexes forward slightly, holding onto the chair allows the student to keep the torso upright. The student can also rest the arms and head on a chair with a pillow on it for relaxation.

weakness or injury—Modify the seated posture to a restorative one such as Viparita Karani (Restorative Legs-Up-the-Wall Pose) where the legs are flat against a wall and the back is on the floor.

KINEMATICS

As the upper body flexes forward, people with tight adductors will oftentimes find that the legs roll into internal rotation. To help make your students aware of this action, give them an additional verbal cue to keep the knees and toes pointing up. Remind students to focus the breath into the groin if they feel any tightness to allow the muscles to release a little more fully.

Upavishtha Konasana

Body segment	Kinematics	Muscles active	Muscles released
Foot and toes	Toe extension	Extensor digitorum and hallucis longus (C, I)	
Lower leg	Ankle dorsiflexion	Anterior tibialis, extensor digitorum longus (C, I)	
Thigh	Knee extension	Quadriceps (C, I)	Hamstrings
Hip and pelvis	Hip flexion over 120 degrees	Iliopsoas, rectus femoris (C, I)	
	Thigh abduction, stability	Tensor fascia lata, gluteus medius and minimus (C, I)	Adductors, gracilis

(continued)

Upavishtha Konasana *continued*

Body segment	Kinematics	Muscles active	Muscles released
Torso	Spinal extension and stability	Erector spinae, quadratus lumborum (C, I)	Pectoralis major
	Rib and chest elevation	Pectoralis minor (C)	
	Trunk stability	Internal and external obliques, transverse abdominis (C, I)	
Shoulder	Scapular adduction	Rhomboids major and minor, mid trapezius (C, I)	
	Humerus horizontal extension	Mid and posterior deltoid, supraspinatus (C, I)	
	External rotation	Infraspinatus and teres minor, posterior deltoid (C, I)	
	Joint stability	Subscapularis, teres minor, infraspinatus	
Upper arm	Elbow extension	Triceps brachii (C, I)	Biceps brachii, brachialis, brachioradialis
Lower arm	Forearm supination	Supinator (C, I)	
Hand and fingers	Finger and thumb flexion	Flexor digiti minimi brevis, interossei dorsales manus and palmaris, opponens digiti minimi, flexor pollicis brevis (C, I)	
Neck	Neck extension and stability	Splenius capitus and cervicis, cervical erector spinae (I)	

C = concentric contraction, E = eccentric contraction, I = isometric contraction.

Parighasana

Kneeling Triangle, or Gate Pose

[par-eegh-AAH-suh-nuh]

In Sanskrit a *parigha* is the crossbar used to lock a gate. When in this posture, the body is shaped like the bar mechanism. Physically, this side stretch lengthens the intercostals (rib muscles) and enables the expansion of the breath. In a metaphysical sense the breath is the gateway that connects the mind, body, and spirit.

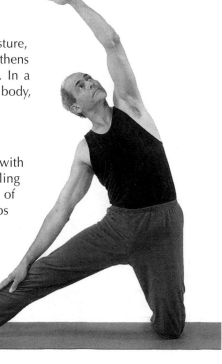

DESCRIPTION

This intense side stretch is generally practiced in a kneeling position with one leg abducted and rotated externally and can be described as a kneeling version of Utthita Trikonasana (Extended Triangle). The deeper variation of this posture requires significant flexibility in the lateral torso, as the hips are on the floor.

BENEFITS

- Applies a deep lateral stretch to the torso and low back
- Loosens the spine
- Stretches the pelvis and chest
- Expands the breath throughout the entire torso
- Strengthens the lateral abdominal muscles
- Aids in digestion

CAUTIONS

knee problems—Practice with modifications.

back problems—Those with back pain or injuries should limit lateral stretch to some degree.

VERBAL CUES

- From a kneeling position, place your knees hip-width apart with the thighs perpendicular to the floor. Rotate your right leg straight out to your right side with the leg in line with the torso. Roll the top of the right thigh out so the knee points up.
- If possible, press your right foot flat against the floor. If this strains the ankle, then allow the toes to lift slightly off the floor.
- Extend your arms out to your sides with the palms facing the floor. Inhale and lengthen your spine, reaching the crown of your head up and your tailbone toward the floor.
- As you exhale, reach your right arm out over your right leg, maintaining length in your low back. When you have reached as far as you can comfortably, slowly drop your right arm down toward the floor. Do not place any weight on your right leg.
- Reach your left arm over your head with your palm facing the floor. Turn your head and look up toward the left arm.
- Continue to focus on your breath.

- As you breathe, notice your breath filling your entire torso. Feel the muscles between your ribs expand as your spine continues to lengthen. Keep your torso aligned over your right leg.
- To exit this posture, press your right foot firmly into the floor and as you inhale feel yourself lifted by your left shoulder. Exhale and lower your arms to your sides. Bring your right knee back under your body and prepare to move to the left side.

ADJUSTMENTS

foot of extended leg—If the student is able to keep the foot aligned with the leg, then the toes should be able to touch the floor. Gently press down on the student's toes with your hand.

extended thigh—Stand or kneel behind the student, and place one hand on the hip of the kneeling leg and the other hand around the mid thigh. Roll the muscles back to rotate the extended leg externally and open the entire pelvic region.

ribcage—If the torso is sinking into the extended thigh, stand behind the student and place your nearest hand on the top portion of the ribcage. Cue the student to lengthen the ribs away from your hand.

shoulders—To help open the chest and shoulders, stand or kneel behind the student and place your nearest hand on the top shoulder and rotate the arm externally. Cue the student to maintain length in the neck.

top arm—If the palm of the student's top hand points forward, place your hand on the upper arm and gently rotate the arm externally so that the palm faces the floor. Also, guide the thumb posterior to the head to open the shoulder and chest more fully.

MODIFICATIONS

knee pain—If the student has difficulty placing the total body weight on the knees, allow the student to lean over a fitness ball. If the floor surface is too hard to remain in the posture comfortably, instruct the student to either double up the mat or place other padding under the knee.

tight hamstrings—Allow the student to keep the extended knee slightly bent.

tight back or sides—If the student is unable to reach the floor with the bottom hand, place a block or ball to the outside of the extended leg. This allows the student to keep weight off of the leg yet remain balanced.

deepen the posture—Instead of having the thigh of the bent knee perpendicular to the floor, the hips can be flexed so that the sits bones are on the floor. The hands reach overhead toward the foot of the straight leg. This variation should only be practiced by those with a range of motion in the hips and knees to allow for deepening the posture comfortably.

KINEMATICS

The upper body and hip mechanics of this posture are similar to those in Utthita Trikonasana (Extended Triangle) except that this is a kneeling posture. Like Trikonasana, the emphasis is to keep the hips and chest moving in the frontal plane and to continue to create length in the spine.

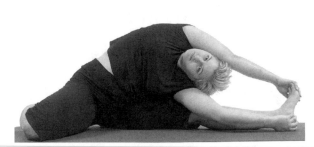

Modifications: tight hamstrings, back, or sides.

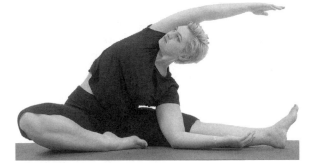

Modification: knee pain.

Modification: deepening the pose.

Parighasana (Leg Abducted to Right Side)

Body segment	Kinematics	Muscles active	Muscles released
Foot and toes (R)	Toe flexion (pressure into ground)	Flexors digitorum and hallucis longus, flexor digitorum brevis (C, I)	
Foot and toes (L)	Toe extension	Extensor digitorum longus, extensor hallucis longus, anterior tibialis (C, I)	
Lower leg (R)	Ankle plantar flexion	Gastrocnemius, soleus (C, I)	Extensor digitorum and hallucis longus, anterior tibialis
Lower leg (L)	Ankle plantar flexion and stability	Anterior tibialis, extensor digitorum longus, peroneals (C, I)	
Thigh (R)	Knee extension	Quadriceps (C, I)	
Thigh (L)	Knee flexion	Hamstrings, gastrocnemius (C, I)	
Hip and pelvis (R)	Hip abduction and external rotation	Tensor fascia lata, deep external rotators,* gluteus medius and minimus (C, I)	Hamstrings, adductors
Hip and pelvis (L)	Hip extension, stability	Hamstrings, gluteus maximus (C, I)	Iliopsoas, quadriceps
	Pelvic stability	Rectus abdominis, hamstrings, quadratus lumborum (I)	
Torso	Trunk stability	Rectus abdominis, internal and external obliques, transverse abdominis (I)	
Torso (L)	Lateral flexion to right	Quadratus lumborum, erector spinae, internal and external obliques (E, I)	Quadratus lumborum, erector spinae, latissimus dorsi, internal and external obliques
Shoulder (R)	External rotation	Infraspinatus and teres minor, posterior deltoid (C, I)	
	Humerus horizontal flexion	Mid, posterior deltoid, supraspinatus (C, I)	
Shoulder (L)	Humerus flexion	Anterior deltoids, pectoralis major, biceps brachii (C, I)	
	External rotation	Infraspinatus, teres minor, posterior deltoid (C, I)	
	Scapular adduction	Rhomboids, mid trapezius (C, I)	
Upper arm	Elbow extension	Triceps brachii (C, I)	
Lower arm (R)	Forearm supination	Supinator (C, I)	
	Forearm extension	Anconeus (C, I)	
Hand and fingers (R and L)	Wrist extension	Extensor carpi radialis longus and brevis, extensor carpi ulnaris (C, I)	
	Finger extension	Extensor digitorum, indicis, and digiti minimi; lumbricales manus; interossei dorsales (C, I)	
Hand and fingers (L)	Finger adduction	Interossei palmaris, adductor pollicis (C, I)	
Neck	Neck extension and stability	Splenius capitus and cervicis (I)	
	Neck stability against gravity	Sternocleidomastoid, scalenes (I)	

*Obturator externus and internus, gemellus superior and inferior, quadratus femoris, and piriformis.

C = concentric contraction, E = eccentric contraction, I = isometric contraction.

Virasana

Hero Pose

[veer-AAH-suh-nuh]

Vira is Sanskrit for hero or champion. In Hindu mythology the thighs are an extremely important part of the body, signifying virility and power.

DESCRIPTION

Virasana is a kneeling posture where the hips reach for the floor between the feet. Variations of this posture are used to sit in certain styles of meditation.

BENEFITS

- Improves circulation in the feet
- Helps alleviate calcaneal (heel) spurs
- Stretches the quadriceps
- Stretches the ankles
- Helps alleviate pain of arthritis in the feet and ankles
- Provides good spinal support for meditation (more so than sitting cross-legged)

CAUTION

acute knee injury—Those with undiagnosed knee pain should not practice this posture. Others with knee injuries should proceed cautiously and with modifications.

VERBAL CUES

- Kneel down on the floor with the knees approximately hip-distance apart. Place the tops of the feet against the floor.
- Exhale as you slowly lower your hips toward the floor. Place your hands on your calves, and rotate the bulk of the calves away from your body. This action helps to relax the knees as you lower down farther.
- Keep the knees together and the spine lifted as you lower the hips onto the floor between your ankles.
- Inhale and lengthen the crown of the head and the chest upward. Roll the shoulders back and down to keep the chest expanding with the breath.
- Rest the hands to your sides or on top of the thighs.
- Continue to focus on your breath.
- To exit the position, place your hands on the floor beside your hips. Slowly lean over onto one hip and extend the opposite leg, then lean to the other side and extend your other leg to sit in Dandasana. Roll the ankles in both directions and loosen the hips.

ADJUSTMENTS

feet—Make sure the student's feet are not pointing out to the sides. If they are, instruct the student to come back into a kneeling position with the tops of the feet onto the floor and ankles against the side of the hips.

knees—Make sure that the student's knees are as close together as possible. Kneel in front of the student, and place your hand between the knee joints. Instruct the student to press against your hand with both knees. Remove your hand but tell the student to keep the pressure constant. Another adjustment is to gently press the tops of the student's knees toward the floor.

shoulders—Remind the student to keep length in the spine and the shoulders rolled back. To help create length, kneel behind the student, and press your knee against the student's spine and press up gently.

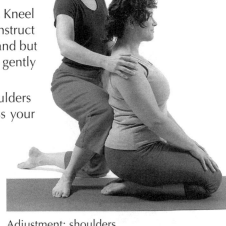

Adjustment: shoulders.

MODIFICATIONS

foot pain or tight ankles—If the student complains of feeling uncomfortable with the tops of the feet against the floor, place a folded blanket under the front of the ankles. Lifting the hips alleviates pain in the foot and ankle.

knee pain—Place a folded blanket or a block under the student's hips to open the angle under the knees. Opening the angle decreases pressure on the knee joints. Another modification is to stretch one thigh at a time, especially if there is pain or injury to one knee. From kneeling position, instruct student to extend one leg forward and lower the hips down to the floor.

deepen the posture—Instruct the student to interlace the fingers and press the palms out. Then, the student inhales and reaches the hands over the head.

KINEMATICS

At times, a student may make the mistake of rotating the lower leg externally in order to rest the pelvis on the ground between the heels. This action places the medial knee structures at risk for injury. Always check to see that the front of the students' shins are resting flat on the floor, and that the feet do not rotate externally.

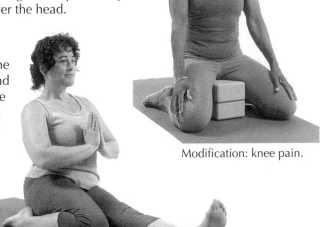

Modification: knee pain.

Modification: knee pain.

Virasana

Body segment	Kinematics	Muscles active	Muscles released
Foot and toes	Toe extension	Extensor digitorum longus (I)	
Lower leg	Ankle plantarflexion	Gastrocnemius, soleus (I, R)	Anterior tibialis, peroneals
	Internal rotation	Posterior tibialis (I)	
Thigh	Knee flexion	Quadriceps (E, R)	Quadriceps
Hip and pelvis	Hip flexion	Hamstrings, gluteus maximus (E, R)	Hamstrings, gluteus maximus
Torso	Spine extension and stability	Erector spinae, quadratus lumborum (C, I)	
	Rib and chest elevation	Pectoralis minor (C, I)	
	Trunk stability	Internal and external obliques, rectus abdominis, transverse abdominis (C, I)	
Shoulder	External rotation of humerus	Infraspinatus and teres minor, posterior deltoid (C, I)	
	Humerus adduction	Latissimus dorsi, pectoralis major (C, I)	
	Scapular adduction	Rhomboids, mid trapezius (C, I)	
Upper arm	Elbow extension	Triceps brachii (C, I)	
Lower arm	Forearm pronation	Pronator teres and quadratus (C, I)	Flexor carpi radialis and ulnaris
	Wrist hyperextension	Extensor carpi ulnaris, radialis longus and brevis (C, I)	
Hand and fingers	Finger extension	Extensor digitorum, indicis, and digiti minimi; lumbricales manus; interossei dorsales (I)	
Neck	Neck extension and stability	Splenius capitus and cervicis, cervical erector spinae (I)	

C = concentric contraction, E = eccentric contraction, I = isometric contraction, R = relaxed.

Bharadvajasana

Bharadvaja's Pose

[bhuh-RUHD-vaah-JAAH-suh-nuh]

In Hindu mythology, Bharadvaja is one of the legendary seven seers. He was also the father of Drona, a great military leader, who fought the war chronicled in the *Mahabharata*.

DESCRIPTION
Bharadvajasana is a gentle, seated twist that can be practiced with the legs in Virasana (Hero Pose) or with one leg in Virasana and the other in Ardha Padmasana (Half-Lotus).

BENEFITS
* Stretches and strengthens the low spine
* Stretches the neck, shoulders, hips, knees, and ankles
* Massages the internal organs
* Helps relieve sciatica pain
* Improves digestion

CAUTIONS

acute knee problems—Those with acute knee issues should only practice the basic variation or use modifications.

acute spinal problems—Students with spinal problems should limit rotation in spine.

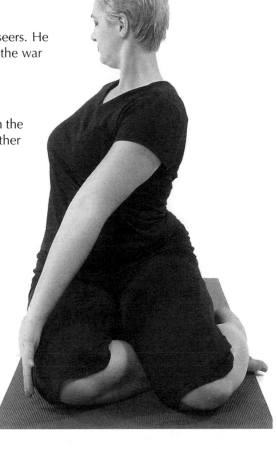

VERBAL CUES
* From Virasana, shift the body weight to the right hip and lower the right hip to the floor. Keep the feet together and close to your left hip.
* Inhale and lengthen the spine as you settle your hips into the floor. Exhale and bring the right hand behind your back. Reach your left hand to the outside of your right knee.
* Work to keep the top of your pelvis level with the ground.
* With each inhalation lengthen the spine, and with each exhalation press the right shoulder toward the back of the body as much as possible.
* Keep the right shoulder pressed back, and then slowly turn the head and look over the left shoulder. Try to align your chin with the shoulder.
* Continue to focus on your breath.
* To exit this posture, exhale and slowly turn your head forward. Then slowly bring your chest forward. Bring your hips back over your heels in Virasana and prepare for the opposite side.

ADJUSTMENTS

feet—Be sure the bottom foot is resting on the ground. Cue the student to relax both feet.

hips—If the top of the student's pelvis is not level with the ground, place a blanket under the lower hip. Kneeling behind the student, gently place your hand on the raised hip and press down. Be aware of the student's comfort level.

spine—Remind the student to lift out of the low spine. Gently place your hand on the rounded spine and encourage lengthening up.

rotation—If the student is having difficulty rotating the shoulder around, stand or kneel behind the student and place one hand on the shoulder closest to you. Gently rotate the shoulder toward you as you press your other hand against the student's ribcage and lift and press forward.

MODIFICATIONS

deepening the posture—The following variation is for those who can sit comfortably in Ardha Padmasana. Instruct the student to bring the bottom leg over the top so that the foot rests in the crease of the opposite thigh in Ardha Padmasana. Reach the hand farthest from the feet around the back and toward the top foot. Grab the big toe and use the connection for leverage in rotation.

tight spine or shoulders in the Ardha Padmasana variation—If the student has difficulty grasping the toe, wrap a strap around the foot and have the student hold on to the other end with the hand behind the back.

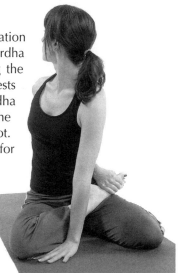

Modification: deepening the posture.

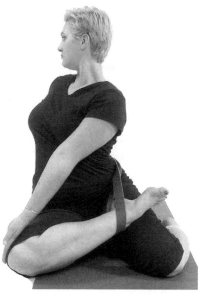

Modification: tight spine or shoulders in the Ardha Padmasana variation.

KINEMATICS

In Bharadvajasana, the spine should remain perpendicular to the floor with all of the natural curves intact. However, because of tight hip extensors and rotators, some students will find that they cannot keep both halves of the pelvis on the floor, and the low back will curve laterally toward the legs to compensate. Another compensation is to exaggerate the forward curve in the low spine (lordosis). For comfort and proper alignment, place a bolster or blanket under the hip farthest from the legs.

Bharadvajasana (Rotating Torso to Right)

Body segment	Kinematics	Muscles active	Muscles released
Foot and toes	Toe extension	Extensor digitorum and hallucis longus (I)	
Lower leg	Ankle stability	Gastrocnemius, soleus, peroneals (I)	
Thigh	Knee flexion	Hamstrings (C, I)	
Hip and pelvis (R)	Hip flexion	Iliopsoas (C, I)	
	External rotation, stability	Adductors (E, I)	
Hip and pelvis (L)	Hip flexion	Iliopsoas (C, I)	
	Internal rotation	Deep external rotators* (E, I)	Deep external rotators,* gluteus medius

Body segment	Kinematics	Muscles active	Muscles released
Torso (R and L)	Spinal stability	Rectus abdominis, transverse abdominis, quadratus lumborum (I)	
	Chest and rib elevation	Pectoralis minor (C, I)	
Torso (R)	Spinal rotation to right	Internal oblique, erector spinae, latissimus dorsi (C, I)	External oblique
Torso (L)	Spinal rotation to right	External obliques (C, I)	Quadratus lumborum, internal oblique, erector spinae
Shoulder (R)	Humeral extension	Posterior deltoid, latissimus dorsi (C, I)	Pectoralis major
	External rotation	Posterior deltoid, teres minor, infraspinatus (C, I)	
Shoulder (L)	Internal rotation and humeral extension (aids in spinal rotation)	Latissimus, posterior deltoid (C, I)	Quadratus lumborum
Upper arm (R)	Elbow extension	Triceps brachii (C, I)	
Upper arm (L)	Elbow extension against resistance, also aids in spinal rotation	Triceps brachii (C, I)	
Lower arm (R)	Supination	Supinator (C, I)	
Lower arm (L)	Forearm pronation	Pronator teres and quadratus (C, I)	
Hand and fingers (R)	Wrist hyperextension	Extensor carpi radialis longus and brevis, extensor carpi ulnaris (C, I)	Wrist flexors
	Finger extension	Extensor digitorum, indicis, and digiti minimi; lumbricales manus; interossei dorsales (C, I)	
Hand and fingers (L)	Wrist flexion	Flexor carpi radialis and ulnaris, palmaris longus (C, I)	
	Finger extension	Extensor digitorum, indicis, and digiti minimi; lumbricales manus; interossei dorsales (C, I)	
Neck (R)	Head rotation to right, stability	Splenius capitus and cervicis, occipitals, cervical erector spinae (C, I)	Sternocleidomastoid
Neck (L)	Head rotation to right	Sternocleidomastoid (C, I)	

*Obturator externus and internus, gemellus superior and inferior, quadratus femoris, and piriformis.

C = concentric contraction, E = eccentric contraction, I = isometric contraction.

Padmasana

Lotus Pose

[puhd-MAAH-suh-nuh]

Padma is Sanskrit for lotus. When meditating in Padmasana, the energy flows through the chakras, which are generally represented as lotus flowers.

DESCRIPTION

Padmasana is generally an upright, seated position where the legs are crossed in front with each ankle resting comfortably on the opposite thigh near the crease of the opposite hip. This is the quintessential seated posture in yoga and East Indian meditation. Many people, especially in the West, have tight hip muscles and cannot easily sit in this posture on their first attempt. To sit comfortably in this position, one needs flexible, open hips. This takes time and practice. Five variations of Padmasana are provided here so that students at every level of flexibility can sit in this restful position.

BENEFITS

- Relieves stiffness in the hips, knees, and ankles
- Strengthens the low spine and abdominal muscles
- Promotes a relaxed, balanced posture
- Increases circulation of interstitial fluids (lymph fluids)
- Boosts energy

CAUTION

acute knee injuries—Those with acute knee issues should only practice the basic variation or use modifications.

VERBAL CUES

Note for all variations: Instruct the students to respect the limits of their bodies! Even if the student normally can come into Padmasana, there may be days when, because of temperature or fatigue, the student may have difficulty. Remind the student to move slowly and to come into the posture only to the point where the body is most comfortably challenged.

First Variation: Baby Lotus

From Dandasana (Staff Pose), cross one ankle over the other with your feet tucked as close to your body as is comfortable. It is fine if your knees are lifted off the floor.

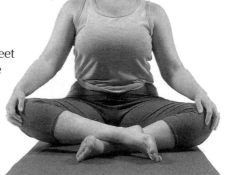

First variation: Baby Lotus.

Second Variation: Sukhasana [soo-KHAAH-suh-nuh] (Easy Pose)

- The legs are not crossed in this position. Instead the knees are bent and rotated out toward the floor. This is generally a precursor to practicing Padmasana.
- From Dandasana, bring your lower right leg in front of your lower left leg with your left heel tucked close to your right hip.

Third Variation

From Sukhasana, bring the right foot on top of the left ankle and calf. To keep the legs in this position more comfortably, wedge your right foot between the left calf and thigh. If you feel comfortable, press down gently on the right thigh to open the hip and groin. Do not place any tension on the knee!

Fourth Variation: Ardha Padmasana (Half-Lotus, also Tailor Sit)

This variation gets to the root of being able to perform Padmasana comfortably and more deeply.

- From Sukhasana, place your right foot and ankle on top of the left calf. Then bring your right knee in more toward the center of the midline of your body. Breathe.

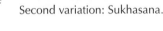

Second variation: Sukhasana.

- Place your right ankle above the left knee so that your right knee hangs toward the ground. Move your left foot away from your body.
- As comfortably as possible, move your knees so that they are in a 90-degree angle. Drop the top (right) knee toward the floor as much as you can in a relaxed manner.
- Turn the sole of the top foot upward; and, if you can, bring your right heel to your navel comfortably. Move the right knee even more toward center.
- Take the top of the right ankle into the crease of the left thigh. Release the right ankle so that the foot hangs over the left thigh. The right hip is stretched and open, allowing for the ankle to relax.

Moving into Ardha Padmasana.

- As you relax the legs and hips in this posture, be sure to keep your spine straight, lengthened, and relaxed.
- To exit this variation, extend the bottom leg, then the top. Loosen the hips, knees, and ankles by rolling the legs from side to side.

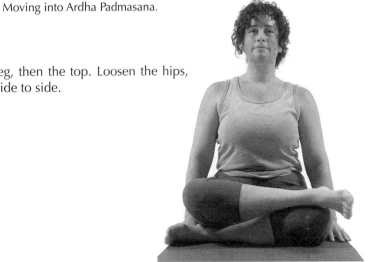

Fourth variation: Ardha Padmasana.

Fifth Variation: Padmasana (Full Lotus)

- From Ardha Padmasana, move the lower leg away from your body so that your top knee comes completely to the floor. As much as you can comfortably, bring your left foot up from the floor and reach your left heel toward your navel. This brings your left knee more forward until you are comfortable and can bring your left ankle into the crease of your right thigh.

- To exit this posture, slowly straighten the left leg. Roll the leg from side to side and rotate the ankle around. With the next breath extend the right leg and loosen the joints. It is always a good idea to practice this posture with the opposite leg positioning to keep both sides of the legs and hips loosened.

ADJUSTMENTS

ankles—Many times students complain of ankle pain when sitting in Ardha Padmasana or other variations where the ankle is on the floor. Place a folded towel under the foot to cushion the bones. Also, make certain that if the feet are crossed over the opposite thigh that the ankles are not inverted (rolling inward). This places undue stress on the lateral ankle muscles. Instruct students to bring the knees more in line with the center, or to move out of the position.

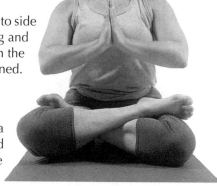

Fifth variation: Padmasana.

knees—If much stress is placed on the knees as the adductors relax, place folded blankets or bolsters under the outside of the thighs as a wedge.

spine—If the student is rounding the back, place a blanket under the hips to lengthen the spine. Place your hand lightly on the spine to cue the student to lift taller through the spine and chest.

MODIFICATIONS

low back or hip tightness; weakness in all variations—Place a folded blanket under the hips. You can also place students with their backs against the wall for support.

hip tightness—Depending on the degree of tightness, instruct the student to keep the legs in the most comfortable and least stressful position.

KINEMATICS

Many students are so determined to come into either Ardha Padmasana or Padmasana that they wind up placing undue stress on all of the leg joints. The most common mistake made is that a person will partially place the ankle across the opposite thigh. If the ankle is not draped over the thigh, the lateral ligaments and tendons are overstretched. Impress on your students the importance of sitting comfortably and without strain.

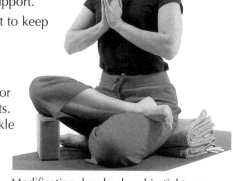

Modification: low back or hip tightness; weakness.

Padmasana

Body segment	Kinematics	Muscles active	Muscles released
Foot and toes	Toe extension	Extensor digitorum and hallucis longus (I)	
Lower leg	Ankle dorsiflexion	Anterior tibialis (C, I)	
Thigh	Knee flexion	Hamstrings (C, I)	Adductors
Hip and pelvis	Hip flexion	Iliopsoas (C, I)	
	External rotation	Adductors (E, R)	Deep external rotators,* adductors
	Flexion and rotation	Sartorius (C, I)	
Torso	Spine extension, stability	Erector spinae, semispinalis, quadratus lumborum, (C, I)	
	Trunk stability	Internal and external obliques, rectus abdominis, transverse abdominis (C, I)	
Shoulder	External rotation of humerus	Infraspinatus and teres minor, posterior deltoid (C, I)	
	Scapular adduction	Rhomboids major and minor, mid trapezius (C, I)	
	Postural support in mid back, downward pull of scapulae	Lower trapezius (C, I)	
Upper arm	Elbow flexion	Biceps brachii, brachioradialis (R)	
Lower arm	Forearm supination	Supinator (R)	
Hand and fingers	Finger flexion	Flexor digiti minimi brevis, interossei palmaris, flexor pollicis brevis (R)	
Neck	Neck extension and stability	Splenius capitus and cervicis, cervical erector spinae, semi-spinalis (I)	

*Obturator externus and internus, gemellus superior and inferior, quadratus femoris, and piriformis.

C = concentric contraction, E = eccentric contraction, I = isometric contraction, R = relaxed.

Tolasana

Scale Pose

[tohl-AHH-suh-nuh]

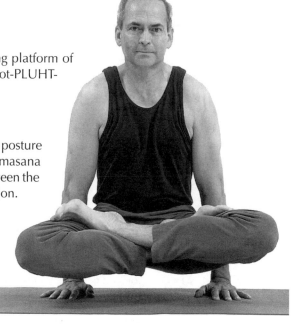

Tola is Sanskrit for scales. This posture resembles the balancing platform of a scale. In Ashtanga practice this posture is called Utpluti (oot-PLUHT-tee).

DESCRIPTION

This arm-balance pose is generally used as a transition from one posture to another. Ideally, this posture is practiced with the legs in Padmasana (Full Lotus) with the body lifted off the ground and balanced between the hands. This posture requires strength, balance, and concentration.

BENEFITS

- Strengthens the abdominal muscles, arms, wrists, and hands
- Increases balance and mental focus
- Increases energy
- Has been shown to help focus people with Attention Deficit Disorder (ADD)
- Stretches hips if legs are in Padmasana

CAUTIONS

pregnancy—Due to the concentrated effort of the lower abdominals, this posture is not recommended beyond the second trimester.

extreme weakness—Practice with modifications to increase strength.

VERBAL CUES

- From the variation of Padmasana that best coordinates with your abilities, place your hands on the ground beside your hips. Squeeze your shoulder blades together and open your chest.
- Inhale and lengthen the spine and focus the breath into your ribcage. Press your palms into the floor.
- Exhale and lift your hips off the floor as you pull the legs up toward the lower abdominal area.
- Keep your breathing smooth and controlled.
- To exit the posture, exhale and slowly lower the hips and legs back to the ground. Uncross the legs and then recross the opposite way and balance again.
- Another option for exiting this posture is to extend the legs either forward or back to move into another asana.

ADJUSTMENTS

arms—Instruct students to be sure the hands are as close to the hips as possible before lifting up. This hand placement makes the balance easier. Also, tell students to keep the elbows straight. To adjust, kneel behind the student and place your hands on the student's forearms and press the arms closer to the body.

neck—Remind the student to look forward and not to drop the head toward the chest in the effort to lift the body.

MODIFICATIONS

building arm strength—To help the student build strength in the arms and shoulders, ask the student to press through the arms and lift the hips while the legs remain on the floor. You can also place a folded blanket under the hips so that the student does not have as far to lift.

building abdominal strength—Have the student keep the palms and the hips on the floor and then lift the legs up toward the abdomen.

long torso—If the student's torso is longer than the arms, the student will generally try to lift up from the fingers instead of the palms of the hands, which places undue stress on the finger joints. Place blocks under the student's hands to "lengthen" the arms.

wrist weakness—If a student complains of wrist pain, there are props available that allow the student to grip an elevated bar so the wrist does not bend.

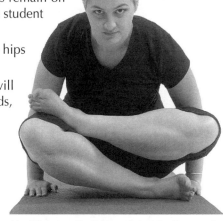

Modification: building abdominal strength.

Modification: long torso.

KINEMATICS

Tolasana is not a "pure" seated posture; however, it is a good transitional posture in the seated category. Additionally, it can build significant strength in the arms, abdominals, and legs even if the legs do not lift off of the ground.

Tolasana

Body segment	Kinematics	Muscles active
Foot and toes	Toe extension	Extensor digitorum and hallucis longus (I)
Lower leg	Ankle dorsiflexion	Anterior tibialis (C, I)
Thigh	Knee flexion	Hamstrings (C, I)
Hip and pelvis	Hip flexion, stability	Iliopsoas (C, I)
	External rotation, stability	Adductors (E, I)
	Flexion and external rotation	Sartorius (C, I)
	Hip stability	Deep external rotators,* gluteus medius (I)
	Pelvic stability	Rectus abdominis, quadratus lumborum (I)
Torso	Flexion	Rectus abdominis (C, I)
	Rib and chest elevation	Pectoralis minor (C, I)
	Trunk stability	Internal and external obliques, rectus abdominis, transverse abdominis (C, I)
Shoulder	External rotation of humerus	Infraspinatus and teres minor, posterior deltoid (C, I)
	Scapular adduction	Rhomboids and mid trapezius (C, I)
	Scapular depression, stability	Serratus anterior (C, I)
	Postural support in mid back, downward pull of scapulae	Lower trapezius (C, I)
	Humerus hyperextension, stability	Latissimus dorsi, posterior deltoids (C, I)
Upper arm	Elbow extension	Triceps brachii (C, I)
	Elbow stability	Biceps brachii, brachialis, brachioradialis (I)
Lower arm	Forearm pronation, stability	Pronator teres and quadratus (C, I)
	Wrist hyperextension, stability, and balance	Wrist flexors and extensors (C, I)
Hand and fingers	Finger abduction	Abductor digiti minimi, interossei (C, I)
	Finger stability, balance	Flexor digitorum profundus and superficialis, flexor digiti minimi brevis, interossei palmaris (C, I)
Neck	Neck extension and stability	Splenius capitus and cervicis, cervical erector spinae, semispinalis, upper trapezius (C, I)

*Obturator externus and internus, gemellus superior and inferior, quadratus femoris, and piriformis.

C = concentric contraction, E = eccentric contraction, I = isometric contraction.

Hanumanasana

Forward-Splits Pose

[huh-noo-maahn-AAH-suh-nuh]

Hanuman was a powerful god of service and the son of Vayu, the god of wind or breath. He was a magical monkey. As an epitome of service, he helped rescue the wife of Lord Ram by making great flying leaps across the seas to fulfill his duties.

DESCRIPTION

This posture is a tribute to Hanuman's giant leap—a forward split. Hanumanasana is another posture that many students may find quite challenging the first time they try it. However, with practice, the lengthening of the hamstrings and hip flexors is most beneficial. When one is able to comfortably practice Hanumanasana, a slight backbend deepens the posture.

BENEFITS

- Stretches the hamstrings and hip flexors
- Stabilizes and balances the deep hip muscles
- Aids in relieving sciatica pain
- Strengthens the spinal and abdominal muscles

CAUTION

hamstring injury—Proceed with modifications.

VERBAL CUES

- Begin in a kneeling lunge (a position in the classical Sun Salutation) with the right leg forward. Slide the left leg back and lower your hips to the floor. Your hands will remain on the floor.
- Square the hips so that they are balanced directly under the shoulders. Press the hips toward the right heel. Point the tailbone down toward the ground.
- Breathe deeply into any area in which you feel resistance.
- Secure your hands on the floor as you slowly stretch your right heel forward. Straighten the right leg as much as possible. Go to your edge of being comfortably challenged. The tailbone should remain pointed toward the ground.

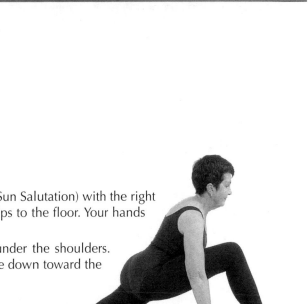

Getting into Hanumanasana.

- Find the place where you feel your balance and remain there as you breathe deeply, allowing your muscles to relax. Lift your ribcage up and away from your hips.
- If you can, lower your hips all the way down to the floor, then begin to raise your arms overhead. Inhale as you raise your arms.

- If you cannot bring your hips to the floor comfortably, work to keep your hips and shoulders in alignment.
- To exit this posture, focus on using your arms and abdominal muscles to eliminate the possibility of straining your low back or groin. Move slowly and press your hands into the floor and lift the hips. Bend your right knee and move your body back into the lunge. Switch legs and prepare to practice on the opposite side.

ADJUSTMENTS

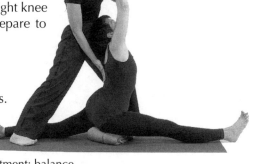

hips—Make sure the student's hips are aligned under the shoulders. Stand or kneel behind the student, and very gently pull the front of the flexed hip back and press the back of the extended hip forward.

Adjustment: balance.

balance—If the student has difficulty balancing in the posture with the arms overhead, stand behind the student and hold onto the person's wrists or upper arms. Gently lift the torso up without bringing the hips off the floor.

MODIFICATIONS

tight hamstrings or hip flexors—If either of these muscle groups are tight, the student will not be able to comfortably lower the hips to the ground, so be sure to place blankets under the hips for support. A block or prop can be used to keep the upper body weight from overly stretching the hamstrings.

knee discomfort—For some students, the pressure of the back knee against the ground will create significant discomfort. Place padding under the knee to alleviate the discomfort.

KINEMATICS

Modification: tight hamstrings or hip flexors.

Like coming into Padmasana, some people can come into this posture naturally and with ease. Most, however, will find that they need to practice modified versions of the posture as they begin to increase the stretch in the hamstrings and hip flexors.

Hanumanasana (Right Leg Forward)

Body segment	Kinematics	Muscles active	Muscles released
Foot and toes	Toe extension	Extensor digitorum and hallucis longus (C, I)	
Lower leg (R)	Ankle dorsiflexion	Anterior tibialis, extensor digitorum longus (C, I)	Gastrocnemius, soleus
Lower leg (L)	Ankle plantar flexion	Gastrocnemius, soleus (I)	Anterior tibialis, extensor digitorum longus
Thigh	Knee extension	Quadriceps	
Hip and pelvis (R)	Hip flexion	Iliopsoas, rectus femoris (C, I, R)	Hamstrings
Hip and pelvis (L)	Hip hyperextension	Hamstrings, gluteus maximus (C, I)	Iliopsoas, rectus femoris
Torso	Slight lumbar hyperextension	Rectus abdominis (E, I)	Rectus abdominis
	Slight lumbar hyperextension and spinal stability	Erector spinae, quadratus lumborum (C, I)	
	Trunk stability	Transverse abdominis, internal and external obliques (I)	
Shoulder	Humeral flexion	Anterior deltoids, pectoralis major, biceps brachii (C, I)	Latissimus dorsi, serratus anterior
	External rotation	Infraspinatus, teres minor, posterior tibialis (C, I)	
	Scapular adduction	Rhomboids, mid trapezius (C, I)	
Upper arm	Elbow extension	Triceps brachii (C, I)	Biceps brachii, brachioradialis
Lower arm	Forearm supination	Supinator (C, I)	
	Forearm extension	Anconeus (C, I)	
Hand and fingers	Finger extension	Extensor digitorum, indicis, and digiti minimi; lumbricales manus; interossei dorsales (C, I)	
	Finger adduction	Interossei palmaris, adductor pollicis (C, I)	
Neck	Neck extension and stability	Splenius capitus and cervicis, suboccipitals, upper trapezius (I)	

C = concentric contraction, E = eccentric contraction, I = isometric contraction, R = relaxed.

Crane Pose

[buhk-AAH-suh-nuh]

Baka is Sanskrit for the crane (a tall, wading bird). Like a tall and graceful crane, Bakasana is a graceful, balancing posture.

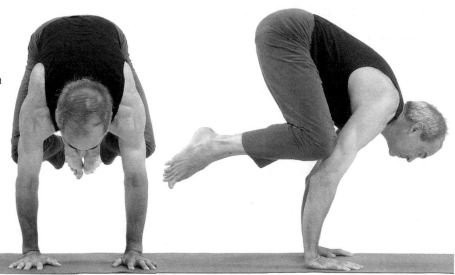

DESCRIPTION

In this squatting arm balance, the bent arms support the weight of the body as the bent knees rest on the backs of the upper arms. Once balanced on the hands, the feet are lifted off the floor. Many students feel somewhat fearful when they first practice this asana that they will fall forward on their faces.

BENEFITS

- Strengthens the arms and wrists
- Improves focus and balance
- Strengthens the abdominal muscles
- Stretches the low back

CAUTIONS

wrist injuries or acute carpal tunnel syndrome—Students with wrist problems should refrain from practicing this posture.

pregnancy—This posture is not recommended after the second trimester.

VERBAL CUES

- From Malasana (Basic Squat Pose), place your hands shoulder-width apart on the floor in front of you.
- Fix your gaze on a focal point slightly forward of your hands. Spread your fingers apart to create a wider base of support.
- Bend your elbows and slowly lift your heels off the floor as you shift your body weight more toward your hands.
- Rest your shins on the backs of your upper arms with your knees as close to your underarms (axillas) as possible.
- Continue to focus on your breath.
- As you lean forward, exhale and slowly lift one foot off the ground. If you do not feel comfortably balanced, slowly lower that leg and lift the other. If you feel balanced, lift both feet off the floor.
- Continue to focus your gaze past your hands. Maintain smooth, steady breathing. Apply abdominal lock (uddiyana bandha) and continue to balance for five to six breaths.
- To exit the posture, exhale and slowly lower the feet back to the floor and rest back in Malasana.

ADJUSTMENTS

aiding balance—Squat or stand behind the student with your hands or a strap wrapped around the student's hips to aid the student in the balance.

hands—Remind the student to place the hands no more than shoulder-width apart and to press the hands firmly into the ground. If the student's palms are lifted, gently press down on the back of the hands with your fingers.

elbows—Remind students to keep the elbows pressed in toward the body.

hips—The hips and low back should be relaxed, and the hips should not be raised much above the level of the head.

MODIFICATIONS

building confidence—Some students will feel much more confident and less fearful with some folded blankets placed in front of them.

strength building—For students who have difficulty lifting both feet off the ground, place blocks or folded blankets under the feet so that they begin the posture in an elevated position. Also, for those recovering from wrist injury, instruct the student to practice putting body weight on the hands, keeping the feet on the floor.

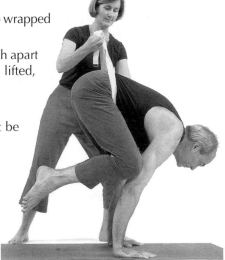

Adjustment: aiding balance.

KINEMATICS

Individuals with tight hips may have the hips significantly higher than the head and generally lose balance more quickly. The more compact students can make their body in this position, the easier it is to remain controlled and balanced. This is a very active posture where once in position, most of the muscles remain in isometric contraction to remain balanced.

Bakasana

Body segment	Kinematics	Muscles active
Foot and toes	Toe extension	Extensor digitorum and hallucis longus (C, I)
Lower leg	Ankle dorsiflexion	Anterior tibialis, extensor digitorum longus (C, I)
Thigh	Knee flexion, stability	Hamstrings, sartorius (C, I)
Hip and pelvis	Hip flexion, stability	Iliopsoas, sartorius, rectus femoris (C, I)
	Hip abduction, stability	Gluteus medius and minimus (C, I)
Torso	Spinal extension and stability	Erector spinae, quadratus lumborum (C, I)
	Sternoclavicular stability	Subclavius (I)
	Torso stability	Rectus abdominis, internal and external obliques, transverse abdominis (I)
Shoulder	Flexion of humerus, stability	Pectoralis major, coracobrachialis, anterior deltoid (C, I)
	Adduction of humerus, stability	Latissimus dorsi, teres major (C, I)
	Stability and external rotation of humerus	Infraspinatus, teres minor, posterior deltoid (C, I)
	Shoulder and scapular stability	Subscapularis, serratus anterior (C, I)
	Scapular stability	Rhomboids and mid trapezius (C, I)
	Supporting posture in mid back, downward pull of scapulae	Lower trapezius (C, I)
Upper arm	Elbow flexion, stability	Triceps brachii (E, I), biceps brachii, brachialis, brachioradialis (I)

(continued)

Bakasana *continued*

Body segment	Kinematics	Muscles active
Lower arm	Forearm pronation, stability	Pronator teres and quadratus (C, I)
	Wrist hyperextension, balance, and stability	Extensor carpi radialis brevis and longus, extensor carpi ulnaris (C, I); flexor carpi radialis and ulnaris, palmaris longus (E, I)
Hand and fingers	Finger abduction	Abductor digiti minimi, interossei (C, I)
	Finger extension, stability, balance	Flexor digitorum profundus and superficialis, flexor digiti minimi brevis, interossei palmaris (C, I)
Neck	Neck hyperextension and stability	Splenius capitus and cervicis, cervical erector spinae, semispinalis, upper trapezius (C, I)

C = concentric contraction, E = eccentric contraction, I = isometric contraction.

chapter 9

Supine and Prone Postures

This chapter comprises 17 postures that render the body face up (supine) or face down (prone) with the bottom of the pelvis (the ischial tuberosities) usually off the floor. Raja Kapotasana (Royal Pigeon Pose) is included in this chapter because it can be practiced with the body in both supine and prone positions. Other positions include backbends, plank poses, positions on the hands and knees, and postures in which the body is lying face up or down (for example, Supta Padangusthasana (Reclining Hand-to-Toe Pose), which borders on being a restorative pose). Vasishthasana (Side Plank Pose) is included here as well, although this posture is neither supine nor prone, because it is related to regular plank poses and does not fit well into the other categories.

Generally, the supine and prone asanas stretch and strengthen the core musculature. Plank poses build stability and strength in the arms and shoulders, and backbends open the chest and strengthen the mid and upper back. Some of the postures in this chapter serve to help warm up the body. Other poses included here are often practiced as closing poses toward the end of class before resting, such as Urdhva Dhanurasana (Upward Bow Pose). Backbends counter forward bends and balance out the total of the six directions of the spine applied during asana sessions.

Although prone postures are not advised after the first trimester of pregnancy due to the pressure on the abdomen, many postures can be practiced with modifications so the belly does not rest on the floor.

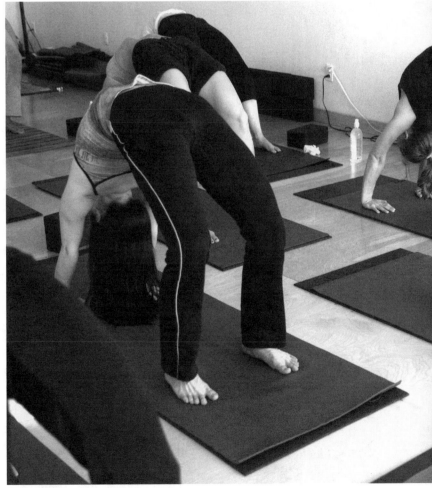

© Levine Roberts

Cat and Cow Pose

[DUR-guh-go]

Cat and Cow pose has no official Sanskrit translation, but we call the pose *Durga-Go*. Durga was a warrior goddess who rode the back of a ferocious tiger and *Go* is Sanskrit for cow.

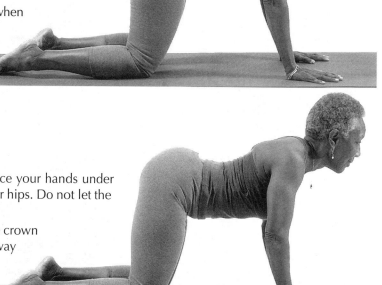

DESCRIPTION

Durga-Go is practiced on the hands and knees. The spine is moved through a gentle range of flexion and hyperextension in the sagittal plane. The rounded, flexed spine refers to the cat portion of the posture, which resembles a cat with its back arched. The hyperextension in the spine is reminiscent of the sway in a cow's back.

BENEFITS

- Warms and stretches the spinal musculature
- Provides safe substitute for other postures when one is pregnant
- Moves the energy with the breath

CAUTION

wrist problems—Those with wrist problems should practice with modifications.

VERBAL CUES

- Begin on your hands and knees, and place your hands under your shoulders and your knees under your hips. Do not let the shoulders collapse toward the ears.

- Inhale and lengthen the spine. Stretch the crown of the head and the tailbone as far away from each other as possible. Feel your breath expand through the entire torso. Imagine your spine is a tabletop.

- Exhale and tuck your pelvis under your body as you lower your chin to your chest. As you squeeze your abdomen in, press the mid spine toward the sky. Relax your shoulders. This is the durga position.

- Inhale and release your spine back into the table position. Lengthen the spine. With the next inhalation, press your hips back as you move your tailbone up. At the same time, lift your chest forward and up, with the chin facing toward the sky. Bend back as far as feels comfortable to you. Feel the front of your body lengthen and stretch as you imagine your navel touching the floor with your abdomen lifted. This is the cow position.

- Exhale and release your spine back to the table position.

- Repeat this cycle two or three times, and then prepare for the next posture.

ADJUSTMENTS

feet—If the student has trouble balancing with the tops of the feet on the floor, instruct the student to curl the toes under for stability.

hands and knees—If the distance between the hands and knees is either too long or too short the student will have trouble flattening the back. Cue the student to adjust the distance accordingly.

shoulders—Remind the student to maintain distance between the ears and shoulders. Gently tap the tops of the shoulders to cue the student to drop the shoulders lower.

spine—To help the student achieve flexion in the spine, place your hand on the middle of the student's back. Encourage the student to press the spine against your hand to lift it. To help the student hyperextend the spine, place your hand to the mid spine and instruct the student to move the spine away from your hand.

breath awareness—When the student is in the durga (rounded back) position, place your hand lightly on the mid spine to cue the student to direct the breath to that area.

MODIFICATIONS

wrist pain—Instead of having the students place the hands on the floor, instruct them to bend the elbows and place the forearms on the floor. Another option is to move a chair in front of the student on which to place the arms. Ideally, the chair should be at shoulder height.

variation for lateral movements of the spine—Cue the students to stay in the same hands-and-knees position with the spine parallel to the floor, exhale, and squeeze the hip and shoulder together. Instruct them to look over the shoulder on the side they are flexing. Inhale and move back to straight spine, then exhale and do the other side.

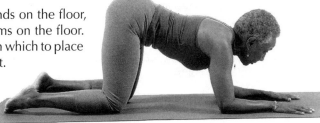

Modification: wrist pain.

KINEMATICS

Hands-and-knees positioning is a transitional position for many other postures. The hands must remain directly beneath the shoulders and the knees directly under the hips to avoid putting undue stress on the joints. It is also important that the elbow joint remains straight but not hyperextended.

Durga-Go

Body segment	Kinematics	Muscles active	Muscles released
Foot and toes	Toe extension	Extensor digitorum longus, extensor hallucis longus (C, I)	
Lower leg	Ankle plantar flexion, stability	Anterior tibialis, extensor digitorum longus, peroneals (C, I)	
Thigh	Knee flexion	Hamstrings (C, I)	
Hip and pelvis	Hip flexion	Iliopsoas (C, I)	
	Hip stability	Gluteus maximus, hamstrings, deep hip rotators (C, I)	
	Pelvic stability	Rectus abdominis, quadratus lumborum, hamstrings (I)	

(continued)

Durga-Go *continued*

Body segment	Kinematics	Muscles active	Muscles released
Torso (Durga phase)	Torso stability	Rectus abdominis, internal and external obliques, transverse abdominis (C, I)	Erector spinae, quadratus lumborum
	Spinal flexion	Rectus abdominis (C, I)	
	Sternoclavicular stability	Subclavius (I)	
Torso (Go phase)	Spinal hyperextension, stability	Erector spinae, quadratus lumborum (C, I)	Rectus abdominis, internal and external obliques, transverse abdominis
Shoulder (both phases)	Flexion of humerus	Pectoralis major, anterior deltoids, coracobrachialis, biceps brachii (C, I)	
	Stability and external rotation of humerus	Infraspinatus, teres minor, posterior deltoid (C, I)	
	Supporting posture in mid back, downward pull of scapulae	Lower trapezius (C, I)	
Shoulder (Durga phase)	Scapular abduction and stability	Subscapularis, serratus anterior (C, I)	Trapezius, rhomboids, latissimus dorsi
	Humerus adduction	Pectoralis major, anterior deltoid (C, I)	
Shoulder (Go phase)	Adduction of scapulae	Rhomboids, mid trapezius (C, I)	
Upper arm	Elbow extension	Triceps brachii (C, I)	
Lower arm	Forearm pronation	Pronator teres and quadratus (C, I)	
	Forearm extension	Anconeus (C, I)	
	Wrist hyperextension, stability	Extensor carpi radialis brevis and longus, extensor carpi ulnaris (C, I)	
Hand and fingers	Wrist stability	Flexor carpi radialis and ulnaris, palmaris longus (C, I)	
	Finger extension, stability	Extensor digitorum, extensor digiti minimi brevis (C, I)	
	Finger abduction	Abductor pollicis longus, opponens pollicis (C, I)	
Neck (Durga phase)	Initial neck flexion	Splenius capitus and cervicis, suboccipitals, semispinalis, upper trapezius (E)	Splenius capitus and cervicis, suboccipitals, semispinalis, upper trapezius
	Neck flexion	Sternocleidomastoid, scalenes (C, I)	
Neck (Go phase)	Neck hyperextension	Splenius capitus and cervicis, suboccipitals, semispinalis, upper trapezius (C, I)	Sternocleidomastoid, scalenes

C = concentric contraction, E = eccentric contraction, I = isometric contraction.

Utthita Chaturanga Dandasana

Plank Pose

[oot-T-HEE-tuh chuh-tour-RUHN-guh duhn-DAAH-suh-nuh]

Utthita is the Sanskrit word for extended, *chatur* means four, and *anga* means limbs. *Danda* is a staff or rod.

DESCRIPTION

This posture is essentially the extended arm positioning of a push-up and is a transitional movement in the Sun Salutations (Surya Namaskaras).

BENEFITS

- Prepares body to perform variations of extended body postures (for example, Chaturanga Dandasana [Four-Limbs Staff Pose], Urdhva Mukha Shvanasana [Upward-Facing Dog])
- Builds strength in the shoulders, arms, back, legs, and abdominal muscles
- Builds stability in the shoulders and core musculature

CAUTION

wrist problems—Those with wrist injuries or pain should use modifications.

VERBAL CUES

- From the Sun Salutation lunge, place your palms on the floor directly under your shoulders.
- Inhale and lengthen the spine as you open the shoulders and chest.
- Exhale and step your front leg back as you lift the back knee off the floor. Curl your toes under. Straighten the legs and press the heels back.
- Breathe deeply and slowly and apply uddiyana bandha, page 52. This helps keep the energy locked in to support your low back.
- Imagine pressing the floor away from your chest. This action helps to keep your upper back straight and your shoulder blades pressed against your spine.

In the Sun Salutations, the body is next lowered toward the floor to continue the vinyasa (flow) although the body is in a position to transition to other postures as well.

ADJUSTMENTS

heels—Make sure students' heels are pressed back to keep the legs active. Remind students to press the heels behind them.

shoulders—If the shoulders are not aligned over the hands, stand to one side or in front of the head. With your hands on the student's shoulders gently pull the student's body weight over the hands.

shoulder blades—If the student's shoulder blades "wing" out (lift away from their back due to weakness), remind the student to press more firmly against the floor. Kneel beside the student and place your hand lightly between the shoulder blades and instruct the student to press the body up against your hand.

neck—Cue the student to look down toward the floor. The ears, shoulders, hips, knees, and ankles should be in alignment. If any of the joints are sinking, gently touch the side of the joint and instruct the student to lift slightly higher.

MODIFICATIONS

problems with alignment—Straddle the student's back and bend your knees as you hold the sides of the student's hips and lift slightly to take some of the body weight.

weakness—If the student is unable to maintain a straight spine in the position, instruct the student to keep the knees bent and on the floor and to focus on keeping the spine straight from the shoulders to the hips.

wrist problems—If the student cannot flex the wrists or put weight on them, instruct them to flex the elbows and place the forearms on the floor. Also, students can use props such as a raised bar if they are unable to flex the wrists.

KINEMATICS

This particular asana works best as a preparatory posture to build strength needed in the arms, legs, and abdominal muscles for arm balances. It also increases the range of motion necessary in the shoulders and chest.

Modification: wrist problems.

Uttitha Chaturanga Dandasana

Body segment	Kinematics	Muscles active	Muscles released
Foot and toes	Toe abduction	Dorsal interossei, abductor digiti minimi brevis, abductor hallucis (C, I)	
	Toe hyperextension	Extensor digitorum and hallucis longus, anterior tibialis (C, I)	
	Forefoot stability	Anterior tibialis, flexor digitorum longus (C, I)	
Lower leg	Ankle stability	Gastrocnemius, soleus, posterior tibialis, flexor digitorum and hallucis longus (I)	Gastrocnemius, soleus
	Ankle dorsiflexion, stability	Anterior tibialis, extensor digitorum longus (C, I)	
Thigh	Knee extension	Quadriceps (C, I)	
	Femur adduction, stability	Adductors (C, I)	
Hip and pelvis	Hip extension, stability	Hamstrings, gluteus maximus (C, I)	
	Hip stabilization	Gluteus medius, deep external rotators (I)*	
Torso	Torso stability	Rectus abdominis, internal and external obliques, transverse abdominis (I)	
	Spinal extension and stability	Erector spinae, quadratus lumborum (I)	
Shoulder	Sternoclavicular stability	Subclavius (I)	
	Flexion of humerus	Pectoralis major, anterior deltoid, coracobrachialis, biceps brachii (C, I)	Rhomboids, mid trapezius
	Stability and external rotation of humerus	Infraspinatus, teres minor, posterior deltoid (C, I)	
	Scapular stability	Rhomboids, mid trapezius	
	Scapular abduction, stability	Serratus anterior, subscapularis (C, I)	

Body segment	Kinematics	Muscles active	Muscles released
Upper arm	Elbow extension	Triceps brachii (C, I)	
Lower arm	Forearm pronation	Pronator teres and quadratus (C, I)	
	Forearm extension	Anconeus (C, I)	
	Wrist hyperextension	Extensor carpi radialis brevis and longus, extensor carpi ulnaris (C, I)	
	Wrist stability	Flexor carpi radialis and ulnaris, palmaris longus (C, I)	
Hand and fingers	Finger extension	Extensor digitorum, extensor digiti minimi brevis (C, I)	
	Finger abduction	Abductor pollicis longus, opponens pollicis (C, I)	
Neck	Neck extension, stability	Splenius capitus and cervicis, suboccipitals, semispinalis, upper trapezius (I)	

*Obturator externus and internus, gemellus superior and inferior, quadratus femoris, and piriformis.

C = concentric contraction, E = eccentric contraction, I = isometric contraction.

Chaturanga Dandasana

Four-Limbs Staff Pose

[chuh-tour-RUHN-guh duhn-DAAH-suh-nuh]

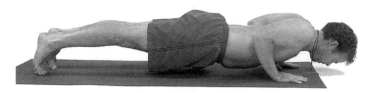

Chatur means four in Sanskrit, and *anga* is a limb.
Danda is a straight staff. The four limbs support the straight staff of the spine in this pose.

DESCRIPTION

This posture is more challenging and similar to the downward phase of a push-up. It is practiced in the Ashtanga Sun Salutations (Surya Namaskara A and B). Unlike Utthita Chaturanga Dandasana (Plank Pose), where the elbows are straight, in this asana the elbows are bent and the body hovers slightly above the ground.

BENEFITS

- Strengthens the shoulders, arms, and wrists
- Strengthens the abdominal muscles and massages the organs

CAUTION

wrist problems—Those with wrist injuries or pain should use modifications.

VERBAL CUES

- From Utthita Chaturanga Dandasana with the palms pressed into the floor and aligned with the shoulders, begin to slowly bend the elbows.
- Exhale and lower the body down toward the floor and remain a few inches above it. The distance will vary from person to person. Go to where you feel you are most comfortably challenged and can still breathe smoothly.
- Squeeze the upper arms in toward the ribs and lengthen the ears away from the shoulders.
- Lower down to the ground and prepare to transition into another posture. (In the Ashtanga vinyasa, students prepare to enter Urdhva Mukha Shvanasana [Upward-Facing Dog].)

ADJUSTMENTS

elbows—If the student's elbows point away from the body, kneel to one side and place your hands just above the person's elbows. Gently press the arms in toward the waist.

hips—Align the student's body so that the hips are neither too high nor too low in relation to the shoulders and knees. If the hips are too low, straddle the student's back and bend your knees as you hold the sides of the hips and lift slightly. If the student's hips are lifted too high, place your hand lightly on the student's low back and instruct the student to move the hips away from your hand.

MODIFICATIONS

strength building—Instead of holding the posture, have the student first work on bending the knees and lowering the chest down to the floor slowly.

wrist problems—If the student cannot flex the wrists or put weight on them, the person can flex the elbows and place the forearms on the floor.

KINEMATICS

To maintain stability in the shoulders, the elbows must be placed close to the body in this posture. This placement maintains the proper alignment of the humerus (upper-arm bone) in the shoulder socket with the body weight on the joint.

Chaturanga Dandasana

Body segment	Kinematics	Muscles active	Muscles released
Foot and toes	Toe abduction	Dorsal interossei, abductor digiti minimi brevis, abductor hallucis (C, I)	
	Toe hyperextension	Extensor digitorum and hallucis longus, anterior tibialis (C, I)	
	Forefoot stability	Anterior tibialis, flexor digitorum longus (C, I)	
Lower leg	Ankle stability	Gastrocnemius, soleus, posterior tibialis, flexor digitorum longus and flexor hallucis longus (I)	Gastrocnemius, soleus
	Ankle dorsiflexion	Anterior tibialis, extensor digitorum longus (C, I)	
Thigh	Knee extension	Quadriceps (C, I)	
	Leg adduction and stability	Adductors (C, I)	
Hip and pelvis	Hip extension	Hamstrings, gluteus maximus (C, I)	
	Hip stabilization	Gluteus medius, deep hip rotators (I)	
Torso	Torso stability	Rectus abdominis, internal and external obliques, transverse abdominis (I)	
	Spinal extension and stability	Erector spinae, quadratus lumborum (I)	
Shoulder	Sternoclavicular stability	Subclavius (I)	
	Humerus extension, stability	Pectoralis major, biceps brachii, anterior deltoid (E, I)	Pectoralis major
	Humerus extension, adduction and stability	Latissimus dorsi (C, I)	
	Stability and external rotation of humerus	Infraspinatus, teres minor, posterior deltoid (C, I)	
	Scapular abduction, stability	Subscapularis, serratus anterior (C, I)	
	Scapular stability	Rhomboids, mid trapezius (C, I)	
	Supporting posture in mid back, downward pull of scapulae	Lower trapezius (C, I)	
Upper arm	Elbow flexion and stability	Triceps brachii, posterior deltoid, biceps brachii, brachialis, brachioradialis (E, I)	
Lower arm	Forearm pronation	Pronator teres and quadratus (C, I)	
	Wrist hyperextension, stability	Flexor carpi radialis and ulnaris, palmaris longus (E, I)	
Hand and fingers	Finger extension	Extensor digitorum, extensor digiti minimi brevis (C, I)	
	Finger abduction	Abductor pollicis longus, opponens pollicis (C, I)	
Neck	Neck extension, stability	Splenius capitus and cervicis, suboccipitals, semispinalis, upper trapezius (I)	

C = concentric contraction, E = eccentric contraction, I = isometric contraction.

A Transitional Pose

[zehn AAH-suh-nuh]

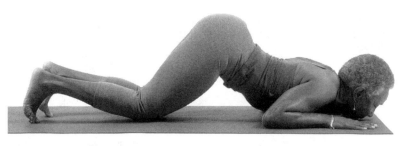

This posture is referred to here as Zen Asana. *Zen* was chosen because the posture is not really a pose. Instead, it is usually practiced only as part of or as a transitional movement during the Classical Sun Salutation. This transitional pose, however, is indeed a valuable and important asana. It does and yet does not exist; therefore, although a name in Sanskrit might not be found, it is appropriate to call this posture Zen Asana.

DESCRIPTION

Zen Asana is a prone pose with the toes, knees, hands, chest, and chin touching the ground. The hips and low back are raised and reaching away from the waist while the elbows are bent close to the ribs.

BENEFITS

Although seldom practiced outside of the Classical Sun Salutation this position provides the following benefits:

- Strengthens the sternum
- Promotes alignment, stability, and flexibility in the spine and shoulders
- Prepares the body for backbends as well as other arm and shoulder weight-bearing postures
- Creates expansion in the neck and low back
- Provides a good substitute pose for modifications as well as a bedrock pose for healthy extension in Urdhva Mukha Shvanasana (Upward-Facing Dog), or Bhujangasana (Cobra Pose), which it often precedes

VERBAL CUES

- From Utthita Chaturanga Dandasana (Plank Pose), exhale and bend your knees to the floor while you slowly begin to drop your chest and chin to the ground.
- Keep your elbows in and close against your ribs.
- Let your chest sink into the earth as you roll your collar bones apart.
- Press your tailbone up and back as far as you possibly can, creating space in your low back.
- Let the inhalation open space, especially in the spine and chest. Let the exhalation release more.
- Transition into Bhujangasana.

ADJUSTMENTS

hips and knees—Some students struggle with the torso in this posture as they find themselves basically flat on the floor instead of with just one part of the body touching the ground. The main reason for this discomfort is that they move forward while lowering down and they lack the arm strength to lower the chest straight down. If the knees are not bent and the hips are not raised then students are not doing the pose correctly. Instruct them to bend their knees while you guide their hips to move up and back. You can straddle or semi-squat above or beside a student and use your hands on the sides of the student's pelvis to guide the direction and distance of the movement.

low back—To support and create space in the student's low back, kneel next to the student and place your hand on the base of the spine. With your palm, fingers pointing toward the student's tailbone, gently push up and away from the waist.

chest—Encourage the student to relax the sternum into the floor. If it seems the student is tense in the upper spine place your hand on the student's mid back; remind the person to breathe and let the spine sink away from your hand. With each breath let your hand get a little heavier while the student further relaxes the spine.

arms and shoulders—Make sure the student's elbows are pressing in and the shoulders are down, away from the ears. If the arms are not close or in alignment with the shoulders, move the student into the more ideal placement. One way to address the positioning of the arms and shoulders is to do an adjustment. You might also apply Bhujangasana—squatting behind the student over the mid to low back region. Hold on to the fronts of the student's shoulders while you move the shoulders open and simultaneously squeeze the arms in by the student's sides.

neck—The adjustment just described also can create more space in the back of the neck because you are moving the student's shoulders down away from the ears as well as opening across the front of the chest. If the student's arms are in a good position but the neck is not lengthened well, kneel by the student and use your hands to push the shoulders down away from the ears. To get the student to elongate the neck a little more actively, gently touch the crown of the student's head and tell the student to push your finger up more with each inhalation.

MODIFICATIONS

pregnancy—During the first half of pregnancy many women might feel comfortable lowering the themselves into this pose, especially if they have been practicing yoga consistently throughout the pregnancy. If not, it is best to substitute Zen Asana with Durga-Go (Cat and Cow Pose). For a woman in her first trimester who feels comfortable, place a pillow or blankets under her abdomen for support. Postpartum, this pose may be a little difficult for women, especially if they breastfeeding. If the student does not wish to substitute the pose then instruct her to keep a folded blanket or pillow under the chest.

low back problems—If a student is uncomfortable in this posture because the low back feels compromised then substitute Balasana (Child's Pose), with the knees spread apart so the chest and chin sink toward the ground as the student releases the spine.

KINEMATICS

Getting into this posture with awareness and control is the key. If the student can lower down slowly while contracting the triceps eccentrically and actively working the posterior shoulder muscles then the student will settle appropriately into the posture. Have the student bend the knees on the floor before the body is halfway down to avoid having to work the back and instead focus on doing the upper-body mechanics correctly. When a student has good low back and core structure support then the other variations of plank (Chaturanga Dandasana [Four-Limbs Staff Pose], for example) and backbends (such as Urdhva Mukha Shvanasana) can be performed more easily.

Zen Asana

Body segment	Kinematics	Muscles active	Muscles released
Foot and toes	Spread toes	Dorsal interossei, abductor digiti minimi brevis, abductor hallucis (C, I)	
	Toe hyperextension	Extensor digitorum and hallucus longus, tibialis anterior (C, I)	
Lower leg	Ankle dorsiflexion	Anterior tibialis, extensor digitorum longus (C, I)	Gastrocnemius, soleus
Thigh	Knee flexion	Hamstrings (E, I)	
	Leg adduction and stability	Adductors (C, I)	
Hip and pelvis	Hip flexion	Hamstrings, gluteus maximus (E, I)	Gluteus maximus
Torso	Torso stability	Rectus abdominis, internal and external obliques, transverse abdominis (I)	Rectus abdominis
	Spinal extension and stability	Erector spinae, quadratus lumborum (I)	
	Sternoclavicular stability	Subclavius (I)	

(continued)

Zen Asana *continued*

Body segment	Kinematics	Muscles active	Muscles released
Shoulder	Humerus extension, stability	Pectoralis major and minor, biceps brachii, anterior deltoid, serratus anterior (E, I)	Pectoralis major, anterior deltoid
	Humerus extension, adduction and stability	Latissimus dorsi, posterior deltoid (C, I)	
	Stability and external rotation of humerus	Infraspinatus, teres minor, posterior deltoid (C, I)	
	Adduction of scapulae	Rhomboids and mid trapezius (C, I)	
	Supporting posture in mid back, and downward pull of scapulae	Lower trapezius (C, I)	
Upper arm	Elbow flexion	Triceps brachii, posterior deltoid (E, I)	
Lower arm	Forearm pronation	Pronator teres and quadratus (C, I)	
	Elbow forearm	Anconeus (C, I)	
	Wrist hyperextension	Flexor carpi radialis and ulnaris, palmaris longus (E, I)	
Hand and fingers	Wrist stability	Flexor carpi radialis and ulnaris, palmaris longus (C, I)	
	Finger extension	Extensor digitorum, extensor digiti minimi brevis (C, I)	
	Finger abduction	Abductor pollicis longus, opponens pollicis (C, I)	
Neck	Neck hyperextension, stability	Splenius capitus and cervicis, suboccipitals, semispinalis, upper trapezius (C, R)	

C = concentric contraction, E = eccentric contraction, I = isometric contraction, R = relaxed.

Vasishthasana

Side Plank Pose

[vuhs-eesht-AAH-suh-nuh]

Vasishtha is Sanskrit for "most excellent." Vasishtha also is the name of a well-known sage associated with good fortune, strength, and dignity. Holding this posture requires strength, and increases poise and confidence.

DESCRIPTION

Vasishthasana is a side plank pose, most often practiced where the body is balanced on the side of one foot and the palm of the hand on the same side. In another variation of this asana, the top leg is lifted in the air above the leg on the ground, as opposed to being stacked on top of the bottom leg, and the big toe of the lifted leg is grasped by the nonweight-bearing hand.

BENEFITS

- Strengthens the arms, abdomen, and legs
- Stabilizes the shoulders
- Stretches and strengthens the wrists
- Opens the chest
- Opens the hips if the top leg is lifted
- Improves concentration and balance

CAUTIONS

wrist problems—Those with wrist problems should practice with modifications.

weakness—This asana should not be practiced by those recovering from serious illness or injury.

pregnancy—After the first trimester, practice with modifications.

VERBAL CUES

- From Utthita Chaturanga Dandasana (Plank Pose), shift the body weight onto the right hand. Lift the left foot off the floor and roll the outside of the right foot against the floor. Rest the left foot on top of the right.
- Rotate the front of the body away from the floor so that the left hip and shoulder are stacked over the right hip and shoulder. Rest the left hand on your left hip.
- Your body weight is supported on the right palm and right foot. Breathe deeply and smoothly. Make sure that your fingers are pointing away from your body.
- Exhale and lift the left arm up. Turn to look at the left hand, aligning your chin with your shoulder as best as you can.
- Lengthen your body as much as possible with the crown of the head moving away from the feet. The more you stretch your feet away from your head, the easier it will be to keep your hips aligned with your knees and shoulders.
- Continue to focus on your breath.
- To exit the posture, exhale and rotate your body back into plank, and prepare to practice the opposite side.

ADJUSTMENTS

feet—Remind students to stack the top foot on top of the bottom foot to aid in balance.

legs and hips—The legs should be straight and active in the posture with the hips lifted and aligned with the knees and shoulders. If the student sinks the hips, stand or kneel behind the student and press your hand against the bottom hip to cue lifting the hips up.

low spine—If a student's low back is in significant lordosis (swayback), stand behind the student and gently press your knee into the student's hips to straighten the back.

shoulders—Make sure that students align the shoulders directly over the weight-bearing hand. If the hand is aligned more toward the head, the shoulder joint will be unstable. If the hand is placed more toward the hips, the wrist joint may be strained.

MODIFICATIONS

weakness or wrist problems—The posture may be practiced with the lower elbow bent and the forearm on the ground. This modification allows the student to gradually build strength in the shoulder and torso.

low back weakness or pregnancy—Instruct the student to bend the lower knee and place the lower leg on the ground.

balance difficulties—If the student cannot balance with the top foot stacked on the lower, allow the student to place the top foot on the floor behind the bottom heel.

deepen the posture—If students are comfortable in the standard side plank, cue them to raise the top leg while keeping the nonweight-bearing arm perpendicular to the floor. To deepen the stretch, cue the students to bend the top knee and grasp the big toe with the first two fingers of the upper hand. Exhale and slowly extend the top foot toward the sky. Gently point the toes down toward the body.

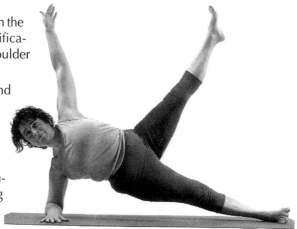

Modification: weakness or wrist problems.

KINEMATICS

This pose requires a coordinated effort between the strength of the torso and the strength of the shoulder on the lower arm. It is important that the student build strength in both areas so that the hips do not drop down toward the floor or allow the bottom shoulder to "collapse" into the side of the head.

Vasishthasana (Weight on Right Side)

Body segment	Kinematics	Muscles active	Muscles released
Foot and toes	Toe extension	Extensor digitorum longus, extensor hallucis longus, tibialis anterior (C, I)	
Lower leg (R)	Lateral ankle stability	Peroneus longus, brevis and tertius (C, I)	
Lower leg (L)	Ankle dorsiflexion	Anterior tibialis, extensor digitorum and hallucis longus (C, I)	
Thigh	Knee extension	Quadriceps (C, I)	
	Adduction and stability	Adductors (C, I)	
Hip and pelvis (R and L)	Hip extension, stability	Hamstrings, gluteus maximus (C, I)	
Hip and pelvis (R)	Hip stability	Gluteus medius, deep external rotators,* tensor fascia lata, quadratus lumborum (C, I)	
Torso	Torso stability	Rectus abdominis, internal and external obliques, transverse abdominis, right latissimus dorsi (I)	
	Spinal extension and stability	Erector spinae, quadratus lumborum (I)	
	Sternoclavicular stability	Subclavius (I)	
Shoulder	Horizontal humerus extension, external rotation and stability	Deltoids, infraspinatus, teres minor (C, I)	
	Scapular adduction	Rhomboids, mid trapezius (C, I)	
Upper arm	Elbow extension	Triceps brachii (C, I)	
Lower arm (R)	Forearm pronation	Pronator teres and quadratus (C, I)	
	Forearm extension	Anconeus (C, I)	
	Wrist hyperextension, stability	Extensor carpi radialis brevis and longus, extensor carpi ulnaris, extensor digitorum, flexor carpi radialis and ulnaris, palmaris longus (C, I)	
Lower arm (L)	Forearm supination	Supinator (C, I)	
Hand and fingers (R)	Finger extension	Extensor digitorum, extensor digiti minimi brevis (C, I)	
	Finger abduction	Abductor pollicis longus, opponens pollicis (C, I)	
Hand and fingers (L)	Finger extension	Extensor digitorum, indicis, and digiti minimi; lumbricales manus; interossei dorsales (C, I)	
	Finger adduction	Interossei palmaris, adductor pollicis (C, I)	
Neck (R)	Head rotation to left	Sternocleidomastoid (C, I)	
Neck (L)	Head rotation, neck stability	Splenius capitus and cervicis, occipitals, cervical erector spinae, upper trapezius (C, I)	Sternocleidomastoid

*Obturator externus and internus, gemellus superior and inferior, quadratus femoris, and piriformis.

C = concentric contraction, E = eccentric contraction, I = isometric contraction.

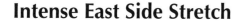

Intense East Side Stretch

[poohr-VOHT-taahn-AAH-suh-nuh]

Purva means the East and relates to the front of the body. *Uttana* means intense. This posture stretches the front of the body intensely.

DESCRIPTION

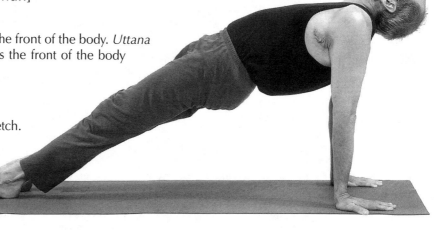

Purvottanasana is a supine plank stretch. In this posture, the hands press into the floor behind the back as the front of the body is lifted up. It is practiced as one of the five major exercises in Tibetan yoga.

BENEFITS

- Deeply stretches the chest and shoulders
- Strengthens the wrists and ankles
- Builds endurance
- Provides a counterstretch to Paschimottanasana (Intense West Side Stretch)
- Strengthens the posterior muscles in the legs and spine

CAUTION

extreme neck weakness—Do not allow students with neck problems to drop the head down below the shoulders. Instruct them to practice modifications if experiencing discomfort.

VERBAL CUES

- From Dandasana (Staff Pose), place the palms on the floor beside the hips. Move the hands six to eight inches (15 to 20 centimeters) behind the hips and shoulder-width apart. Point the fingers toward or away from the feet, depending on the student's shoulder comfort.
- Press through the arms, opening the chest as you tuck your pelvis under. Breathe deeply, lengthening the spine.
- Exhale and lift the hips and legs off the floor, bringing your body weight onto your arms. Press the soles of your feet into the floor. Feel the length of the body.
- Your arms should be perpendicular to the floor. If your shoulders and chest are open and the level of the chest is above the shoulders, exhale and slowly drop the head back, stretching the neck.
- Continue to focus on your breath.
- To exit the posture, exhale and slowly lower the hips down to the floor. Keep the head relaxed back. As the hips touch the floor, slowly roll up the spine from the bottom to the top, moving back into an upright position. Inhale and slowly raise the head upright.

ADJUSTMENTS

feet—If the student's toes are almost touching the floor, gently press down on the top of the foot.

hips—Assist the student in lifting the hips by standing to the side and placing your hands on either side of the student's hips. You can also straddle the student, with one calf on each side of the student's hips. Lift the pelvis until it is aligned between the shoulders and knees.

shoulders and chest—Remind the student to keep the chest lifted. You can lightly tap the chest while instructing the student to push through the arms and move the chest toward the sky. You can also place your hand on the student's chest and cue the student to move your hand up.

neck—Make certain that the student places the neck in a comfortable position. If the student feels strain caused by hyperextension then instruct the student to keep the ears aligned with the shoulders and to look straight ahead, or to press the chin into the chest.

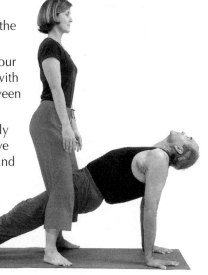

Adjustment: hips.

MODIFICATIONS

weakness or discomfort—Instruct the student to keep the knees bent with the feet flat on the floor. The body will be in a table position. This position reduces the workload by redistributing the center of mass.

weak or tight shoulders—Instruct the student to rotate the shoulders externally so that the fingers point away from the body rather than pointing toward the feet. If the student is unable to lift the chest higher than the shoulders then instruct the student to rest the chin toward the chest. Encourage the student to work on lifting the chest to eventually touch the chin. See Kinematics for the reasons this modification is important.

KINEMATICS

If students sag in the shoulders and chest, they tend to overcompensate for the weakness by hyperextending the neck to such a degree that they "pinch" the neck rather than maintain length throughout the entire spine. This overcompensation tends to decrease circulation and expansion in the region, which leads to tension and can create injury to the vertebrae and supporting structures, rather than increasing the circulation and creating more length and strength.

Purvottanasana

Body segment	Kinematics	Muscles active	Muscles released
Foot and toes	Toe flexion (pressure into ground)	Flexors digitorum and hallucis longus, flexor digitorum brevis (C, I)	
Lower leg	Plantar flexion	Gastrocnemius, soleus (C, I)	Anterior tibialis, extensor digitorum longus
Thigh	Knee extension	Quadriceps (C, I)	
Hip and pelvis	Hip extension or hyperextension	Hamstrings, gluteus maximus (C, I)	Iliopsoas, rectus femoris
Torso	Trunk stability	Internal and external obliques, transverse abdominis (I)	Rectus abdominis
	Hyperextension	Erector spinae, semispinalis (C, I)	
Shoulder	Scapular adduction, stability	Rhomboids, mid trapezius (C, I)	Anterior deltoid, pectoralis major and minor
	Humeral hyperextension	Latissimus dorsi, teres major (C, I)	
	Hyperextension, stability	Posterior deltoid (I)	
Upper arm	Elbow extension	Triceps brachii (C, I)	Biceps brachii, brachialis, brachioradialis
Lower arm	Forearm pronation	Pronator teres and quadratus (C, I)	
	Wrist hyperextension	Extensor carpi radialis brevis and longus, ulnaris (I)	
Hand and fingers	Finger extension	Extensor digitorum, indicis, and digiti minimi; lumbricales manus; interossei dorsales (I)	Flexor digitorum profundus and superficialis, flexor digiti minimi, interossei
	Finger abduction	Abductor digiti minimi, abductor pollicis brevis, opponens pollicis (C, I)	
Neck	Neck hyperextension	Sternocleidomastoid, scalenes (E, I)	Sternocleidomastoid

C = concentric contraction, E = eccentric contraction, I = isometric contraction.

Bhujangasana

Cobra Pose

[bhoo-juhn-GAAH-suh-nuh]

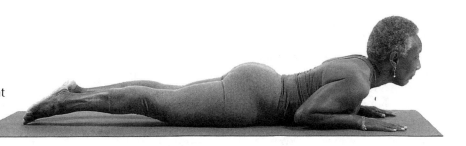

Bhujanga is Sanskrit for a serpent or snake. This pose is often translated in the West as Cobra because the chest is lifted in the same way that a cobra raises up its head.

DESCRIPTION

Bhujangasana is a prone back-bending posture with numerous variations. In its simplest form, the chest is lifted off the floor with the arms at the sides. A deeper variation brings the head and the feet together. This posture is part of the Classical Sun Salutation.

BENEFITS

- Increases range of motion in the spine
- Strengthens and stretches the spine
- Opens the chest and shoulders
- Increases circulation through the lungs and abdomen
- Energizes the legs
- Can be utilized to relieve pain from herniated disks and sciatica

CAUTION

pregnancy—Women past the first trimester should use a substitute posture.

VERBAL CUES

- From a prone position with your chin resting on the floor, bring your hands under your shoulders. Point your fingers forward and press your upper arms into your sides.
- Move your shoulder blades toward your hips and tuck your pelvis under to lengthen the spine.
- Press your hips into the floor and keep your legs active and pressing toward your toes.
- Inhale and lift the chest forward and up. Feel your ribcage move away from your hips. Reach the crown of your head up.
- As you inhale, feel the spine lengthen; and, as you exhale, feel your shoulders sink down away from your ears. Keep your hips on the ground.
- Notice your body slowly lift as you inhale deeply and lower as you exhale.
- To exit the position, exhale and slowly lower the abdomen and chest back to the floor from the bottom of your torso to the top.

ADJUSTMENTS

feet—The tops of the feet should be flat against the floor. If the student's toes are curled under, instruct the student to relax the top of the foot on the floor.

legs—The legs should remain active in this position, stretching down away from the hips. Tap the backs of the legs gently to cue the student to activate the muscles.

hips—If the student's hips are off the ground, gently press down on the low back and remind the student to push the hips into the floor.

low back—If the student has trouble lengthening through the back, place your hand on the student's sacrum and press away from the direction of the head. You can also straddle the student's back and sit on the lower sacrum so that the weight of your body anchors the pelvis and allows the student to lift the chest away from the hips.

elbows—If the student's elbows point away from the body, gently press the outside of each elbow toward the body. If you sit on the hips you can place your hands to the front of the shoulders and rotate the shoulders externally and lift the torso slightly.

shoulders—Make sure that the student's shoulders do not lift up near the ears. Lightly tap the tops of the shoulders to cue the student to create more space between the ears and shoulders, and to position the head so the ears remain aligned with the shoulders.

Adjustment: elbows.

MODIFICATIONS

tight back—Instruct the student to use the arms for support instead of the back muscles.

pregnancy—From the second trimester on, pressure on the abdomen is generally uncomfortable and contraindicated. Instead of Bhujangasana, pregnant women should substitute Durga-Go (Cat and Cow Pose).

KINEMATICS

The MacKenzie press-up in physical therapy is a variation of Bhujangasana. The MacKenzie version is a passive spinal arch where the arms press the spine into a gentle backbend to increase the range of motion in the spine. Bhujangasana is a much more active pose, where the erector spinae muscles aid in lifting the chest and arching the back, building strength as well as increasing the range of motion in the spine.

Bhujangasana

Body segment	Kinematics	Muscles active	Muscles released
Foot and toes	Toe abduction	Dorsal interossei, abductor digiti minimi brevis, abductor hallucis (C, I)	
	Toe hyperextension	Extensor digitorum longus, extensor hallucis longus, tibialis anterior (C, I)	
Lower leg	Ankle plantar flexion	Gastrocnemius, soleus (C, I)	Anterior tibialis, extensor digitorum longus
Thigh	Knee extension	Quadriceps (C, I)	
	Leg adduction	Adductors (C, I)	
Hip and pelvis	Hip hyperextension	Hamstrings, gluteus maximus (C, I)	Iliopsoas
Torso	Spinal hyperextension	Erector spinae, quadratus lumborum (C, I)	Rectus abdominis
	Torso stability	Internal and external obliques, transverse abdominis (I)	
	Sternoclavicular stability	Subclavius (I)	
Shoulder	Extension and adduction of humerus	Latissimus dorsi, teres major (C, I)	Pectoralis major
	Stability and external rotation of humerus	Infraspinatus, teres minor, posterior deltoid (C, I)	
	Scapular stability	Subscapularis, serratus anterior (C, I)	
	Adduction of scapulae	Rhomboids and mid trapezius (C, I)	
	Supporting posture in mid back, downward pull of scapulae	Lower trapezius (C, I)	
Upper arm	Elbow flexion	Triceps brachii, posterior deltoid (E, I)	
Lower arm	Forearm pronation	Pronator teres and quadratus (C, I)	
	Wrist hyperextension	Extensor carpi radialis brevis and longus, extensor carpi ulnaris (C, I)	
Hand and fingers	Wrist stability	Flexor carpi radialis and ulnaris, palmaris longus (C, I)	
	Finger extension	Extensor digitorum, extensor digiti minimi brevis (C, I)	
	Finger abduction	Abductor pollicis longus, opponens pollicis (C, I)	
Neck	Neck extension	Splenius capitus and cervicis, suboccipitals, semispinalis, upper trapezius (I)	

C = concentric contraction, E = eccentric contraction, I = isometric contraction.

Urdhva Mukha Shvanasana

Upward-Facing Dog

[oohr-dhuh-vuh moo-KUHSH-vuhn-AAH-suh-nuh]

Urdhva in Sanskrit means upward, *mukha* is face, and *shvana* is a dog. The stretch in this pose resembles the way a dog stretches its hindquarters.

DESCRIPTION

While this posture resembles Bhujangasana (Cobra Pose), it is different in that the entire body is lifted off the ground and supported on the palms and tops of the feet. The spinal extension is deeper in Urdhva Mukha Shvanasana and more strength is needed to maintain the openness in the chest and shoulders.

BENEFITS

- Strengthens the spine, arms, and wrists
- Opens the chest
- Increases circulation to the lungs and abdomen
- Increases spinal range of motion
- Improves posture
- Stretches the abdomen and hip flexors
- Strengthens the legs and hips

CAUTIONS

pregnancy—Women past the first trimester should use a substitute posture such as Durga-Go (Cat and Cow Pose).
low back or injury—Students with low back pain or injuries should use Bhujangasana as a substitute pose.
wrists—If a student has a history of wrist problems or complains of wrist pain, use a prop or modify the pose.

VERBAL CUES

- From a prone position with the chin resting on the floor, or from Chaturanga Dandasana (Four-Limbs Staff Pose), stretch the legs away from the hips. Bring the hands down closer to the waist, spread your fingers, and press the palms into the floor.
- Inhale and press the tops of the feet down as you begin to lift the chest and shoulders off the floor.
- Straighten the arms and lift the crown of the head toward the sky. Lift the hips and legs off the floor.
- Continue to focus on your breath.
- Roll the front of the shoulders open by squeezing the shoulder blades together, and keep as much length as possible through the low back. Draw the shoulder blades down toward the hips.
- Maintain length in the neck and take your focus upward. Do not drop the back of the head onto the back.
- To exit this position, bend the elbows and slowly lower the body back to the floor while lengthening through the crown of the head.

ADJUSTMENTS

feet—Remind the student not to curl the toes under, but to flatten the top of the feet on the floor.

legs—The legs should remain close together, active, and lifted off the floor. If the student's hips, knees, and calves (legs) are touching the floor, straddle the student's legs and place your hands under the thighs. Support the student's weight and instruct the student to contract the leg muscles.

pelvis—If the pelvis is not tucked under, the low back will be in a great deal of lordosis (swayed low back). Squat behind the student and place your hands on the sides of the torso or the ribcage. Guide the ribcage gently upward and slightly back toward you to help create more space in the low back.

hands—Remind students to align the hands under the shoulders.

chest—The chest should be positioned forward of the arms. Squat to one side of the student and place one hand between the shoulder blades. Encourage the student to press forward and up through the chest.

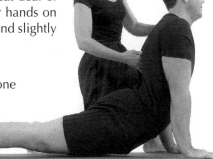

Adjustment: chest.

neck—If the student's shoulders are hunched up toward the ears the student should not attempt to look up. Cue the student to lower the shoulders and then stretch the chin up toward the sky. You can place one hand with the palm against the base of the student's skull and your fingers pointed toward the spine to encourage more length through the back of the neck.

MODIFICATIONS

extreme weakness—To build strength, have students practice Bhujangasana before attempting this pose.

building strength—Allow the student to keep the lower legs on the floor and work on lengthening the spine.

tight hip flexors or low back—Place blankets or a bolster under the student's hips and encourage the student to press the hips and upper thighs down while lengthening the spine upward.

KINEMATICS

Many students new to yoga confuse this posture with Bhujangasana. They will extend the arms fully but keep the legs and hips on the floor. Generally, this position creates too much hyperextension in the lumbar spine, so suggest they come down to Bhujangasana and work on lengthening the spine.

Urdhva Mukha Shvanasana

Body segment	Kinematics	Muscles active	Muscles released
Foot and toes	Toes in extension against floor	Extensor digitorum longus and hallucis, anterior tibialis, flexor digitorum and hallucis longus, posterior tibialis (C, I)	
Lower leg	Ankle in plantar flexion but actively dorsiflexing	Anterior tibialis, extensor digitorum longus, peroneals (C, I)	
Thigh	Knee extension	Quadriceps (C, I)	
Hip and pelvis	Hip extension and hyperextension	Hamstrings, gluteus maximus (C, I)	Iliopsoas, rectus femoris
	Hip stability	Deep external rotators,* adductors (C, I)	
Torso	Torso stability	Rectus abdominis, internal and external obliques, transverse abdominis (I)	Rectus abdominis, obliques
	Spinal hyperextension	Erector spinae, quadratus lumborum (C, I)	

(continued)

Urdhva Mukha Shvanasana *continued*

Body segment	Kinematics	Muscles active	Muscles released
Shoulder	Flexion of humerus, stability	Pectoralis major, coracobrachialis, biceps brachii (C, I)	
	Arm stability	Latissimus dorsi, teres major (C, I)	
	Stability and external rotation of humerus	Infraspinatus, teres minor, posterior deltoid (C, I)	
	Adduction of scapulae	Rhomboids and mid trapezius (C, I)	
	Supporting posture in mid back, downward pull of scapulae	Lower trapezius (C, I)	
Upper arm	Elbow extension	Triceps brachii (C, I)	Biceps brachii, brachialis, brachioradialis
Lower arm	Forearm pronation	Pronator teres and quadratus (C, I)	
	Elbow extension	Anconeus (C, I)	
	Wrist hyperextension	Extensor carpi radialis brevis and longus, extensor carpi ulnaris (C, I)	
	Wrist stability	Flexor carpi radialis brevis and longus, extensor carpi ulnaris (C, I)	
Hand and fingers	Finger extension	Extensor digitorum, extensor digiti minimi brevis (C, I)	
	Finger abduction	Abductor pollicis longus, opponens pollicis (C, I)	
Neck	Slight neck hyperextension and stability	Splenius capitus and cervicis, suboccipitals, semispinalis, upper trapezius (I)	Sternocleidomastoid, scalenes

*Obturator externus and internus, gemellus superior and inferior, quadratus femoris, and piriformis.

C = concentric contraction, E = eccentric contraction, I = isometric contraction.

Shalabhasana

Locust Pose

[shuh-luhb-HAAH-suh-nuh]

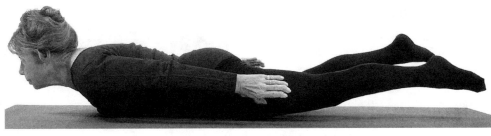

Shalabha is Sanskrit for locust or grasshopper. The posture is said to resemble a locust as it rests on the ground, with the legs higher than the front of the body.

DESCRIPTION

In Shalabhasana, the body is prone with the legs lifted off the floor. There are two major variations of this posture and both strengthen the back of the body.

BENEFITS

- Strengthens the low spine
- Strengthens the posterior hip and thigh muscles
- Stretches the abdominal cavity
- Opens the shoulders and chest
- Stimulates circulation in the abdomen and chest

CAUTION

pregnancy—Because the belly is on the ground, this posture should not be practiced after the second trimester of pregnancy.

VERBAL CUES

- From a prone position with the chin resting on the floor, extend the tops of the feet against the floor. Arms are at your sides.
- Feel the crown of the head lengthen away from the feet. Stretch the arms down toward the feet.
- Exhale and lift the head, chest, and legs off the floor. The abdomen and front of the pelvis remain on the floor.
- Press the chest forward and stretch the feet away from the body. Feel your body lift and lengthen slowly as you breathe deeply. Keep length in the low spine.
- Breathe deeply and feel the muscles throughout the back half of your body working to maintain the lift in the legs and torso.
- To exit the position, exhale and slowly lower the chest, head, and legs back to the floor.

ADJUSTMENTS

feet—If the student is not pressing through the feet actively, tap the ball of the foot to cue the student to stretch out through the ends of the toes.

legs—The knees should be extended and the hips slightly hyperextended. Remind the student to contract the muscles of the legs and stretch the legs down away from the hips.

shoulders—Stand behind the student, straddling the back, and place your hands on the upper arms. Rotate the student's shoulders externally, and remind the student to lengthen the spine.

MODIFICATIONS

building strength—Have students practice Ardha Shalabhasana (Half-Locust). The chin remains on the floor and one leg is lifted up at a time.

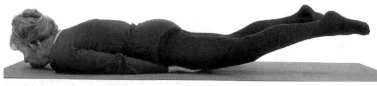
Modification: deeper variation.

deeper variation—Cue students to start in Shalabhasana, and to keep the chin on the ground and place the forearms under the front of the hips and thighs for support. Lift one or both legs into the air as high as is comfortably challenging.

KINEMATICS

The degree of hyperextension in the spine is dependent on the strength of the spinal and hip extensor muscles as well as the flexibility of the oppositional abdominal and hip flexor muscles.

Shalabhasana

Body segment	Kinematics	Muscles active	Muscles released
Foot and toes	Toe abduction	Dorsal interossei, abductor digiti minimi brevis, abductor hallucis (C, I)	
	Toe flexion	Flexor digitorum longus and brevis, flexor hallucis longus (C, I)	
Lower leg	Ankle plantar flexion	Gastrocnemius, soleus (C, I)	Anterior tibialis, extensor digitorum longus
Thigh	Knee extension	Quadriceps (C, I)	
	Slight thigh adduction	Tensor fascia lata (C, I)	
Hip and pelvis	Hip hyperextension	Hamstrings, gluteus maximus (C, I)	Iliopsoas, rectus femoris
Torso	Spinal hyperextension	Erector spinae, quadratus lumborum (C, I)	Rectus abdominis, obliques
	Rib and chest elevation	Pectoralis minor (C, I)	
	Torso stability	Internal and external obliques, transverse abdominis (I)	
Shoulder	Arm hyperextension	Latissimus dorsi, posterior deltoid, triceps brachii	Pectoralis major, anterior deltoid
	External rotation	Infraspinatus, teres minor, posterior deltoid (C, I)	
	Scapular adduction	Rhomboids and mid trapezius (C, I)	
Upper arm	Elbow extension	Triceps brachii (C, I)	Biceps brachii, brachialis, brachioradialis
Lower arm	Forearm supination	Supinator (C, I)	
	Arm extension	Anconeus (C, I)	
	Wrist extension	Extensor carpi radialis brevis and longus, extensor carpi ulnaris (C, I)	
Hand and fingers	Finger extension	Extensor digitorum, indicis, and digiti minimi; lumbricales manus; interossei dorsales (C, I)	
	Finger adduction	Interossei palmaris, adductor pollicis (C, I)	
Neck	Neck extension and stability	Splenius capitus and cervicis, suboccipitals, semispinalis, upper trapezius (I)	

C = concentric contraction, E = eccentric contraction, I = isometric contraction.

Bow Pose

[dhuh-noor-AAH-suh-nuh]

Dhanu is a bow in Sanskrit, like a bow and arrow. The torso represents the bow, and the arms signify the action of the bowstring by pulling the head and the feet closer together.

DESCRIPTION

Dhanurasana is a moderate to deep backbend. The knees are bent and the arms reach back toward the lifted feet.

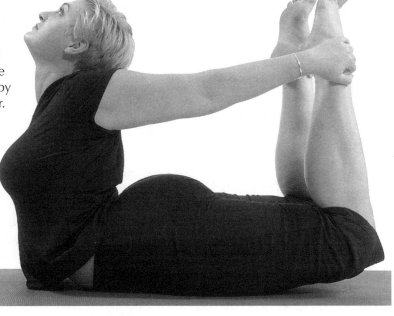

BENEFITS

- Stretches the entire front of the body
- Strengthens the spine
- Opens the shoulders, chest, and throat
- Stimulates circulation in the abdomen and anterior of the pelvis
- Strengthens the lungs

CAUTIONS

pregnancy—This pose is not recommended for women after their first trimester.

acute low back injuries, high blood pressure, heart problems—Students with these health problems are not advised to practice this pose.

VERBAL CUES

- From a prone position with the chin resting on the floor, bend the knees so the lower legs are perpendicular to the floor.
- Inhale and extend the hands back toward the feet while lifting the chest off the floor. Wrap the hands around the outside of the feet or ankles. Press the front of the pelvis toward the floor to lengthen the low back.
- Squeeze the shoulder blades together to open the front of the shoulders and chest.
- Exhale and lift the front of the thighs off the floor as you reach the feet toward the sky. Maintain the lift and openness in the chest and shoulders.
- With each inhalation, lift the crown of the head up, pressing the chest forward and lengthening the low back.
- Feel your breath as your abdomen presses against the floor.
- To exit the position, exhale and release the hands gently from the feet and lower the legs and chest back to the floor.
- Balasana (Child's Pose), is a good counter stretch.

ADJUSTMENTS

feet—If the student's toes are not pointed down toward the knees, lightly tap the feet to cue the student to activate them more.

knees—The knees should be no wider than hip-width apart. If the student points the knees too far out to the sides, gently press the knees toward each other. Also, the knees should not be flexed more than 90 degrees. If they are, generally the elbows are flexed as well, so remind the student to keep the arms straight.

shoulders—If the student has difficulty lifting through the front of the chest, stand behind the student and rotate the shoulders externally as you gently lift the student's upper torso.

MODIFICATIONS

strength building—Have students first practice Ardha Dhanurasana (Half-Bow) by lifting one leg at a time while keeping the torso on the ground. This helps build strength gradually in the legs and low spine. As the students build strength over time, they can begin to practice lifting both legs and then move to lifting the torso as well.

tight shoulders—If the student cannot reach back to the feet comfortably, place the end of a strap in each hand and wrap it around the front of the ankles.

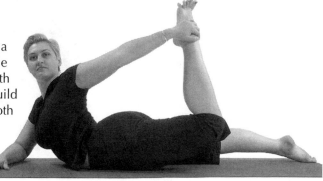

Modification: strength building.

deepen the shoulder stretch—Instead of placing the palms around the outsides of the ankles or feet, instruct the student to place the palms against the arches of the feet with the thumbs aligned with the big toes. This position increases the external rotation of the shoulders more actively.

KINEMATICS

Because the entirety of the body weight is borne by the abdominal cavity in Dhanurasana, individuals new to practicing the posture may find that the heart rate increases because of the increased pressure on the deep blood vessels such as the vena cava. For students able to grasp their ankles, lifting the thighs off the floor is accomplished more by contracting the quadriceps concentrically, than from the concentric contraction of the hip extensors. The two sets of opposing muscles work together to create the "bow".

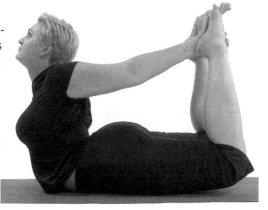

Modification: deepen the shoulder stretch.

Dhanurasana

Body segment	Kinematics	Muscles active	Muscles released
Foot and toes	Toe extension	Extensor digitorum longus, extensor hallucis longus, tibialis anterior (C, I)	
Lower leg	Ankle plantarflexion	Gastrocnemius, soleus	Anterior tibialis, extensor digitorum longus (C, I)
Thigh	Knee flexion	Hamstrings (C, I)	Quadriceps
Hip and pelvis	Initial hip hyperextension	Hamstrings, gluteus maximus (C, I)	Iliopsoas, rectus femoris
	Active hip hyperextension	Quadriceps (C, I)	
Torso	Spinal hyperextension	Erector spinae, quadratus lumborum (C, I)	Rectus abdominis
	Rib and chest elevation	Pectoralis minor (C, I)	
	Torso stability	Internal and external obliques, transverse abdominis (I)	
Shoulder	Humerus hyperextension	Latissimus dorsi, posterior deltoid, triceps brachii (C, I)	Pectoralis major, anterior deltoid
	External rotation	Infraspinatus, teres minor, posterior deltoid (C, I)	
	Scapular adduction	Rhomboids and mid trapezius (C, I)	
Upper arm	Elbow extension	Triceps brachii (C, I)	
Lower arm	Forearm pronation	Pronator teres and quadratus (C, I)	
	Elbow extension	Anconeus (C, I)	
Hand and fingers	Wrist extension	Extensor carpi radialis brevis and longus, extensor carpi ulnaris (I)	
	Finger flexion	Flexor digitorum, extensor digiti minimi brevis, dorsal interossei (I)	
	Finger adduction	Interossei palmaris, adductor pollicis (I)	
Neck	Neck hyperextension	Splenius capitus and cervicis, suboccipitals, semispinalis, upper trapezius (C, I)	

C = concentric contraction, E = eccentric contraction, I = isometric contraction.

Bridge Pose

[sey-TOO buhn-DHAAH-suh-nuh]

Setu is a Sanskrit term for a bridge or dam. A *bandha* is a lock. The shape of the body resembles a bridge.

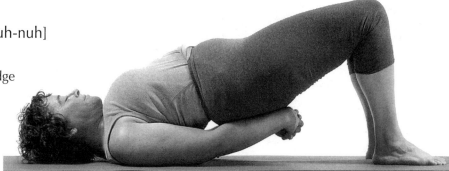

DESCRIPTION

Setu Bandhasana is a relatively easy back-bending posture because the head, neck, and top edges of the shoulders remain on the floor while the knees are flexed with the feet flat on the floor. The body resembles a bridge, and the energy in the body is locked in because the neck and chin press together (jalandhara bandha) to lock in the energy much like a dam acts to lock in water.

BENEFITS

- Opens and expands the chest
- Strengthens the mid and upper spine
- Helps alleviate symptoms of mild depression
- Stretches the torso
- Increases circulation to the thyroid gland
- Energizes the legs
- Relieves low back tightness
- Aids in alleviating menstrual and menopausal discomfort

CAUTION

neck pillows—The use of neck pillows should be avoided in this posture.
pregnancy—This pose should not be practiced after the second trimester.

VERBAL CUES

- From a supine position, bend the knees and bring the heels toward the hips, with the feet hip-width apart and parallel. Reach the hands toward the heels.
- Tuck the pelvis under to lengthen the low back against the floor. Press the backs of your shoulders against the floor, and lengthen the back of your neck.
- Inhale to lengthen and energize the body. Exhale, peel the hips and back off the floor. Lift the front of the hips and abdomen up toward the sky. Press your chest up toward your chin.
- Interlace your fingers together under your back. Squeeze your elbows and shoulder blades together, lifting the chest even higher.
- Continue to focus on your breath.
- With each inhalation, feel the chest and ribs open more fully. On each exhalation, press the feet more firmly against the floor.
- To exit the position, unclasp the fingers and bring the arms back to the sides. Exhale and slowly lower the spine back to the floor, one vertebrae at a time, from the top to the bottom. Rest the spine against the floor and allow all the muscles to relax.

ADJUSTMENTS

feet—The feet should be hip-width distance apart and parallel to each other. If the toes turn in or out, gently tap the outsides of the student's feet to cue the student to align the feet properly.

knees—If the student points the knees laterally from the body, lightly move the knees closer to parallel with your hands.

hips and low back—If the hips are not lifted higher than the chest and knees, place a strap around the student's hips at the sacral level. Stand facing the student's knees in a slight lunge with your front

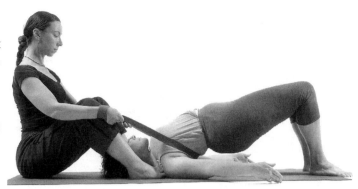

Adjustment: chest.

foot between the student's feet. As you hold on to the ends of the strap, lean back, straightening your front leg and gently lifting the student's hips upward.

chest—If the chest sinks down between the shoulders, place a strap around the student's upper torso under the scapulae. Hold the ends of the straps in your hands and semisquat a few inches away from the student's head. Lean back and lift the student's chest and ribcage up and toward you. For more comfort on your part, sit down on the floor in front of the student's head, and place your feet against the person's shoulders. As you pull the student's chest toward your body with the strap, your feet anchor the person's shoulders to the floor.

If no strap is available, instruct the student to take the feet slightly wider than hip width. Sit facing the student's calves with your knees bent and place your hips just between their feet, or close enough to reach the wrists. Place the balls of your feet between the student's shoulder blades and press gently as you lean back, drawing their hands toward you slightly. Make certain the movement is slow and smooth.

MODIFICATIONS

pregnancy or weakness—Place folded blankets under the student's low back and hips. You also can place a block under the sacrum for the student to rest on. This allows the abdomen and chest to stretch, but without the work.

low back discomfort—If the student has some slight tightness in the lumbar area, instruct the student to lift the heels off the floor to relieve some of the muscular activity in the back.

deepen the pose—Instruct the student to draw the heels closer to the hips and grasp the ankles. This increases the stretch through the thighs as well as allows for a greater arc throughout the length of the spine.

KINEMATICS

Because the neck remains on the floor in this posture, it can be used as a preliminary step in building the range of motion in the neck and shoulders that is necessary for Salamba Sarvangasana (Supported Shoulderstand).

Setu Bandhasana

Body segment	Kinematics	Muscles active	Muscles released
Foot and toes	Toe abduction	Dorsal interossei, abductor digiti minimi brevis, abductor hallucis (I)	
	Toe flexion (pressure into ground)	Flexor digitorum and hallucis longus, flexor digitorum brevis (C, I)	
Lower leg	Ankle dorsiflexion, stability	Anterior tibialis, extensor digitorum and hallucis longus (I)	
Thigh	Knee flexion	Hamstrings (C, I)	Quadriceps
	Slight adduction	Adductors (I)	
Hip and pelvis	Hip hyperextension	Gluteus maximus, hamstrings (C, I)	Iliopsoas, rectus femoris
Torso	Spinal hyperextension	Erector spinae, quadratus lumborum (C, I)	Rectus abdominis
	Rib and chest elevation	Pectoralis minor (C, I)	
	Torso stability	Internal and external obliques, transverse abdominis (I)	
Shoulder	Humerus hyperextension	Latissimus dorsi, teres major, posterior deltoid, triceps brachii (C, I)	Pectoralis major and minor, anterior deltoid, serratus anterior
	External rotation	Infraspinatus, teres minor, posterior deltoid (C, I)	
	Scapular adduction and depression	Rhomboids and mid and lower trapezius (C, I)	
Upper arm	Elbow extension	Triceps brachii (C, I)	
Lower arm	Forearm pronation	Pronator teres and quadratus (C, I)	
	Elbow extension	Anconeus (C, I)	
Hand and fingers	Finger adduction	Adductor pollicis, flexor pollicis longus and brevis, interossei (C, I)	
	Finger flexion	Flexor digitorum, extensor digiti minimi brevis, dorsal interossei (C, I)	
Neck	Neck flexion, jalandhara bandha	Sternocleidomastoid, scalenes, hyoids (C, I)	Cervical erector spinae, splenius capitus and cervicis, upper trapezius

C = concentric contraction, E = eccentric contraction, I = isometric contraction.

Urdhva Dhanurasana

Upward Bow Pose

[oohr-dhuh-vuh dhuh-noor-AAH-suh-nuh]

Urdhva means upward or backward in Sanskrit, and *dhanu* is bow. The name signifies an upward bow and is sometimes also called Urdhva Mukha Dhanurasana (Upward-Facing Bow). Another much-used name for this position is Chakrasana [chuk-RAAH-suh-nuh]. *Chakra* is a wheel (also the name for the energy centers in the body in chapter 5). The shape of the body in Urdhva Dhanurasana can be said to resemble the roundness of a wheel. However, generally, Chakrasana signifies a backward somersault, which is used in a vinyasa flow.

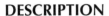

DESCRIPTION

Urdhva Dhanurasana is a full backbend where the hands and feet support the body, and the abdomen faces up toward the sky.

BENEFITS

- Increases flexibility and range of motion in the spine
- Strengthens the shoulders, arms, wrists, legs, and spine
- Opens the chest and shoulder girdle
- Relieves symptoms of asthma by expanding the lungs
- Increases energy

CAUTIONS

shoulder or wrist problems, low back injury—Students with these health concerns should practice with modifications.

glaucoma or high blood pressure—Those with glaucoma or high blood pressure are advised against practicing this pose.

VERBAL CUES

- From a supine position on the floor, bend the knees and bring the heels as close as comfortable toward the hips. Bend your elbows and squeeze them toward each other so that they are parallel and pointing up. Place the palms of your hands on the floor under your shoulders with your fingers pointing toward your feet.
- Lengthen the spine against the floor for two to three breaths.
- Feel your feet and hands pressing firmly against the floor. As you inhale, lift the body slightly and place the crown of your head to the floor. Place as much weight on your head as is comfortable, no more.
- Inhale to open the chest and lengthen the low back. Exhale and straighten your arms, lifting your head and upper torso from the floor. Maintain the alignment in your elbows.
- Continue pressing through your arms and lift your hips off the floor, coming into a full backbend.

- Continue to focus on your breath.
- Feel your spine lengthen and maintain equal balance between your feet and hands.
- To exit the posture, exhale and slowly lower your body back to the floor, vertebra by vertebra, by bending the knees and then the elbows.

ADJUSTMENTS

feet—Make certain that the student's feet are hip-width apart and parallel to each other. Remind the student to keep the feet active.

knees—The knees should have a slight bend in them. If the knees point laterally from the body, lightly move the student's knees closer to parallel with your hands. The student must not allow the knees to touch each other.

hips and low back—If the hips are not lifted, place a strap around the student's hips at the sacral level. Stand facing the student's knees in a slight lunge with your front foot between the student's feet. As you hold on to the ends of the strap, lean back, straightening your front leg and gently lifting the student's hips upward.

mid and upper spine and chest—The chest should be lifted and positioned opposite the lower legs. If the chest sinks down between the shoulders, place a strap around the student's scapulae (shoulder blades). Stand facing the student's head and begin in a lunge position, holding the ends of the strap in your hands. Lean back and lift the student's chest and ribcage up and forward. Use caution with this adjustment so as not take the student off balance.

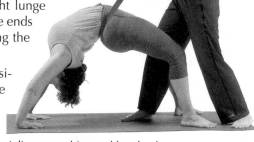
Adjustment: hips and low back.

shoulders—Use extreme caution when adjusting students' shoulders in Urdhva Dhanurasana! The shoulders should be rotated externally; however, because the student's body is upside down and facing away from you it sometimes is confusing as to which direction you should attempt to roll the student's arms. Face the student's head and place your hands on the upper arms, with your thumbs closest to the head. Roll the student's arms so that your thumbs move toward you and the student's elbows move toward the student's body. Moving the arms in the opposite direction can cause injury to the student's shoulders.

neck—Do not touch the student's neck in this posture. Verbally cue the student to relax the neck and to keep length between the ears and shoulders.

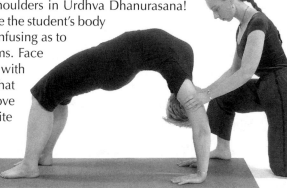
Adjustment: shoulders.

MODIFICATIONS

arm weakness—If the student has difficulty straightening the elbows, allow the student to remain with the head on the floor and work to maintain parallel elbows. To focus more energy into pressing through the arms, a strap can be placed around the arms just above the elbows to keep the arms together.

limited spinal range of motion and significant weakness—Lay the student over an exercise ball with the feet and hands on the floor. This prop supports the spine and lengthens the torso.

deepening the posture—Students can deepen the posture by entering the asana from a standing position. This also builds strength in the abdominal muscles.

KINEMATICS

The closer the hands are to the feet, the more challenging the posture will be. Sufficient range of motion is needed through the torso to remain comfortable in the posture. Also, external rotation in the shoulder joint is very important in retaining joint stability.

Urdhva Dhanurasana (Lifting Up From a Supine Position)

Body segment	Kinematics	Muscles active	Muscles released
Foot and toes	Toe abduction	Dorsal interossei, abductor digiti minimi brevis, abductor hallucis (I)	
	Toe flexion (pressure into ground)	Flexor digitorum and hallucis longus, flexor digitorum brevis (C, I)	
Lower leg	Ankle plantarflexion, stability	Gastrocnemius, soleus, anterior tibialis, extensor digitorum and hallucis longus (I)	
Thigh	Knee flexion	Hamstrings, stability (C, I)	Quadriceps
	Thigh adduction, stability	Adductors (C, I)	
Hip and pelvis	Hip hyperextension	Gluteus maximus, hamstrings (C, I)	Iliopsoas, rectus femoris
Torso	Spinal hyperextension	Erector spinae, quadratus lumborum, rectus abdominis (C, I)	
	Torso stability	Internal and external obliques, transverse abdominis (I)	Rectus abdominis
	Sternoclavicular stability	Subclavius (I)	
Shoulder	Humerus hyperflexion, stability	Pectoralis major, anterior deltoid (I)	Latissimus dorsi, pectoralis major and minor
	External rotation	Infraspinatus, teres minor, posterior deltoid (C, I)	
	Scapular stability	Serratus anterior, subscapularis (C, I)	
	Scapular adduction	Rhomboids and mid trapezius (C, I)	
Upper arm	Elbow extension, stability	Triceps brachii (C, I)	Biceps brachii, brachialis, brachioradialis
Lower arm	Forearm pronation	Pronator teres and quadratus (C, I)	
	Forearm extension	Anconeus (C, I)	
	Wrist hyperextension	Extensor carpi radialis brevis and longus, extensor carpi ulnaris (C, I)	
Hand and fingers	Finger extension, stability	Extensor digitorum, extensor digiti minimi brevis (C, I)	
	Finger abduction	Abductor pollicis longus, opponens pollicis (C, I)	
Neck	Neck hyperextension	Sternocleidomastoid, scalenes (E)	Sternocleidomastoid, scalenes

C = concentric contraction, E = eccentric contraction, I = isometric contraction.

Raja Kapotasana

Royal Pigeon Pose

[RAAH-juh kuh-poht-AAH-suh-nuh]

Raja means royal in Sanskrit. *Kapota* is a pigeon or dove. The pose is named for the way the chest "puffs" out like a pigeon.

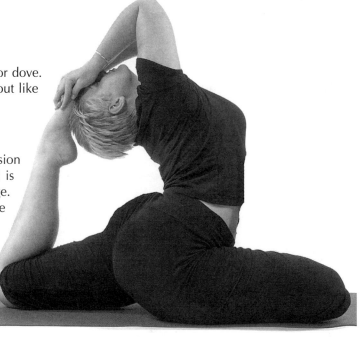

DESCRIPTION

Raja Kapotasana has three basic variations. The version practiced most commonly is "Baby Pigeon" and is more of a prone posture that comes after a lunge. The outside of the front leg is placed with the knee flexed against the floor and the trailing leg is extended straight back with the front of the leg on the floor. The torso is folded forward over the bent knee.

The second variation begins in the same position as "Baby Pigeon;" however, instead of folding forward over the front leg, the torso is upright and arching back and the head and hands reach back toward the back foot. This variation is generally called Raja Kapotasana or Eka Pada Raja Kapotasana (One-Legged Royal Pigeon).

Although it is not illustrated in this book, the third variation of Kapotasana is practiced in the second series of Ashtanga practice. This posture is a completely supine backbend where the lower legs, elbows, and head remain on the floor; the hips and torso are lifted in a backbend; and the hands reach for the feet under the body.

BENEFITS

- Opens the hips and chest
- Lengthens the hip flexors and external rotators
- Stabilizes the hips
- Stimulates and stretches the abdominal organs

CAUTION

knee or hip injuries—Those with knee or hip problems should not practice this posture.

VERBAL CUES

Variation 1: "Baby Pigeon"

- Starting with the weight on the hands and knees, inhale and lengthen the spine. Move the crown of the head and tailbone as far from each other as possible.

- Exhale and bring your right knee to your chest. Place your right foot on the floor to the outside of your left leg and bring your right knee to the outside of your right hand. Lower the outside of the right leg down to the floor.

- Stretch your left leg back behind you and lower your hips to the ground. Point the tailbone down toward the floor to lengthen the low back.

- Inhale and stretch the chest and head toward the sky. Look up.
- Exhale and begin to move your hands forward away from your body. Your hands should be shoulder-width apart, and the right knee should extend to the outside of the right shoulder. This helps release the hip muscles without straining the knee.
- Continue lengthening the upper body forward, breathing deeply to release the muscles.
- To exit from this position, press your hands into the floor and slowly walk your hands back toward your body as you raise your torso. When your hands are under your shoulders, press down and lift the hips off the floor and move back onto your hands and knees.

Variation 2: Raja Kapotasana (Royal Pigeon)

- From Baby Pigeon, with the torso perpendicular to the floor, focus on lengthening the spine and lifting the ribcage away from the hips.
- Bend your left knee to lift the left foot off the floor. Exhale and reach your hands back and grasp the left foot or ankle.
- Inhale deeply and puff your chest out like a pigeon to lift your ribcage even more. Gaze upward and arch back as much as you feel comfortable.
- Continue to focus on your breath.
- Maintain the length in your low back as you continue to lift the chest.
- To exit this position, slowly release the left foot. Maintain control of the left leg so the foot does not drop quickly to the floor. Bring the hands back to the floor and press down to lift the hips off the floor and move back onto your hands and knees.

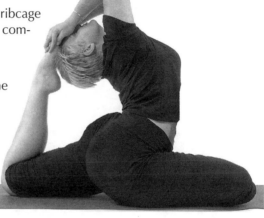

ADJUSTMENTS

feet—The foot behind the student should be relaxed, with the top of the foot against the floor. Instruct students to relax both feet.

knees—The extended knee should be square to the ground and not rotating outward. If the knee rotates externally, it is generally because the bent-leg hip is tight (see modifications). If the student is able to keep the hips on the floor but feels discomfort on the knee, place a folded towel under the knee for support.

hips—If the student's hips are not level, place your hands on the hips while kneeling behind the student. Guide the hips gently into alignment with the shoulders. If the top of the pelvis is not level, place a blanket under the bent-leg hip.

lumbar spine—Cue the student to press the tailbone toward the floor. Kneel beside the student, and place your hands on the low spine and press gently in the direction of the sacrum to encourage length in the back.

shoulders—Remind the student to create length between the shoulders and ears. Place your hand gently on the shoulders to cue the student to lower them down.

MODIFICATIONS

tight hips—Place a rolled blanket or a block under the hip of the bent leg to bring the top of the pelvis level.

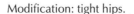

Modification: tight hips.

deepen Raja Kapotasana into Parivrtta Kapotasana (Twisted Pigeon)—Cue students as follows: From Baby Pigeon with the right leg bent forward, cross the left elbow to the outside of the right thigh. Press both palms together in front of the chest and turn the head to look over the right shoulder. The hips should maintain contact with the floor during the twist. Adjust by kneeling behind the student with one hand on the closest shoulder and your other hand on the student's ribcage. Use your hands to gently help the student rotate around farther.

Modification: deepen into Parivrtta Kapotasana.

KINEMATICS

A significant number of people have overly tight external hip rotators and have difficulty sitting comfortably in Raja Kapotasana. The posture can be modified with some type of bolster under the bent-leg hip; otherwise, the student is placed at risk for injuring the knee. The risk is even greater if the student places the weight of the upper body on the bent-leg thigh.

The following table illustrates the kinematics of Raja Kapotasana. In this version of Kapotasana, the stretch in the torso and back quadriceps is more intense.

Raja Kapotasana (Right Knee Bent)

Body segment	Kinematics	Muscles active	Muscles released
Foot and toes	Toe extension	Extensor digitorum and hallucis longus, anterior tibialis (C, I)	
Lower leg (R)	Ankle dorsiflexion, inversion	Anterior tibialis, extensor digitorum longus (C, I)	
Lower leg (L)	Ankle plantar flexion, stability	Anterior tibialis, extensor digitorum longus, peroneals (C, I)	
Thigh (R)	Knee flexion	Hamstrings, sartorius (C, I)	
Thigh (L)	Knee flexion	Hamstrings (C, I)	
Hip and pelvis (R)	Hip flexion	Iliopsoas (C, I)	Adductors, gracilis
	Femoral abduction	Gluteus medius and minimus (C, I)	
	Initial femoral external rotation	Adductors, sartorius (E, R)	
	Femur external rotation	Deep external rotators* (I, R)	
Hip and pelvis (L)	Hip hyperextension	Hamstrings, gluteus maximus (C, I)	Iliopsoas, quadriceps
Torso	Spinal hyperextension	Erector spinae, quadratus lumborum (C, I)	Rectus abdominis
	Rib and chest elevation	Pectoralis minor (C, I)	
	Torso stability	Rectus abdominis, internal and external obliques, transverse abdominis (E, I)	
Shoulder	Humerus flexion	Pectoralis major, anterior deltoids (C, I)	
	Stability and external rotation of humerus	Infraspinatus, teres minor, posterior deltoid (C, I)	
	Scapular stability	Subscapularis, serratus anterior (C, I)	
	Scapular adduction	Rhomboids, mid trapezius (C, I)	
	Supporting posture in mid back, downward pull of scapulae	Lower trapezius (C, I)	
Upper arm	Elbow flexion	Biceps brachii, brachialis, brachioradialis (C, I)	Triceps brachii
Lower arm	Wrist flexion	Flexor carpi radialis and ulnarus, palmaris longus (C, I)	
Hand and fingers	Finger flexion	Flexor digitorum profundus and superficialis, flexor pollicis longus (C, I)	
Neck	Neck hyperextension	Sternocleidomastoid, scalenes (E)	

*Obturator externus and internus, gemellus superior and inferior, quadratus femoris, and piriformis.

C = concentric contraction, E = eccentric contraction, I = isometric contraction, R = relaxed.

Ushtrasana

Camel Pose

[oosh-TRAAH-suh-nuh]

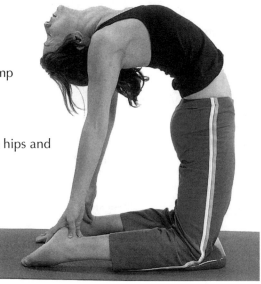

Ushtra is Sanskrit for camel. The arch of the body represents the hump of a camel's back.

DESCRIPTION

Ushtrasana is a kneeling backbend. The openness that occurs in the hips and shoulders is a good precursor to more demanding backbends.

BENEFITS

- Opens the shoulders and chest
- Strengthens the mid back and posterior shoulder muscles
- Stretches the abdominal cavity
- Increases circulation to the throat area
- Lengthens the hip flexors
- Stretches the fronts of the ankles
- Increases awareness of alignment

CAUTIONS

back or neck problems—Students with back or neck difficulties should practice modifications.

high blood pressure—Those with high blood pressure are advised to use modifications.

VERBAL CUES

- Start in a kneeling position with the knees hip-width apart. Curl the toes under so the heels are lifted.
- Place your hands on your hips and squeeze the elbows and shoulder blades together. Press your hands against the top of your pelvis to push the hips slightly forward. Your thighs should be perpendicular to the floor.
- Inhale and lift the ribs and chest as you press your pelvis forward a little more.
- Reach your right hand behind you toward your right heel. Slowly reach your left hand to your left heel. Your thumbs should point away from your body.
- Continue to focus on your breath.
- Press your hands into your heels. With your next inhalation, relax your neck, allowing your head to drop back. Continue to maintain length in the neck as you gaze upward.
- If you are comfortable in this position, lower the tops of your feet flat against the floor.
- To exit this position, inhale deeply and imagine being lifted up by your chest. Move slowly and bring the torso upright. Bring your hips to your heels and your upper body to the floor into Balasana (Child's Pose).

ADJUSTMENTS

feet—Remind students to curl the toes under and lift the heels. This positioning also stretches the arches.

knees—If the student begins with the knees wider than hip-width apart, instruct the student to move the knees closer together before moving into the posture.

hips—The hips must be aligned directly over the knees. As students reach for the feet, they often neglect to press the pelvis forward. Stand or kneel beside the student and place your closest hand on the student's spine at the level of the lower ribs. Press the ribcage and spine upward while moving the student's pelvis into alignment with the knees. Another option is to place a strap around the base of the student's spine. Then, while standing in front of the student, pull the student toward you with the strap.

spine—If the student's low spine is collapsing, place your hand on the student's low back and instruct the student to move the body away from your hand.

shoulders—The shoulders should be rotated externally and down away from the ears. Instruct the student to press firmly through the arms for length. To aid in external rotation, stand or kneel behind the student and place your hands on the shoulders with your thumbs closest to you. Roll the student's arms so that the shoulders come closer together.

chest—The chest should be higher than the shoulders. Stand beside the student and place your hand between the shoulder blades; instruct the student to lift up away from your hand.

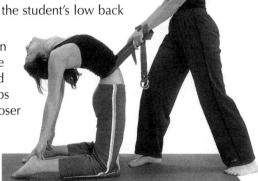

Adjustment: hips.

MODIFICATIONS

neck discomfort—If the student is not comfortable dropping the head back, instruct the student to tuck the chin into the chest. This modification should be used for those with high blood pressure.

tight hip flexors—If the student has difficulty bringing the hands to the feet without dropping the hips back, cue the student to place the hands on the back of the pelvis and squeeze the elbows and shoulder blades in while pressing the pelvis forward. This modification aids in building more flexibility in the tops of the thighs.

upper spine weakness and tight chest—You may need to assist the student in lifting the upper spine and ribcage. Before the student arches back, sit behind the student and place the ball of one of your feet on the mid to upper back. Clasp the student's wrists in your hands and instruct the student to grasp your wrists. As the student inhales, gently press forward against the back while holding the student's arms. As the student exhales, instruct the student to move the pelvis forward and relax the shoulders and neck. This action is a Thai-yoga therapy technique to open the student's chest and shoulders while the instructor supports the weight.

Modification: tight hip flexors.

abdominal weakness—Assist the student in exiting the posture. Standing in a semisquat position behind the student, place your hands between the student's shoulder blades with your fingers pointing down. As the student inhales, gently press up on the shoulder blades as the student lifts up.

KINEMATICS

With the toes hyperextended, the arch of the foot is stretched as the body weight is moved over the heels. Some students may find such positioning fairly uncomfortable at first, but you should encourage them to practice this positioning to benefit the structures of the feet.

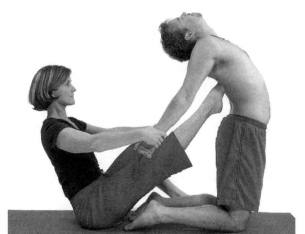

Modification: upper-spine weakness and tight chest.

Ushtrasana

Body segment	Kinematics	Muscles active	Muscles released
Foot and toes	Toe hyperextension	Extensor digitorum longus and hallucis, anterior tibialis, flexor digitorum and hallucis longus, posterior tibialis (C, E, I)	Plantar fascia, flexor digitorum and hallucis longis, posterior tibialis
	Foot stability	Extensor digitorum longus and hallucis, anterior tibialis, flexor digitorum and hallucis longus, posterior tibialis (I)	
Lower leg	Ankle in dorsiflexion, stability	Anterior tibialis, extensor digitorum longus, peroneals (C, I)	Gastrocnemius and soleus
Thigh	Knee flexion, stability	Hamstrings (C, I)	Quadriceps
Hip and pelvis	Hip hyperextension, stability	Iliopsoas, rectus femoris (E, I)	Iliopsoas, rectus femoris
	Hip stability	Hamstrings, gluteus maximus (C, I)	
	Stability	Deep external rotators,* gluteus medius (I)	
Torso	Torso stability	Rectus abdominis, internal and external obliques, transverse abdominis (E, I)	Rectus abdominis, obliques
	Spinal stability	Erector spinae, quadratus lumborum (I)	
Shoulder	Adduction of scapulae	Rhomboids, mid trapezius (C, I)	Pectoralis major and minor, anterior deltoid, subscapularis, serratus anterior
	External rotation and stability	Infraspinatus, teres minor, posterior deltoid (C, I)	
	Hyperextension and adduction of humerus	Latissimus dorsi, teres major (C, I)	
Upper arm	Elbow extension (also aids in hyperextending humerus)	Triceps brachii (C, I)	Biceps brachii, brachialis, brachioradialis
Lower arm	Forearm supination	Supinator (C, I)	
	Wrist hyperextension	Extensor carpi radialis brevis and longus, extensor carpi ulnaris (C, I)	
Hand and fingers	Finger flexion	Flexor digiti minimi brevis, interossei palmaris, flexor pollicis brevis (C, I)	
Neck	Neck hyperextension	Sternocleidomastoid, scalenes (E, I)	Sternocleidomastoid, scalenes

*Obturator externus and internus, gemellus superior and inferior, quadratus femoris, and piriformis.

C = concentric contraction, E = eccentric contraction, I = isometric contraction.

Supta Virasana

Reclining Hero Pose

[SOOP-tuh veer-AAH-suh-nuh]

Supta in Sanskrit means reclining or lying down. *Vira* is a hero, chief, warrior, or champion. In Latin, *virilis* means man. It is interesting to note that in the great Hindu epic, the *Mahabharata,* and in the *Legend of King Arthur,* a man's secret strength, power, and virility resides symbolically in the thighs.

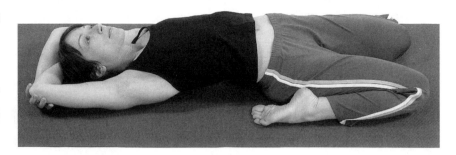

DESCRIPTION

Supta Virasana is a supine posture where the knees are bent and the lower legs are tucked under or to the outside of the thighs. This posture provides an excellent stretch for the quadriceps.

BENEFITS

- Lengthens the quadriceps and iliopsoas
- Increases circulation in the legs
- Can help prevent varicose veins
- May help alleviate sciatica
- Gently stretches the abdomen and helps with digestion
- Opens the chest
- Increases flexibility in the ankles and feet
- Helps relieve menstrual discomfort

CAUTIONS

serious knee or back problems—This pose may be practiced with modifications if the student is uncomfortable in the pose.

pregnancy—Due to the hormone-induced laxity in the tendons and ligaments in pregnancy, the reclining version of Virasana should not be practiced past the first trimester.

VERBAL CUES

- From a kneeling position with the shins and tops of the ankles against the floor, slowly lower your hips down between your ankles. Make certain that you find a comfortably challenging position and do not go deeper than that.
- Place your hands on the floor in front of your toes. Inhale and press down firmly through your arms to lengthen the torso.
- Exhale and slowly bend one elbow at a time so your forearms come to the ground. As you breathe, continue to lengthen the ribcage away from your hips. Lower your chin to your chest if you are comfortable.
- As your legs relax, extend one arm at a time out to your sides, lowering your torso a little closer to the floor. Your breath should be smooth and steady.
- If you are comfortable, lower your shoulders and head to the floor. Listen to your body and be sure to avoid any strain in your knees or back.

- Continue to focus on your breath.
- If you are comfortable with your entire back and head resting on the floor, reach your hands over your head, interlacing your fingers.
- To exit this posture, bring your elbows in to the sides of your waist. Press your elbows into the ground and lift your shoulders off the floor. Keep your neck relaxed. Press your hands into the floor and straighten one arm at a time. Leading from your chest, slowly lift the torso upright, from the bottom to the top, and raise your head last.

ADJUSTMENTS

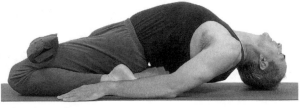

ankles—If the student cannot comfortably rest the tops of the feet on the floor, place a small cushion or rolled-up towel under the ankles.

Adjustment: knees.

knees—Before the student lowers the body to the floor, be sure that the knees are no more than hip-width distance apart. Wrap a strap around the legs to keep the knees together, or place a rolled towel between the knees and instruct the student to squeeze the towel. Another adjustment is to face the student and place your hands on the student's mid thighs and rotate the muscles externally to help the knees align and relax. If the student's knees lift up from the floor slightly, place a weighted sandbag or other weighted prop on the lower thighs to hold the knees down.

low back—If the student's back arches up away from the floor, instruct the student to stretch the tailbone down toward the knees. Ask the student to lift the knees off the floor and press the low back to the floor. Then instruct the student to slowly lower the knees back down.

abdomen—If a student's abdomen is sinking, place a lightweight sandbag prop on the abdomen and instruct the student to keep the bag lifted.

chest—The chest should remain lifted up and not collapsed. Lightly touch the student's upper sternum with one finger, and instruct the student to push your hand up.

MODIFICATIONS

building flexibility and awareness—Have the student practice Ardha Supta Virasana (Half-Reclining Hero Pose). In this variation, only one knee is flexed under the body; the other is extended forward. Practice each side.

tightness in the feet, ankles, or knees—Place blankets or a block under the student's hips to support the body weight, taking pressure off the feet, ankles, and knees.

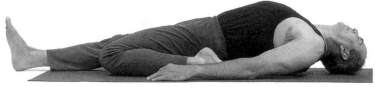

overly arched lumbar spine—Place blankets under the student's hips and shoulders to encourage the low back to relax.

tight hip flexors—If the student is unable to rest the torso on the floor without the knees lifting

Modification: building flexibility and awareness.

off the floor, place blankets under the shoulders to raise the student's chest and encourage the legs to relax.

KINEMATICS

It may appear to be contraindicated to practice Supta Virasana with knee conditions because of the extreme flexion of the knee and the pull of the body weight. However, with the guidance of a qualified yoga therapist or instructor, practice may actually help alleviate some of these conditions. The focus of the posture is to increase the strength and flexibility in the knee joint by way of modifications and props.

Supta Virasana

Body segment	Kinematics	Muscles active	Muscles released
Foot and toes	Toe extension	Extensor digitorum longus (I)	
Lower leg	Ankle plantarflexion	Gastrocnemius, soleus (I, R)	Anterior tibialis, peroneals
	Ankle inversion	Posterior tibialis (C, I)	
Thigh	Knee flexion	Quadriceps (E, R)	Quadriceps
Hip and pelvis	Hip and pelvis extension	Iliopsoas, rectus abdominis (E, R)	Iliopsoas, rectus femoris
Torso	Trunk stability	Internal and external obliques, transverse abdominis (E, I)	Rectus abdominis
Shoulder	External rotation	Infraspinatus, teres minor, posterior deltoid (C, I)	Pectoralis major
	Humeral flexion (initial)	Anterior deltoid, pectoralis major (C, I)	
	Humeral flexion (final)	Posterior deltoid, triceps brachii (E)	
Upper arm	Elbow extension	Triceps brachii (C, I)	
Lower arm	Forearm pronation	Pronator teres and quadratus (C, I)	
	Elbow extension	Anconeus (C, I)	
Hand and fingers	Finger adduction	Adductor pollicis, flexor pollicis longus and brevis, interossei (C, I)	
	Finger flexion	Flexor digitorum, extensor digiti minimi brevis, dorsal interossei (C, I)	
Neck	Neck flexion, jalandhara bandha	Sternocleidomastoid, scalenes, hyoids (C, I)	Cervical erector spinae, splenius capitus and cervicis, upper trapezius

C = concentric contraction, E = eccentric contraction, I = isometric contraction, R = relaxed.

Matsyasana

Fish Pose

[muht-see-YAHH-suh-nuh]

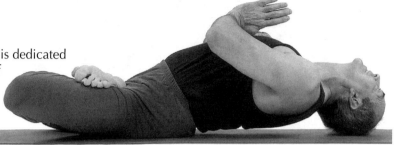

Matsya is a Sanskrit term for fish. This asana is dedicated to Matsya who was the fish incarnation of Vishnu and saved the first man (Manu) and the seven sages from a great flood.

DESCRIPTION

Matsyasana is a supine back-bending posture where the legs, hips, and crown of the head remain on the floor and the chest and ribs are lifted. Traditionally, Matsyasana is practiced with the legs in Padmasana (Lotus Pose). In another, more challenging variation, the arms and legs are lifted in the air.

BENEFITS

- Opens the ribcage and chest
- Aids respiratory ailments
- Gently strengthens the neck
- Increases circulation in the throat
- Stretches the abdomen
- Strengthens the back
- Improves digestion

CAUTIONS

high blood pressure or migraines—Those with high blood pressure or migraines should refrain from practicing this pose.

insomnia—Students who suffer from insomnia should not practice this posture before trying to sleep.

neck injury or severe low back pain—Those with muscle injuries may practice this pose with modifications.

VERBAL CUES

If the student is comfortable practicing Padmasana, begin in that position and rest the back on the floor. If not, follow the instructions from a straight-leg position.

- From an active supine position, with the legs extended and your arms at your sides, bend your elbows and press down into the ground.
- Exhale and lift the chest and shoulders off the floor, supported by the arms. Arch the head back and rest the crown of your head on the floor.
- If your spine is comfortable in this position, place your palms together over the center of your chest in anjali mudra (prayer position).
- Continue to focus on your breath.
- Feel the chest continue to lift and lengthen with your breath. Make sure that the weight on the head is minimal and that the spinal muscles support the upper body.
- To exit the position, bring your arms back to your sides. Exhale and slowly relax the neck and bring the back of the head to the floor. Lower the rest of the torso to the ground slowly.

ADJUSTMENTS

hips—The hips should remain on the floor. If the student presses against the floor and lifts the hips, instruct the student to use the legs as anchors to keep the hips down.

chest—If the chest or ribcage collapses, stand over the student with your feet on either side of the hips. Wrap a strap around the student's back at the level of the shoulder blades. Gently pull up on the strap to lift the student's chest.

head—The crown of the head should be touching the floor, not the back of the head. Instruct the student to press down strongly with the arms to create more lift in the chest and to extend the neck farther until the crown rests on the floor.

MODIFICATIONS

discomfort—If the student is not comfortable in Padmasana, the student can bring the legs into Baddha Konasana (Bound Angle Pose), which helps to open the hips.

straining in posture—If the student's face is strained or red and the breath is labored, place the student in a less demanding posture such as the Setu Bandhasana (Bridge Pose).

neck or low back pain—Place folded blankets or bolsters under the student's shoulders to relieve the back muscles.

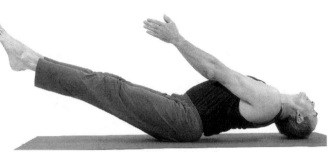

Modification: deepen the posture.

deepen the posture—If the student is comfortable, deepen the posture by lifting the legs and arms up while keeping the crown of the head on the floor. You may need to provide assistance by helping the student to hold the limbs in this position.

KINEMATICS

The crown of the head, not the back of the head, should rest on the floor to eliminate the possibility of straining the neck muscles.

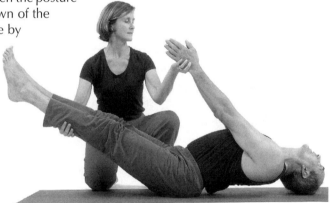

Assist the student in deepening the posture.

Matsyasana

Body segment	Kinematics	Muscles active	Muscles released
Foot and toes	Toe flexion	Flexor digitorum and hallucis longus, flexor digitorum brevis (C, I)	
Lower leg	Plantar flexion	Gastrocnemius, soleus (C, I)	Anterior tibialis, extensor digitorum longus
Thigh	Knee extension	Quadriceps (C, I)	
Hip and pelvis	Hip flexion	Lumbar erector spinae, quadratus lumborum (C, I)	Iliopsoas, rectus femoris
Torso	Trunk stability	Internal and external obliques, transverse abdominis, quadratus lumborum (I)	Rectus abdominis
	Spinal hyperextension	Erector spinae, semispinalis (C, I)	
Shoulder	Scapular adduction	Rhomboids, mid trapezius (C)	Anterior deltoid, pectoralis major and minor
	Humeral hyperextension	Latissimus dorsi, posterior deltoid (C, I)	
Upper arm	Elbow flexion	Biceps brachii, brachialis, brachioradialis (C, I)	
Lower arm	Forearm pronation	Pronator teres and quadratus (C, I)	
	Wrist extension, stability	Flexor digitorum profundus and superficialis (I)	
Hand and fingers	Finger extension and stability	Flexor digitorum profundus and superficialis, flexor digiti minimi, interossei (C, I)	
Neck	Neck hyperextension, stability	Sternocleidomastoid, scalenes (E, I)	Sternocleidomastoid, scalenes
	Neck stability	Cervical erector spinae, splenius capitus and cervicis, upper trapezius (C, I)	

C = concentric contraction, E = eccentric contraction, I = isometric contraction.

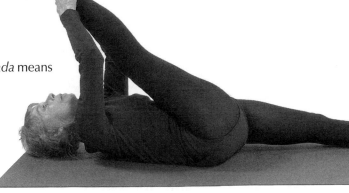

Reclining Hand-to-Toe Pose

[SOOP-tuh paah-daahng-oost-AHH-suh-nuh]

Supta in Sanskrit means reclining, *pada* means foot, and *angustha* means big toe.

DESCRIPTION

Supta Padangusthasana is a supine position where one leg is flexed at the hip and the big toe of that foot is grasped by the same-side hand. This is a transitional asana, performed to move from the more active positions into the relaxing and restorative postures near the end of a session.

BENEFITS

- Stretches the hamstrings and hips without any strain to the back
- Relaxes the spine
- Aids in digestion

CAUTION

pregnancy—Instruct pregnant women to lie on their side instead of their back, and flex the top leg toward the chest.

VERBAL CUES

- From a supine position with the arms to the sides and the legs straight, inhale and lift the right foot up toward the sky. The knee should remain as straight as possible without locking, but be mindful of any discomfort in the low back.

- Reach up with your right hand and grab as close to the right toes as possible, wherever you can reach comfortably. Your shoulders and hips should remain on the floor. Feel your back pressing down and lengthening along your mat.

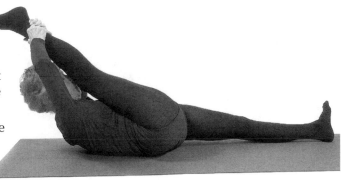

Phase two.

- Inhale deeply. As you exhale next, lift your chest and head up toward your right foot. Send energy through the right heel and point your toes toward your head (phase two).

- As you breathe, allow your abdomen to soften and relax your shoulders.

- Continue to focus on your breath.

- To exit the position, exhale and slowly lower your spine back to the floor. On your next exhalation, release your hands to your sides and slowly lower your leg back to the floor. Notice that your right leg feels longer and more relaxed than your left. Rest for a few breaths, and then prepare to practice on the left side.

ADJUSTMENTS

feet—If the heel of the lifted leg is not higher than the toes, instruct the student to point the toes down toward the head more fully. You can gently press down on the ball of the foot to guide the toes lower.

knee—If the student bends the knee in an effort to grasp the toes, adjust the hands to a position where the student can hold on comfortably or wrap a strap around the foot while maintaining as much knee extension as possible.

hips—If the leg extended on the floor is comfortable, but the leg lifts off the ground, kneel beside the student and press gently on the top of the thigh, near the hip. Do not press near the knee joint. Another option is to instruct the student to hold onto the calf rather than reaching up toward the foot. Then place your foot on the student's upper thigh and apply gentle pressure.

shoulders—The shoulders should remain drawn down away from the ears. Especially when the torso is lifted, students have a tendency to round the shoulders and bring them up toward the ears. Gently place your hands on the tops of the shoulders and guide the shoulders back and down.

neck—Remind the student to keep the ears aligned with the shoulders and not to drop the head back or to bring the chin to the chest. The chin should be held in a neutral position.

MODIFICATIONS

tight hamstrings—If the student is unable to reach the hand to the foot without bending the knee, wrap a strap around the ball of the foot and place the loose ends in the student's hand. Instruct the student to find the place where the student is comfortably challenged, yet still extending the knee.

overly tight spine—Instruct the student to bend the knee of the leg on the ground to take any strain off the low back.

spinal weakness—Place the student with the back on the floor, the hips touching a wall, and the backs of the legs resting against the wall. Instruct the student to move one leg down toward the chest, keeping the knee extended. This reduces the strain on the back while still allowing the hamstring to stretch.

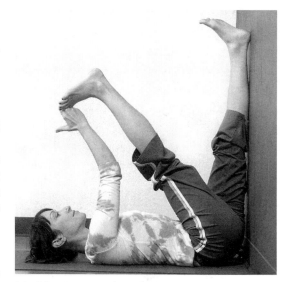

Modification: spinal weakness.

KINEMATICS

The torso resting on the floor at the beginning and ending phase of the posture allows the focus to remain on stretching the hamstrings and hips while the spine remains lengthened. When the posterior shoulder muscles are pressed into the floor, a true measure of hamstring and posterior hip-muscle flexibility is seen, as no flexion occurs in the torso to distort the range of motion, as happens in seated and standing forward bends.

Supta Padangusthasana (Right Hip Flexed)

Body segment	Kinematics	Muscles active	Muscles released
Foot and toes (R)	Toe abduction	Dorsal interossei, abductor digiti minimi brevis, abductor hallucis (C, I)	
	Toe dorsiflexion	Extensor digitorum and hallucis longus, anterior tibialis (C, I)	
Foot and toes (L)	Toe extension	Extensor digitorum and hallucis longus, anterior tibialis (C, I)	
Lower leg (R)	Ankle dorsiflexion	Anterior tibialis, extensor digitorum and hallucis longus (C)	Gastrocnemius, soleus
Lower leg (L)	Ankle dorsiflexion	Anterior tibialis, extensor digitorum and hallucis longus (C, I)	Gastrocnemius, soleus
Thigh (R)	Knee extension	Quadriceps, gracilis (C, I)	
Thigh (L)	Knee extension	Quadriceps (C, I)	
Hip and pelvis (R)	Hip flexion	Iliopsoas, rectus femoris, pectineus (C, I)	Hamstrings, gluteus maximus
Hip and pelvis (L)	Hip extension, stability	Hamstrings, gluteus maximus (C, I)	
Torso	Trunk stability	Rectus abdominis, internal and external obliques, transverse abdominis, quadratus lumborum (C, I)	
Shoulder (R)	Shoulder flexion	Anterior deltoid, pectoralis major (C, I)	
	External humeral rotation	Infraspinatus, teres minor (C, I)	
	Scapular adduction	Rhomboids, trapezius (C, I)	
Shoulder (L)	Shoulder abduction	Deltoids (C, I)	
Upper arm (R)	Elbow extension	Triceps brachii (C, I)	
Upper arm (L)	Elbow flexion	Biceps brachii, brachioradialis (C, I)	
Lower arm (R)	Forearm supination	Supinator (C, I)	
	Elbow extension	Anconeus (C, I)	
Lower arm (L)	Forearm pronation	Pronator teres (C, I)	
Hand and fingers (R)	Wrist extension	Extensor carpi radialis brevis and longus, extensor carpi ulnaris (I)	
	Finger flexion	Flexor digitorum, extensor digiti minimi brevis, dorsal interossei (C, I)	
Hand and fingers (L)	Finger adduction	Interossei palmaris, adductor pollicis (C, I)	
Neck	Neck extension and stability	Splenius capitus and cervicis (I)	

C = concentric contraction, E = eccentric contraction, I = isometric contraction.

chapter 10

Inverted Postures

Inversions are postures not only in which the head is placed below the heart and the weight of the body but also, in whole or in part, is supported by the upper body (shoulders, arms, or head). For this reason, Uttanasana (Intense Forward Bend) is considered a standing pose rather than an inversion. However, keep in mind that many poses share characteristics of more than one category. Inversions demand not only strength but also openness in the shoulders. It is advisable, therefore, to teach students who are not already familiar with inversions a modified version of the posture. You can also instruct students who are new to inversions to hold the posture for only brief periods and then gradually increase the work and time in the position.

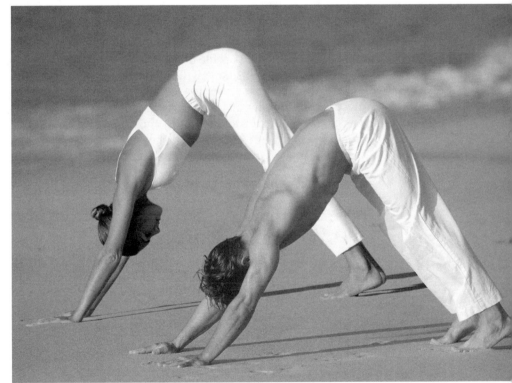

© Jumpfoto

Being upside down provides physical and emotional benefits. It strengthens the veins by increasing demands on the heart and strengthens the integrity of the neck, arms, and torso by requiring the body weight to be supported by the upper body. With proper training and consistent practice a healthy student eventually will gain the ability to support the entire weight of the body on the head, which results in an incredibly strong neck and spine. Balance improves and the effects of gravity, such as sagging, are relieved. Perhaps one of the most profound reasons for practicing inversions beyond simply doing Adho Mukha Shvanasana (Downward-Facing Dog) is for the metaphor of being comfortable when turned upside down! Often the biggest obstacle to learning Salamba Shirshasana (Headstand) is fear, exacerbated by the disorientation that first accompanies being inverted.

Listed next are cautions specific to inversion postures that you must be aware of with regard to certain medical conditions of your students. If other cautions are specific to a particular asana, they are listed in the description section for that asana.

- **glaucoma and detached retinas**—Most of the inversions have some risks for students with glaucoma and detached retinas. If a student is not accustomed to being upside down, the pressure of the circulation suddenly flooding into the head could place pressure on the blood vessels surrounding the eyes. Salamba Sarvangasana (Supported Shoulderstand) and Halasana (Plow Pose) are two inversions where

the head and neck are in a neutral position, and therefore the blood is concentrated in the throat area versus generating pressure in the head and subsequently the eyes.

- **high or low blood pressure**—The inverted postures that raise blood pressure and are therefore contraindicated for students with high blood pressure are as follows: Salamba Shirshasana, Adho Mukha Vrkshasana (Handstand), Pincha Mayurasana (Scorpion), and to some extent Adho Mukha Shvanasana. Postures contraindicated for people with low blood pressure include Salamba Sarvangasana and Halasana.

- **menstruation**—As mentioned in chapter 5, inversions are usually modified during menstruation because during this time part of the woman's energy needs to flow downward.

- **neck and shoulder injuries, extreme spinal weakness**—Depending on the severity of injury to the neck and shoulders, some students might not have the strength to use the muscles that would support the students safely in inversions. If a student cannot muster the strength to use the ideal muscles, then the student will try to compensate with other muscles and injuries can be exacerbated. This concept is true for all the poses, but especially in some of the inversions the results of compensating with the incorrect muscles may be more dramatic. It is more injurious, for example, for a student to twist the neck while falling than to twist the ankle.

Adho Mukha Shvanasana

Downward-Facing Dog

[uhd-HOE moo-KUHSH-vuhn-AAH-suh-nuh]

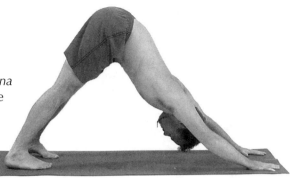

Adho in Sanskrit means downward, *mukha* means face, and *shvana* is dog. This posture is named Downward-Facing Dog because it looks like the pose that a dog strikes when instinctively stretching and sometimes when in a playful mood.

DESCRIPTION

Adho Mukha Shvanasana is practiced on the mat lengthwise with the feet and the hands pushing against the ground and the hips lifted high in the air. This posture is actually considered a resting posture, but for many just starting out in yoga it can be quite challenging because it requires a considerable amount of strength in both the upper and lower body. The restful, rejuvenating effects become apparent after practice. This posture is part of the Sun Salutations (Surya Namaskaras) series.

BENEFITS

- Builds strength and stability in the shoulders
- Stretches the hamstrings and deeper calf muscles that other stretches usually cannot
- Stretches, strengthens, and improves circulation in the legs, making this posture especially beneficial for runners
- Rejuvenates the whole body
- Builds foundation for other inversion postures
- Relaxes the heart
- Can balance menstrual and menopausal discomfort

CAUTIONS

shoulder dislocation—If a student has a tendency to dislocate the shoulders, do not emphasize the external rotation of the shoulders. Instruct the student to focus on keeping the arms as straight and comfortable as possible. See modifications for ways to build stability and strength.

wrist injury—Those with injury or weakness in the wrists should practice this posture with modifications.

pregnancy—Women past the first trimester or new to the pose and pregnant should practice with modifications.

VERBAL CUES

- From Bhujangasana (Cobra Pose), curl your toes under and as you exhale straighten your arms to lift your upper body. Then press your hips up and back as far as possible.
- Relax your neck or look up at your belly. Press your shoulders away from your hands and your ears toward your hips.
- Press your hands into the floor so as to push the earth away from you. Your hands should be shoulder-width apart with the fingers spread.
- Turn the backs of your upper arms toward the ground. Feel the shoulders and chest open and the spine lengthen with greater traction. Create more space between the vertebrae with each breath.
- Press your thighbones back and reach your heels away from your toes, then toward the floor. Do not worry if they cannot touch the floor, just focus on lengthening your legs and lifting your tailbone.
- As you breathe in, feel your chest and spine lengthen toward the apex of your tailbone. Feel the work of your hands and arms along with the weight of your head provide traction to your spine, creating more space between each vertebrae.

- To exit this position in the Classical Sun Salutation, step one foot forward between your hands, coming into a lunge.
- To exit this position in an Ashtanga Sun Salutation, walk or jump both feet forward between your hands into Uttanasana (Intense Forward Bend).
- Otherwise, flow into another posture. If you need to rest, bend your knees to the ground and relax in Balasana (Child's Pose).

ADJUSTMENTS

hips—Stand behind the student and place each of your hands to the outsides of the hip joint where the legs and hips connect. Stand in a semilunge to use your legs instead of your back or arms, and lift the student's hips higher and pull or lean back. The whole torso of the student's body should elongate. The arms will be relieved of some workload and they will feel more relaxed. Make certain that your own body mechanics are sound; bend your knees and use your body weight rather than the strength of your back to pull the student's body.

spine—If the student's upper spine is rounded, perform the adjustment just described for the hips. You can also stand to the student's side and place your palm lightly between the student's shoulder blades with your fingers pointed toward the hips. Gently move your hand in and up in the direction of the pelvis, encouraging the student to lengthen the spine.

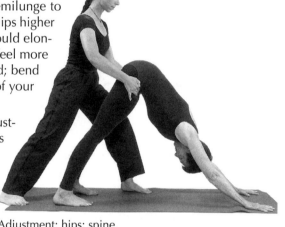

Adjustment: hips; spine.

neck—Make sure the student's neck is relaxed. Cue the student to lower the crown of the head toward the floor. Place a hand gently on the back of the neck to encourage the student to lower the head. This adjustment is frequently needed. Brush your fingers gently along the neck to the shoulders imparting the message that the shoulders should stay far away from the ears thus keeping the neck long.

shoulders—Encourage the student to rotate the shoulders externally. Note: Because the student is upside down, it may be challenging for you to recognize the correct direction in which to adjust. It is crucial that you rotate the arms in the correct direction. Stand or squat down facing the student's head. Place your hands on the student's upper arms (distal) just below the shoulders with your thumbs closest to the head. Very slowly rotate both of the student's arms so your thumbs move away from each other. Make certain that the student keeps pressing the palms firmly and securely into the floor.

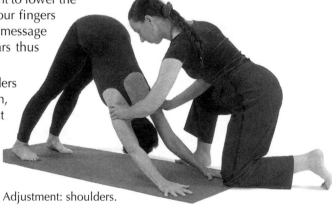

Adjustment: shoulders.

hands—The student must have the hands shoulder-width apart with the fingers spread and pointed away from the body. Cue the student to press the palms down by lightly pressing on the tops of the student's hands with your hands or toes.

fingers—Each finger should be spread and as active as possible. Check to see that students' fingers are level with the ground. Some students' fingers may seem to be rolling or rotating (usually when this occurs the fingers and hands are rolling outward from the middle). Lightly brush or straighten those fingers to a point where the student still feels comfortable and the fingers are rolled down evenly and square. Often, it is effective to tell the student to press down more with the thumbs and index fingers. This action will allow the student to work the hands and arms in a more balanced way versus keeping the entire arm rotated. By pressing down on the thumbs and index fingers the lower arms almost turn in while the upper arms externally rotate.

MODIFICATIONS

arm, wrist, or shoulder weakness—Instruct the student to bend the elbows and place the forearms on the floor. This positioning is actually more challenging for the shoulder joint, but for anyone who cannot support the body weight fully with the arms, this is a good modification. This position is often considered a pose in and of itself, and is called Dolphin Pose.

hip, hamstring, or back tightness—Allow the student to bend the knees slightly while still pressing the hips up. Bending the knees slightly makes it easier to lift the hips. You can also have the student move the feet wider apart, which helps with balance.

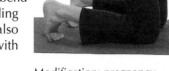
Modification: pregnancy.

pregnancy, extreme weakness or tightness in the upper extremities—Have the student face a wall with the hands on the wall at shoulder height. The student then moves the body arms-length away from the wall while keeping the hands in place. Instruct the student to bend at the hip joint so the hips are over the feet. Tell the student to push (or you can pull) the hips behind the student as far as is comfortable. The spine is now free to suspend, opening the shoulders and chest. The head can be relaxed between the upper arms. Another alternative pose is Durga-Go (Cat and Cow Pose).

fatigue—Because this posture is physically demanding, many students will not be able to stay in the posture for long. Encourage such students to rest in Balasana (Child's Pose).

KINEMATICS

The arms and legs gain considerable strength from practicing this posture. Tightness in the anterior-shoulder muscles and chest combined with weakness in the posterior-shoulder muscles and upper back lead to a constriction of the nerve and blood vessel plexus supplying the arms and wrists. Therefore, if a student complains of carpal tunnel syndrome and numbness or pain in the wrists, a major contributing factor may be due to the imbalance in the upper body. Adho Mukha Shvanasana is an excellent posture to balance the shoulders and back and also open the chest.

Adho Mukha Shvanasana

Body segment	Kinematics	Muscles active	Muscles released
Foot and toes	Toe extension, stability	Extensor digitorum and hallucis longus, flexor digitorum longus, and flexor hallucis longus (C, I)	
	Toe abduction, stability	Dorsal interossei, abductor digiti minimi brevis, abductor hallucis (C, I)	
Lower leg	Ankle dorsiflexion	Anterior tibialis, extensor digitorum, and hallucis longus (C, I)	Gastrocnemius, soleus
Thigh	Knee extension	Quadriceps (C, I)	Hamstrings
Hip and pelvis	Hip flexion	Iliopsoas, rectus femoris (C, I)	Gluteus maximus, deep external rotators*
	Hip internal rotation	Adductors, gluteus medius, gluteus minimus (C, I)	
	Pelvic stability	Rectus abdominis, quadratus lumborum, hamstrings (I)	
Torso	Trunk stability	Internal and external obliques, rectus abdominis, transverse abdominis, quadratus lumborum, erector spinae (I)	Erector spinae, quadratus lumborum

(continued)

Adho Mukha Shvanasana *continued*

Body segment	Kinematics	Muscles active	Muscles released
Shoulder	Humerus flexion and hyperflexion, stability	Pectoralis major, coracobrachialis, deltoids, biceps brachii (C, I)	Pectoralis major, latissimus dorsi, levator scapulae
	Scapular stability and external rotation of humerus	Infraspinatus, teres minor, posterior deltoid (C, I)	
	Joint stability	Subscapularis, supraspinatus (C, I)	
	Scapular stability	Rhomboids, mid trapezius (I)	
	Scapular stability and downward pull of scapulae	Lower trapezius (C, I)	
	Scapular stability and abduction	Serratus anterior, teres major (C, I)	
	Sternoclavicular stability	Subclavius (I)	
Upper arm	Elbow extension, stability	Triceps brachii (C, I)	Biceps brachii, brachialis, brachioradialis
Lower arm	Forearm pronation, stability	Pronator teres, quadratus (C, I)	Flexor carpi radialis and ulnaris, palmaris longus
	Wrist hyperextension, stability	Flexor carpi radialis and ulnaris, palmaris longus (E, I)	
Hand and fingers	Finger extension, stability	Extensor digitorum, extensor digiti minimi brevis (C, I)	
	Finger abduction	Abductor pollicis longus, opponens pollicis (C, I)	
Neck	Neck relaxed	None	Cervical erector spinae, splenius capitus and cervicis

*Obturator externus and internus, gemellus superior and inferior, quadratus femoris, and piriformis.

C = concentric contraction, E = eccentric contraction, I = isometric contraction.

Supported Shoulderstand

[saah-LUM-buh sahr-vaahng-AAH-suh-nuh]

Sa is Sanskrit for with, and *alamba* means support. *Sarva* means all, and *anga* means limb. This pose is one where almost all of the body weight is supported by the upper body. The shoulders and upper spine support the legs (limbs) instead of the legs giving firm support to the back, which is normal in standing upright poses like Tadasana (Mountain Pose). Salamba Sarvangasana has variations that are unsupported such as Niralamba [neer-aah-LUM-buh]. Shoulderstand is often considered the queen of all asanas because it is active and restorative at the same time.

DESCRIPTION

In Salamba Sarvangasana, the student's shoulders are on the floor or a prop with the arms behind the student and the hands on the back to provide greater lift to the body. The neck remains resting on the floor.

The queen of poses

BENEFITS

- Soothes the nervous system and the mind and helps relieve stress and mild depression
- Stimulates the thyroid
- Aids in digestion
- Stretches the shoulders and neck
- May relieve menopausal symptoms
- Can reduce fatigue and alleviate insomnia
- May be therapeutic for asthma, infertility, and sinusitis

- reversed gravity.
- varicose veins/spider veins
-

CAUTION

acute neck or shoulder injuries—Practice with modification or substitute another asana.

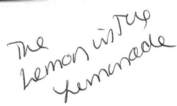

The lemon in the lemonade

VERBAL CUES

- From a supine position, exhale and bend your knees to your chest. Roll back, if you can, so that your hips lift up in alignment with your shoulders.
- Keep your elbows shoulder-width apart on the ground. Place your hands on your back as close to the floor or prop as possible.
- Straighten the legs up in the air and bring your legs, hips, and shoulders into alignment as much as possible by pressing your chest in toward your chin.
- With each inhalation, open the chest and shoulders more so that the spine continues to lift.
- Tuck your tailbone and feel your legs working as if you were in Tadasana.
- To exit this pose, bend your knees and roll down slowly onto the floor onto your back. Use your hands and arms against the ground and do not tense or lift your neck.
- Another option is to bend from your hips into Halasana (Plow Pose), then slowly lower to the floor.

never turn the neck in this pose!

ADJUSTMENTS

chest—Many students can get into the pose but are not able to get the body straight or to lift well. If the student's chest is collapsing, stand to the student's back and hold on to the legs. Wrap your arms around the student's hips or upper legs, or grasp the ankles with both hands. Lift the student's legs straighter while pressing your lower leg into the student's back to lengthen it.

elbows—To aid in straightening the spine the elbows should be as close together as possible. You can assist the student by holding onto the legs as they squeeze the elbows closer. Stand behind the student and use your feet to help slide the arms together.

MODIFICATIONS

difficulty lifting torso—Place folded blankets under the student's shoulders so that the head touches the floor and the shoulders rest on the blankets. This modification helps lift the spine higher and helps stretch the neck more effectively.

balance problems—If the student has difficulty balancing and lengthening the spine, place folded blankets against a wall so that the student's torso is on the floor and the hips and legs are against the wall. Instruct the student to place the feet flat against the wall and "walk" up so that the body weight is placed at the top of the shoulders. When comfortable, the student can move the legs away from the wall.

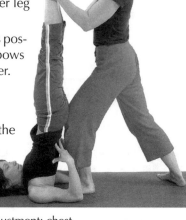

Adjustment: chest.

assistance with shoulderstand prop—The student rests supine on the shoulderstand prop with the back of the head on the floor. There are grips in the prop where the student can hold on to help the student lift the body from the leverage of the arms and shoulders.

KINEMATICS

Salamba Sarvangasana is an excellent posture to gently loosen the neck and shoulder joints. In addition, because of the gentle pressure on the thyroid gland, this asana helps to balance the function of the gland and also helps to lower blood pressure.

Modification: assistance with shoulderstand prop.

Salamba Sarvangasana

Body segment	Kinematics	Muscles active	Muscles released
Foot and toes	Toe extension	Extensor digitorum and hallucis longus, anterior tibialis (C, I)	
Lower leg	Plantar flexion	Gastrocnemius, soleus (C, I)	Anterior tibialis, extensor digitorum longus
Thigh	Knee extension	Quadriceps (C, I)	
	Femur adduction	Adductors (C, I)	
Hip and pelvis	Hip extension	Hamstrings, gluteus maximus (C, I)	
	Hip stability	Iliopsoas (I)	
Torso	Torso stability	Rectus abdominis, internal and external obliques, transverse abdominis (I)	
	Spinal extension and stability	Erector spinae, quadratus lumborum (C, I)	
Shoulder	Humerus hyperextension, stability	Posterior deltoid, triceps brachii, latissimus dorsi, teres major (C, I)	Pectoralis major and minor, anterior deltoid, serratus anterior
	External rotation	Infraspinatus, teres minor, posterior deltoid (C, I)	
	Scapular adduction, depression and stability	Rhomboids, mid and lower trapezius (C, I)	
Upper arm	Elbow flexion	Biceps brachii, brachioradialis, brachialis, (C, I)	
	Arm stability	Triceps brachii (I)	
Lower arm	Forearm supination, stability	Supinator (I)	
	Wrist hyperextension	Extensor carpi radialis brevis and longus, extensor carpi ulnaris (I)	Flexor carpi radialis and ulnaris, palmaris longus
Hand and fingers	Finger extension	Extensor digitorum, extensor digiti minimi brevis (C, I)	
	Finger abduction	Abductor pollicis longus, opponens pollicis (C, I)	
Neck	Neck flexion, stability, jalandhara bandha	Sternocleidomastoid, scalenes, hyoids (C, I)	Cervical erector spinae, splenius capitus and cervicis, upper trapezius

C = concentric contraction, E = eccentric contraction, I = isometric contraction.

Pincha Mayurasana

Scorpion, or Peacock Feather

[PIN-chuh may-oohr-AAH-suh-nuh]

Pincha Mayurasana is generally called Scorpion in English because of the shape of the body in the asana. However, the translation from Sanskrit to English is Peacock Feather. *Pincha* is a feather, and *mayura* is a peacock. The posture also resembles a peacock with its tail feathers spread before its mating dance.

DESCRIPTION

This arm balance works the shoulder-stabilizing muscles as in Salamba Shirshasana (Supported Headstand), but unlike Salamba Shirshasana, the head and neck do not support any body weight. This pose has two common variations: one where the legs are extended straight and one where the spine arches and the legs bend to bring the feet to the head.

BENEFITS

- Strengthens and stabilizes the shoulders and the mid and upper back
- Maintains shoulder flexibility
- Strengthens the low spine
- Stretches and tones the abdominal muscles
- Increases circulation and concentration

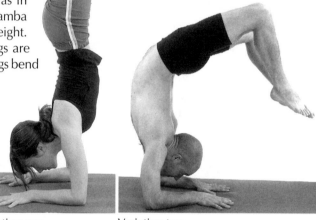

Variation one.   Variation two.

VERBAL CUES

- From Adho Mukha Shvanasana (Downward-Facing Dog), bring your forearms to the ground. Place your palms flat against the floor. Maintain the alignment of your elbows with your shoulders.
- Press firmly down through your elbows. Squeeze your shoulders in the direction of your hips. This action lifts and expands the chest and activates the muscles needed to help you balance.
- Find a gazing point on the ground in front of your hands.
- Remain focused on your gazing point as you begin to walk your feet forward slightly. As your torso moves forward, do not allow your shoulders to move beyond your elbows. Be sure to keep your upper arms perpendicular to the floor.
- Continue to press through the arms and maintain length in your neck. Exhale and slowly raise one leg in the air at a time. Do not kick the legs up; raise them in a controlled manner. This is variation one.
- Continue to focus on the breath.
- For variation two, if you are comfortable in variation one, you can bend your knees and arch your back slightly so that your feet move closer to your head. Maintain the length in your low back. Do not let your chin drop toward your chest. Keep focus on your drishti (gazing point).
- To exit this position, exhale and bring your legs slowly back to the ground. Fold your body into Balasana (Child's Pose) and relax.

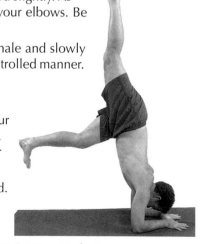

Entering Pincha Mayurasana.

268

ADJUSTMENTS

elbows—Make sure the student's elbows are shoulder-width apart and not splaying out to the sides. Before the student begins to balance, squeeze the elbows toward each other with your hands or wrap a strap around the upper arms. A block against the wall can be used for the first few times if a students is struggling with this pose (see modifications).

head and neck—Remind the student to maintain the head position so that the balance and stability in the shoulders are not compromised.

spotting—Stand to the student's side and catch the legs as the student comes up. Ideally, you want to act like a training wheel for the student not a crutch. Do *not* stand behind the student! The possibility that the student will come crashing down onto your body is very high. Always spot from the side. Assist the student to find and then independently maintain the balance instead of supporting the student in the posture.

MODIFICATIONS

balance issues—Unlike in Salamba Shirshasana, it is appropriate to practice Pincha Mayurasana using the wall as a training wheel.

difficulty maintaining arm positioning—Place a block against the wall and instruct the student to kneel facing the wall with the thumbs pressed against the near side of the block and the index fingers on the lateral sides.

KINEMATICS

If the student positions the elbows wider than the shoulders the foundation of the posture is compromised. A house balanced on stilts that are placed wider than the base of the building will collapse, as will a body on an unstable base.

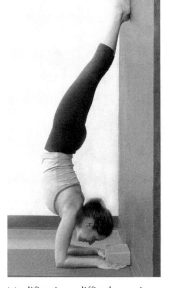

Adjustment: spotting.

Modification: difficulty maintaining arm positioning.

Pincha Mayurasana

Body segment	Kinematics	Muscles active	Muscles released
Foot and toes	Toe extension	Extensor digitorum and hallucis longus, anterior tibialis (I)	
Lower leg	Plantar flexion	Gastrocnemius, soleus (C, I)	
Thigh	Knee flexion	Quadriceps (E, I)	Quadriceps
Hip and pelvis	Hip extension	Hamstrings, gluteus maximus (C, I)	Iliopsoas
	Hip stability	Iliopsoas (E, I)	
Torso	Torso stability, spinal hyperextension	Rectus abdominis, internal and external obliques, transverse abdominis (E, I)	Rectus abdominis, internal and external obliques
	Spinal stability	Erector spinae, quadratus lumborum (C, I)	

(continued)

Pincha Mayurasana *continued*

Body segment	Kinematics	Muscles active	Muscles released
Shoulder	Humerus flexion, shoulder stability	Pectoralis major, coracobrachialis, deltoids, biceps brachii (C, I)	Latissimus dorsi
	Stability	Latissimus dorsi (I)	
	Stability and external rotation of humerus	Infraspinatus, teres minor, posterior deltoid (I)	
	Joint stability	Subscapularis (I)	
	Scapular depression	Subclavius (I)	
	Scapular stability	Rhomboids, and mid trapezius (I)	
	Supporting posture in mid back and downward pull of scapulae	Lower trapezius (C, I)	
	Scapular stability	Serratus anterior (I)	
Upper arm	Elbow flexion	Biceps brachii, brachialis, brachioradialis (C, I)	
	Elbow stability and balance	Biceps and triceps brachii (I)	
Lower arm	Forearm pronation	Pronator quadratus and teres (C, I)	
	Elbow stability	Triceps brachii (I)	
Hand and fingers	Finger extension, stability	Extensor digitorum, extensor digiti minimi brevis (I)	
	Finger abduction	Abductor pollicis longus, opponens pollicis (I)	
	Hand and wrist stability and balance	Flexor carpi radialis and ulnaris, palmaris longus (I)	
Neck	Neck hyperextension	Splenius capitus and cervicis, suboccipitalis, semispinals, upper trapezius (C, I)	Sternocleidomastoid

C = concentric contraction, E = eccentric contraction, I = isometric contraction.

Adho Mukha Vrkshasana

Downward-Facing Tree, or Handstand

[uhd-HOE moo-KUH vrick-SHAAH-suh-nuh]

Adho means downward in Sanskrit, and *mukha* means face. *Vrksha* is a tree. The length and strength in the body resembles that of a tree with the hands as the roots.

DESCRIPTION

Adho Mukha Vrkshasana is the basic handstand, that is, an arm balance where the hands are placed on the ground with the rest of the body straight up in the air. This posture can be practiced against a wall to begin with for those new to the pose or those who feel initially fearful. Once a student has success in the posture, the person should practice without the aid of a wall.

BENEFITS

- Strengthens the shoulders, arms, and wrists
- Opens the chest and ribcage
- Strengthens the abdominal and spinal muscles

VERBAL CUES

- Stand facing a wall approximately two to four feet (about one half to one meter) away. Exhale and fold forward from the hips, placing your hands flat on the floor approximately one to three feet (no more than a meter) from the wall. Make certain that your hands are shoulder-width apart.

- Keep your arms straight as you look toward the floor in front of you, focusing your gaze on a spot between your hands and the wall.

- Exhale and slowly swing the legs up one at a time. If your feet kick into the wall, slowly move them in line with your hips as you balance on your hands.

- Continue gazing toward the wall as you work to spread your toes. Your breath should be as smooth and deep as possible.

- If you feel comfortable in this position, experiment by slowly bringing one foot away from the wall and then the other. Find the edge of your balance by using the wall as a training wheel. Do not strain, but stay with the breath.

- To exit, slowly lower the legs back to the floor one at a time.

ADJUSTMENTS

hand alignment—Make certain that the student's hands are shoulder-width apart. The arms in Adho Mukha Vrkshasana act like stilts under a house. If the arms are aligned with the shoulders the support structure is solid, but if the arms are wider than the shoulders the body above collapses just as a house with stilts would if the stilts were wider than the frame of the house.

assisting or spotting—Stand to the side of the student and use the inside of your arm as a "leg-stop" so that the student does not lose the

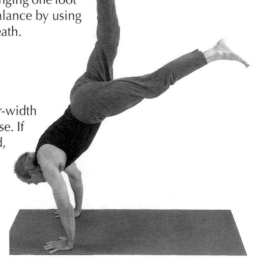

Entering Adho Mukha Vrkshasana.

balance. Do not hold the student's legs so that the student can feel where the proper alignment is. Instead of holding the legs, place your hand in between the student's knees or calves and direct the student to squeeze your hand. As in Pincha Mayurasana (Scorpion), always stand to the side of the student for your own protection.

low back—If the low back is arching, instruct the student to squeeze your hand between the knees (technique described above) and to lift your hand up. Tell the student to feel as if the floor were being pushed away with the hands.

MODIFICATIONS

difficulty maintaining balance—Instruct the student to keep the feet resting against the wall and to focus on gaining the strength in the shoulders and spine to maintain balance.

variations of exit—Instead of bending the hips and lowering the legs to the floor in front of the body, the student may lower the legs behind into a backbend. This variation is only applicable if the student practices away from the wall.

KINEMATICS

Maintaining the elongated hyperextension in the neck helps preserve the openness in the upper chest and also helps to keep the legs from dropping forward.

Adjustment: assisting or spotting.

Adho Mukha Vrkshasana

Body segment	Kinematics	Muscles active	Muscles released
Foot and toes	Toe extension	Extensor digitorum and hallucis longus, anterior tibialis (I)	
Lower leg	Plantar flexion	Gastrocnemius, soleus (C, I)	
Thigh	Knee extension	Quadriceps (C, I)	
Hip and pelvis	Hip extension	Hamstrings (C, I)	
	Hip stability	Iliopsoas (C, I)	
	Hip adduction	Adductors (C, I)	
Torso	Torso stability	Rectus abdominis, internal and external obliques, transverse abdominis (I)	
	Spinal extension and stability	Erector spinae, quadratus lumborum (C, I)	
Shoulder	Humerus flexion, stability	Pectoralis major, coracobrachialis, deltoids (C, I)	Latissimus dorsi
	Stability and external rotation of humerus	Infraspinatus, teres minor, posterior deltoid (C, I)	
	Joint stability	Subscapularis (I)	
	Scapular depression, stability	Subclavius (I)	
	Scapular stability	Rhomboids, and mid trapezius (C, I)	
	Supporting posture in mid back and downward pull of scapulae	Lower trapezius (C, I)	
	Scapular stability	Serratus anterior (C, I)	
Upper arm	Elbow extension, stability	Triceps brachii (I)	
	Arm stability	Biceps brachii, brachialis, brachioradialis (I)	
Lower arm	Forearm pronation	Pronator teres and quadratus (C, I)	
	Forearm extension	Anconeus (C, I)	
Hand and fingers	Wrist hyperextension, stability	Extensor carpi radialis brevis and longus, extensor carpi ulnaris	
	Wrist stability	Flexor carpi radialis and ulnaris, palmaris longus (E, I)	
	Finger extension, stability	Extensor digitorum, extensor digiti minimi brevis (C, I)	
	Finger abduction, stability	Abductor pollicis longus, opponens pollicis (C, I)	
Neck	Neck extension	Splenius capitus and cervicis, suboccipitalis, semispinals, upper trapezius (I)	

C = concentric contraction, E = eccentric contraction, I = isometric contraction.

Headstand

[saah-LUM-buh sheer-SHAAH-suh-nuh]

Salamba Shirshasana is a supported headstand. *Salamba* means with support, and *shirsha* is the head.

DESCRIPTION

Shirshasana is considered the king of all the asanas and, as such, one of the most important asanas in yoga. This supported version of Shirshasana puts the least amount of stress on the head and neck because the forearms and shoulders support the majority of the body weight. The crown of the head is cradled between the hands, and the back of the head rests against the fingers. There are numerous variations of headstands; however, this version is best for building the strength and stamina for all others.

BENEFITS

- Increases stamina and strength in the shoulders, neck, abdominals, and upper spine and helps prevent bone degeneration in these areas
- Creates good posture
- Improves circulation
- Massages the lungs and builds resistance to illness
- Increases energy and body heat
- Increases concentration and balance as it stimulates the pressure points at the sahasrara chakra (crown of the head)

VERBAL CUES

Explain to students that there is a possibility that they will lose balance when they practice Salamba Shirshasana. If they happen to lose balance, the fall is not nearly as painful as they might imagine, especially if they simply allow their bodies to relax on the way down. If, or when, a student begins to fall, cue the student to immediately tuck the chin to the chest. The most important, albeit most difficult, thing they can do is to relax. Also, ask students to make sufficient space between themselves and those around them before they begin.

- From a hands-and-knees position, bring your forearms to the ground in front of your knees. Align your elbows with your shoulders and loosely interlace your fingers. Place the top of your little finger and ring finger against the floor. Release the thumbs so that they do not touch but rest on your index fingers.
- Bend forward and place the crown of your head in your palms. Keep length in your neck so that your shoulders do not hunch toward your ears.
- Straighten your knees, bringing your hips into the air. Your body positioning now resembles Adho Mukha Shvanasana (Downward-Facing Dog) with the forearms on the floor. Pause here for a few breaths and create length in your spine, moving your chest and ribcage away from your arms. See photo 1.
- Lift your heels off the floor and begin to slowly walk your feet toward your face. Maintain the lift and length in the spine, feeling your hips move toward alignment over your shoulders.
- Continue to focus on your breath.
- When your hips are stacked over your shoulders, bend one of your knees to your chest and as you breathe deeply, find your balance on your arms. Gradually, as you are comfortable, bring your other knee toward your chest. Keep both knees bent and balance here. See photo 2.

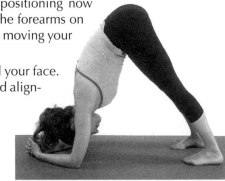

Photo 1.

- When you can remain comfortably balanced with your knees into your chest for five to six breaths, you are ready to extend your legs. For most students this will be after a number of consistent practice sessions. Once a student has sufficient strength, the student can enter the position by slowly raising and straightening both legs up simultaneously.

- Exhale and very slowly straighten your legs. *Do not* kick your legs up! Move slowly and purposefully to maintain your balance. Straighten one leg up at a time if it helps you remain balanced.

- As you breathe in this position, focus on aligning your body in an upside down Tadasana. Roll your thighs in toward each other slightly. Straighten your spine with each inhalation. Press firmly through your elbows to bring strength and stability to your shoulders.

- To exit from this posture, exhale and slowly bring your legs down to the floor. Fold yourself into Balasana (Child's Pose) and rest.

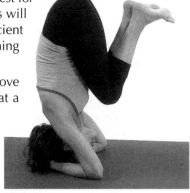

Photo 2.

ADJUSTMENTS

Again, emphasize the importance of moving slowly. Control comes from building strength and coordination in the muscles and using them to lift the legs, rather than using momentum, which generally takes the student out of alignment.

elbows—Make sure the student's elbows are shoulder-width apart and not splaying out to the sides. Before the student begins to balance, squeeze the student's elbows toward each other if necessary.

spine—If the back starts to round as the student brings the feet toward the face while raising the legs, instruct the student to stop in that position. Stand beside the student and place your hand to the rounded spine, and instruct the student to move the spine away from your hand. Cue the student to lengthen the back with each breath.

assisting in the initial balance—Stand to the side of your student in a semisquat position for your own comfort and safety. As the student brings one or both of the knees into the chest, catch the leg(s) to keep the student from rolling over. When you feel that the student is balanced on the arms, slowly remove your hands.

assisting in straight-leg balance—For your protection, stand to the student's side and use the inside of your arm as a "leg-stop" so that the student does not lose balance and roll forward. It is important that you do not hold the legs so that the student can get a feel for where the proper alignment is.

building strength—To aid the student's alignment and strength, place your hand between the knees and cue the student to squeeze your hand as the student lifts your hand up toward the sky. This adjustment teaches the student to lengthen and lift more actively in the posture.

MODIFICATIONS

determined, yet slightly fearful students—If a student is truly building the strength for the balance but feels disappointed in not yet being able to balance in the posture, place the student's back against a wall. Use this modification sparingly so that students do not become dependent on the wall for the balance.

tight shoulders—If the student has difficulty keeping the elbows aligned, a strap can be wrapped around the upper arms to keep the elbows from moving apart. This should be done in the preliminary stages of building the strength and flexibility for this posture.

building more upper-body strength—As the student builds strength in the upper body, the student can practice finding balance by bringing the knees into the chest and focusing on the balance. If the person loses balance, the forward roll comes naturally.

extreme weakness—Instruct the student to practice Adho Mukha Shvanasana to build the strength needed for this posture.

KINEMATICS

It is a common practice for people new to Shirshasana to practice with the back against a wall. Unfortunately, it is highly possible to become dependent on the support the wall provides and never build the proper muscular coordination and balance needed to practice without the wall. With patience and practice, learning to enter and exit this asana not only builds the muscles of the body but also helps to eliminate the fear factor many students feel when they first attempt the asana.

This is an excellent posture to build and maintain vertebral strength in the neck region. Some may argue that the neck is not designed to carry the load of the body; however, in many cultures throughout the world, women carry heavy loads balanced on their heads. Proper postural alignment keeps the load balanced and strengthens the vertebrae and surrounding musculature. In addition, with proper alignment, the intensity of isometric contractions in the torso and legs lessens so the pose becomes more relaxing.

Salamba Shirshasana

Body segment	Kinematics	Muscles active	Muscles released
Foot and toes	Toe extension	Extensor digitorum and hallucis longus, anterior tibialis (I)	
Lower leg	Plantar flexion	Gastrocnemius, soleus (C, I)	Anterior tibialis, extensor digitorum longus
Thigh	Knee extension	Quadriceps (C, I)	
	Femur adduction	Adductors (C, I)	
Hip and pelvis	Hip extension	Hamstrings, gluteus maximus (C, I)	
	Hip stability	Iliopsoas (I)	
Torso	Torso stability	Rectus abdominis, internal and external obliques, transverse abdominis (I)	
	Spinal extension and stability	Erector spinae, quadratus lumborum (C, I)	
Shoulder	Humerus flexion, stability	Pectoralis major, coracobrachialis, deltoids (C, I)	Latissimus dorsi
	Stability and external rotation of humerus	Infraspinatus, teres minor, posterior deltoid (C, I)	
	Scapular abduction and stability	Subscapularis, serratus anterior (I)	
	Scapular depression, stability	Subclavius (I)	
	Scapular stability	Rhomboids, and mid trapezius (C, I)	
	Supporting posture in mid back and downward pull of scapulae	Lower trapezius (C, I)	
Upper arm	Humeral flexion, and shoulder stability	Biceps brachii, brachioradialis, brachialis (I)	
	Stability and balance	Triceps brachii (I)	
Lower arm	Forearm pronation	Pronator quadratus and pronator teres (I)	
Hand and fingers	Wrist stability	Flexor carpi radialis and ulnaris, palmaris longus (E, I)	
	Finger flexion	Flexor digitorum superficialis and profundus; lumbricales manus, interossei palmaris (C, I)	
	Finger adduction	Interossei palmaris, adductor pollicis (C, I)	
Neck	Neck extension and stability	Splenius capitus and cervicis, suboccipitals, semispinals, sternocleidomastoid, scalenes, levator scapulae, upper trapezius (I)	

C = concentric contraction, E = eccentric contraction, I = isometric contraction.

Plow Pose

[huhl-AAH-suh-nuh]

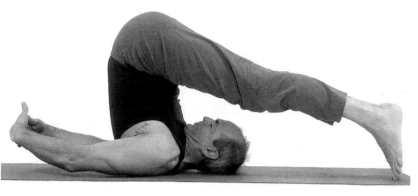

Hala is the Sanskrit word for plow.

DESCRIPTION

In this asana, the tops of the shoulders and neck are on the ground as in Salamba Sarvangasana (Supported Shoulderstand). The spine is as straight as possible but can be rounded in some variations. For the greatest benefit, the spine is totally straight. The hips are flexed with the legs outstretched as the feet rest on the ground behind the head.

BENEFITS

- Stretches the back and shoulders
- Can relieve indigestion
- Promotes sound sleep
- Stimulates the thyroid gland, abdominal organs, and digestion
- Helps relieve menopausal symptoms
- May be therapeutic for certain backaches, headache, infertility, and insomnia

CAUTIONS

asthma and high blood pressure—Practice Halasana with the legs supported on props such as a chair.

pregnancy—Students experienced with this pose may continue to practice it late into pregnancy using props for support. However, it is contraindicated to begin initial practice once pregnant.

back pain or problems—Those with a history of back pain or problems should practice this pose with modifications.

VERBAL CUES

- From Salamba Sarvangasana, exhale and bend one leg from your hip joint, like a hinge, to slowly lower your foot toward the floor beyond your head. Then lower the second leg in the same manner. If you feel completely comfortable and strong, lower both legs at the same time.
- Keep your torso straight and perpendicular to the ground with your legs fully extended as if your legs are in Tadasana (Mountain Pose).
- With your toes on the floor, lift your tailbone toward the ceiling.
- If you feel comfortable in your low back, release your arms from your back and straighten them behind you. Clasp your hands and roll your shoulders open.
- Lift your chest toward your chin (jalandhara bandha).
- Continue to focus on your breath.
- To exit this posture, bring your hands down against the floor. Keep your head and neck completely relaxed. Do not lift your head or tense your neck. Move and breathe slowly.
- Bend your knees and gently begin to roll down the spine while you use the leverage in your arms to help keep your shoulders and head against the ground.
- Pause when your hips first contact the floor and take a couple breaths making sure your whole body is sinking into the ground underneath you.
- Relax your legs the rest of the way to the floor. Take a breath or two and prepare for a counterpose or Shavasana (Corpse Pose).

ADJUSTMENTS

neck and shoulders—Make sure the student's chest is not collapsing, which is prevalent when the upper back is weak or the shoulders and neck are tight. Allow the student to use props (see modifications). Do not let the student have a pillow under the head as this compromises the neck by allowing it to overstretch or strain.

hips—If the hips are rounded and positioned toward the feet rather than aligned with the shoulders, stand behind the student and place your leg against the student's back to guide the student to move the hips more into alignment. You can also use a pole, or even a broomstick to illustrate the length in the spine.

spine—If the back is rounded, sit behind the student facing the student's spine. Hold the student's hands (wrists to wrists works well). Place one of your feet on the student's mid to upper back. Pull the arms back toward you while you push the spine away from you. This action will help elongate and lift the back.

MODIFICATIONS

tight hips or back—If the student has difficulty reaching the feet to the floor, instruct the student to practice this pose with an appropriate prop such as a block, chair, or stacked blankets. If using a chair, brace the back of a chair against a wall. You might need to place a folded sticky mat under the chair legs or on the seat to prevent slipping. The exact distance between the prop and the wall will depend on the student's height (taller students will be farther away, shorter students closer). Instruct the student to lie down on the floor with the head toward to the wall and the prop.

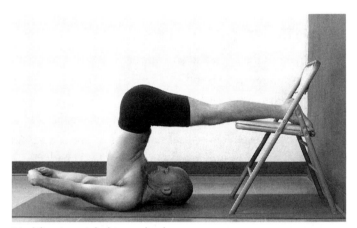

Modification: tight hips or back.

weak shoulders and back—The extra support of a folded blanket under the shoulders, as in Salamba Sarvangasana, is helpful and adds comfort. A strap around the arms to keep the arms shoulder-width apart can also be used.

KINEMATICS

Often students will allow the back to round in order to stretch the entire spine. It feels great! However, do not allow the student to remain in this position for more than a breath or two because the misalignment of having the hips placed posterior to the shoulders and head will place undue strain on the neck over time.

Halasana

Body segment	Kinematics	Muscles active	Muscles released
Foot and toes	Toe (hyper)extension	Extensor digitorum and hallucis longus, anterior tibialis (I)	Flexor digitorum longus and brevis, flexor hallucis longus
Lower leg	Ankle dorsiflexion	Anterior tibialis, extensor digitorum and hallucis longus (C, I)	Gastrocnemius, soleus
Thigh	Knee extension	Quadriceps (C, I)	
	Femur adduction	Adductors (C, I)	
Hip and pelvis	Hip flexion	Hamstrings, gluteus maximus (E)	Hamstrings, gluteus maximus
	Pelvic stability	Rectus abdominis, quadratus lumborum, hamstrings (C, I)	
Torso	Trunk stability	Internal and external obliques, rectus abdominis, transverse abdominis, quadratus lumborum, erector spinae (C, I)	
	Spinal extension and stability	Erector spinae, quadratus lumborum (C, I)	
Shoulder	Arm hyperextension	Posterior deltoid, triceps brachii, latissimus dorsi, (C, I)	Pectoralis major and minor, anterior deltoid
	External rotation	Infraspinatus, teres minor, posterior deltoid (C, I)	
	Scapular adduction	Rhomboids, and mid trapezius (C, I)	
Upper arm	Elbow extension	Triceps brachii (C, I)	Biceps brachii, brachioradialis, brachialis
Lower arm	Forearm pronation	Pronator teres and quadratus (C, I)	
	Elbow extension	Anconeus (C, I)	
Hand and fingers	Finger adduction	Adductor pollicis, flexor pollicis longus and brevis, interossei (C, I)	
	Finger flexion	Flexor digitorum, extensor digiti minimi brevis, dorsal interossei (C, I)	
Neck	Neck flexion, jalandhara bandha	Sternocleidomastoid, scalenes, hyoids (C, I)	Cervical erector spinae, splenius capitus and cervicis, upper trapezius

C = concentric contraction, E = eccentric contraction, I = isometric contraction.

chapter 11

Restorative Postures

deally, all asanas are practiced with comfort and a sense of ease. It may be difficult to relax while trying to balance on one foot or on your head, but it can be done. Birds often sleep standing on one foot and bats hang upside down, which for most humans would be considered a form of physical torture. Any posture done in a way that allows for the release of tension rather than the buildup of work is in the restorative realm. These postures are restorative because little physical energy is needed to enter and maintain the pose. Therefore, the restorative effects of the asana permeate the experience more than does any struggle to hold the posture.

Adho Mukha Shvanasana (Downward-Facing Dog) is classified as a restorative pose for students who have practiced it consistently enough to feel rested and recharged in the posture rather than challenged by tight shoulders or legs. But, there is a pose students generally embrace to escape the work of Downward-Facing Dog and other more strenuous postures that is one of the most highly practiced restorative asanas. Balasana (Child's Pose) is a wonderful resting asana because it requires no muscular activity. All true restorative postures require extremely little or no work of the muscles whatsoever. They are usually totally passive other than the act of getting into and out of them. Some are uniquely restorative like Shavasana (Corpse Pose) and Balasana, and many are passive variations of other poses. For example, using a fitness ball to do a backbend transforms a rather challenging posture into a restorative one.

In addition to making yoga accessible to students who may be physically tired or weak, restorative poses offer a way to release deep

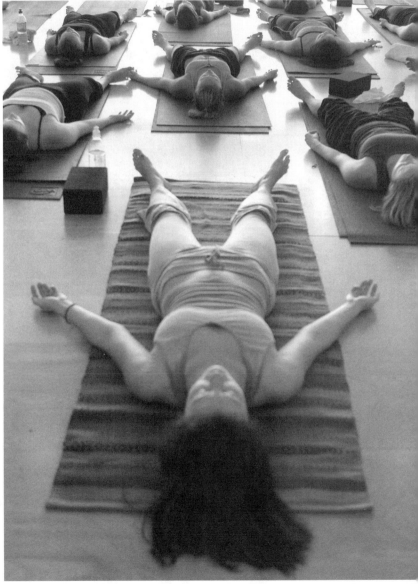

© Levine Roberts

281

habitual tensions. For instance, people often hold tension unconsciously in the shoulders and neck. When the neck and shoulder muscles have absolutely no work to do in a posture, they generally begin to relax after a few breaths. Restorative poses are often practiced with pillows or blankets supporting the body, which feels safe and nurturing to students. Encourage your students to relax into these poses as fully and deeply as possible. Although restorative poses do not build bones or enhance muscle strength, they enable the release of the imbalanced holding patterns the body has carried for years. Many students report they feel the hips relax back into alignment just as much as if they had experienced a chiropractic adjustment or acupuncture treatment. Relaxation scripts, such as those found in appendix A, can be utilized to help guide students into a state of restive relaxation.

Balasana

Child's Pose

[buhl-AAH-suh-nuh]

Bala is the Sanskrit word for child. Balasana resembles the fetal position in the womb. This asana is very restorative and calming and evokes a feeling of safety and security.

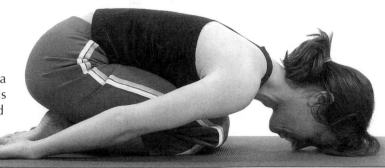

DESCRIPTION

Balasana is a kneeling, prone position where the lower legs are tucked under and the chest rests on the thighs. The arms may be extended over the head, resting on the floor, or wrapped around the outside of the body and resting beside the ankles. This pose rests the body and replaces energy after vigorous, challenging postures. It should be practiced after backbends and inversions.

BENEFITS

- Restores energy
- Stretches and releases the low back
- Relaxes the neck and shoulders
- Stimulates digestion

CAUTION

knee pain—Practice with modifications, or supine with the knees drawn in toward the chest.

VERBAL CUES

- From a kneeling position, sink your hips down on to your heels.
- Exhale and fold forward from your hips. Relax your upper body down so that your torso rests on your legs and your head rests on the floor.
- Feel your shoulders sink down toward the floor as you relax your neck.
- With each inhalation, feel your shoulder blades move apart. As you exhale, allow your body to completely relax down toward the floor. Draw your tailbone gently down toward the floor to lengthen and relax your back.
- Adjust your hips and legs so you are as comfortable as possible. You may need to open the space between your knees.
- Really focus on your breath. Feel each breath open your ribcage and lengthen your spine. Relax your neck and shoulders more and more.
- To exit from this posture, place your palms on the floor under your shoulders. As you inhale, press through your arms and lift your torso upright.

ADJUSTMENTS

feet—The feet should be relaxed. However, if the student experiences discomfort in the feet or ankles, instruct the student to curl the toes under.

knees—To relax the most, instruct the student to move the knees a little wider than hip-width apart. This positioning is easier for the knees to relax because it opens the hips more.

spine—To help the student lengthen the low back, the best adjustment is to press down on the sacrum. Kneel beside the student and place your hand closest to the hips flat against the pelvis, with your hands pointing away from the student's head. Place your other hand between the shoulder blades with your fingers pointing toward the student's head. Press your hands down and away from each other firmly as the student exhales. Another option is to stand behind the student's hips, facing away from the student

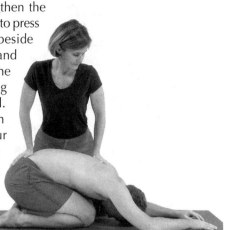

Adjustment: spine; breath.

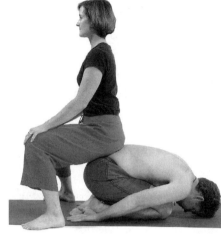

Adjustment: spine.

and sit very lightly on the student's pelvis. Make certain you connect with the pelvis and not higher up onto the low spine. With both of these adjustments, it is important to ask students if they are comfortable.

breath—To help enhance the student's breathing, kneel beside the student and place one hand on the pelvis and the other between the shoulder blades. Instruct the student to breathe deeply into the hand at the pelvis then move the breath up the spine into the hand at the shoulders. Ask the student to exhale in the opposite direction from the shoulders down to the pelvis.

MODIFICATIONS

tight hips and knees—If the student is not comfortable with the knees fully flexed, place a rolled-up towel or blanket under the student's abdomen or between the hamstrings and calves.

tight shoulders—If the student has difficulty relaxing the shoulders, instruct the student to stretch the hands overhead and roll the palms upward resting on the floor.

KINEMATICS

Balasana is essentially a resting and restorative posture that stretches the front of the calf muscles, thighs, and hips as well as the spinal musculature. With the arms resting alongside the body, the shoulder blades gently stretch away from each other as the student focuses on deepening the breath. Because this is a passive pose, all the muscles are relaxed. The muscles indicated on the following chart are those that are additionally stretched when practicing this pose.

Modification: tight shoulders.

Balasana

Body segment	Kinematics	Muscles released
Foot and toes	Plantar flexion	Quadriceps
Lower leg	Knee flexion	
Thigh	Hip flexion	
Hip and pelvis	Legs slightly abducted	Gluteals, deep external rotators*
Torso	Extended or slightly flexed	Erector spinae
		Pectorals if arms are outstretched
Shoulders	Slightly internally rotated if arms are at the sides	Rhomboids, trapezius, posterior deltoid
	Overhead extension if in this position	Latissimus dorsi, serratus anterior
Upper arm	Relaxed in either position	Biceps brachii, brachioradialis, triceps brachii
Lower arm	Extended	
Hand and fingers	Relaxed	
Neck	Forward flexion	Splenius capitus and cervicis, suboccipitals, semispinals, sternocleidomastoid

*Obturator externus and internus, gemellus superior and inferior, quadratus femoris, and piriformis.

Supta Urdvha Dhanurasana

Restorative Backbend

[SOOP-tuh oohr-dhuh-vuh dhuh-noor-AAH-suh-nuh]

Supta Urdvha Dhanurasana is a restorative, supported backbend. *Supta* is Sanskrit for sleeping, or reclining, and *Urdvha Dhanurasana* means upward-facing bow.

DESCRIPTION

This posture is a modification of the more strenuous backbends with the use of a supportive prop. A fitness ball, chair, or numerous folded blankets provide support for the spine in this backbend. Because this posture is actually a modification of more strenuous backbends, no further modifications are provided.

BENEFITS

- More easily accessible to students with weakness or physical challenges
- Opens the chest
- Increases flexibility in the spine

VERBAL CUES

Cues for a Fitness Ball

- Sitting on a fitness ball with the feet flat on the floor, hip-width distance apart, place your hands to your hips or against the side of the ball—wherever you need them for balance.
- Walk your feet forward and slowly roll your hips forward on the ball. Roll the ball to your low back. Tuck your chin to your chest and slowly lower your spine onto the ball.
- Inhale and slowly lower the back of your head to the ball.
- If you feel comfortable and balanced, reach your arms out to your sides or overhead.
- Breathe here and feel your shoulders and chest stretch open and relax.
- To exit from the position, tuck your chin to your chest and slowly walk the legs backward as the ball rolls down the spine until your torso is back in an upright position. You can either lower your hips to the floor, or you can walk your feet back toward the ball and roll your hips back to the top of the ball. Bring your head up last.

Cues for a Chair

- Sit sideways at the edge of a chair that is heavily padded with blankets or pillows.
- Tuck your chin to your chest and exhale as you slowly lower your torso backward. Draping your body over the chair, slowly lower your head toward the floor.
- If you are comfortable, reach your arms overhead. Breathe and relax the chest and shoulders.
- To exit the position, tuck your chin and roll your spine upright slowly and bring your head up last.

Cues for Blankets

- Fold a number of blankets so they stack at least 6 but not more than 12 inches (15-30 cm) high.
- Place your hips on the floor and slowly lower your torso back onto the blankets. Let your head lower down toward the floor. The blankets should be pressed into the curve of your spine.
- Breathe and relax the entire body.
- To exit this position, press your hands to the floor, tuck your chest to your chin, and inhale as you slowly lift the body upright.

ADJUSTMENTS

spine—The apex of the ball should rest comfortably against the student's back. Help the student roll the ball along the spine to wherever the student is balanced and can completely relax into the posture.

shoulders—Make certain the student's shoulders are relaxed away from the ears.

KINEMATICS

The relative softness of the blankets and ball provides support along the contours of the spine, thus allowing for relaxation throughout the entire body.

Supta Urdvha Dhanurasana

Body segment	Kinematics	Muscles active	Muscles released
Foot and toes	Toe extension		
Lower leg	Ankle plantar flexion (and stability if on ball)	Gastrocnemius, soleus (I)	Anterior tibialis, extensor digitorum longus
Thigh	Relaxed knee flexion		Quadriceps
Hip and pelvis	Hip hyperextension (stability if on ball)	Hamstrings (I)	Iliopsoas, rectus femoris
Torso	Spinal hyperextension		Internal and external obliques, rectus abdominis, transverse abdominis, quadratus lumborum, erector spinae
Shoulder	Humeral external rotation		Pectoralis major and minor, deltoids
	Horizontal hyperextension		
Upper arm	Elbow extension		Biceps brachii, brachioradialis, triceps brachii
	Forearm supination		
Lower arm	Wrist hyperextension		
Hand and fingers	Finger extension		
Neck	Neck hyperextension		Splenius capitus and cervicis, suboccipitals, semispinals, sternocleidomastoid

C = concentric contraction, E = eccentric contraction, I = isometric contraction.

Jathara Parivartanasana

Belly Twist

[juht-HAR-uh par-ee-VAR-tuhn-AAH-suh-nuh]

Jathara is the Sanskrit word for stomach, or belly. *Parivartana* means to roll or turn around.

DESCRIPTION

In this supine posture, the hips are flexed and the legs are rotated to one side. The torso remains as flat on the ground as possible. This posture is generally used in a finishing sequence at the end of class. For a restful and restorative posture, as in this example, the knees are bent with one leg crossing over the other. For a more active yet still restorative posture, the legs remain straight.

BENEFITS

- Cools and relaxes the body
- Stretches the spine gently
- Requires little strength in the back
- Opens the chest
- Relaxes the neck
- Aids digestion

CAUTION

hip replacement—Those with hip replacements should not cross the thighs across the midline of the body, so should practice with modification.

VERBAL CUES

- From a supine position, bend your knees and bring your heels as close to your hips as is comfortable, with the soles of your feet on the floor.
- Exhale and cross your right leg over your left above the knee. If you are flexible enough, hook the top of your right foot behind your left calf.
- Reach your arms out to your sides at shoulder height. Turn and look toward your right hand on the floor.
- Inhale deeply and feel your spine lengthen against the floor. Press your shoulder blades against your mat and feel your chest expand.
- Exhale and shift your hips slightly so that your left hip moves back toward the right and aligns with the midline of the body. Slowly lower your knees to the left. Your right hip should be stacked over your left hip as much as is comfortable.
- Continue to focus on your breath.
- With each breath, feel your knees and shoulders sink deeper into the floor.
- To exit the posture, inhale and slowly bring your knees and head back to center. Uncross your legs and prepare for the other side.

ADJUSTMENTS

twist direction—The legs and the head should be pointing in opposite directions. Whichever leg is on top rotates to the opposite side. Sometimes a student will roll to the side of the top leg. Simply touch the outside leg and instruct the student to inhale as they rotate to the opposite side.

knees—If the distance from the knees to the shoulders is great, the twist is less intense in the low back. If the student has the flexibility and is comfortable, instruct the student to draw the knees more toward the chest.

spine—The spine should not round while rotating. Assist the student in finding the appropriate place for the knees to rest while the spine remains lengthened and straight. To aid the student in deepening the twist, slowly and gently press the outside of the top knee toward the floor. Press down gently as the student exhales.

shoulders—If the shoulder farthest from the twisted knees is lifting off the floor, kneel beside the student and press gently on the front of the shoulder while anchoring the hips with your other hand. Using light pressure, and if the student gives you permission, you can press down slightly more each time they exhale.

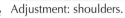

Adjustment: shoulders.

neck—If the student's neck is not lengthened, lightly sweep your fingers against the back of the neck from the base of the shoulders to the back of the skull to cue for length.

MODIFICATIONS

tight spine or hips—Support the student's knees by placing folded blankets between the floor and the legs. Another modification is to instruct the student to place the soles of the feet flat against a wall.

hip pain or hip replacement—If crossing the legs stresses the top hip, then instruct the student to drop the knees to the sides and press the insides of the legs together. Also, instruct the student not to lower the knees to the ground completely. Place blankets under the legs if necessary.

deepening the posture—If the student can comfortably rest the lower leg and opposite shoulder on the floor then the student can straighten the knees and bring the feet closer to the hands. This deepening occurs in the straight-leg version as well.

KINEMATICS

The closer the knees are to the shoulders, the deeper the stretch is in the hips, low back, and shoulders. However, the closer they are together, generally, the harder it is to keep the opposite shoulder relaxed on the ground. This is a nice asana to measure the progress of increasing flexibility in the spine.

Jathara Parivartanasana (Legs Rotated Left)

Body segment	Kinematics	Muscles active	Muscles released
Foot and toes	Toe extension	Extensor digitorum and hallucis longus, anterior tibialis (C, I)	
Lower leg	Foot dorsiflexion	Anterior tibialis, extensor digitorum and hallucis longus (C, I)	Gastrocnemius, soleus
Thigh (R/L)	Knee flexion	Hamstrings (C, I, R)	
Thigh (R)	Thigh adduction	Adductors (C, I, R)	
Hip and pelvis (R/L)	Hip flexion	Iliopsoas (C, I)	Gluteus maximus
Hip and pelvis (R)	Internal rotation	Gluteus medius and minimus, adductors (C, R)	Gluteus medius and maximus, tensor fascia lata, deep external rotators*
Torso (R)	Pelvis rotation	External oblique, quadratus lumborum, lattisimus dorsi (E, R)	Quadratus lumborum, external oblique, erector spinae, latissimus dorsi
Torso (L)	Stability	Rectus abdominis, transverse abdominis, erector spinae (I, R)	Erector spinae, quadratus lumborum
Shoulder	Adduction of scapulae	Rhomboids, mid trapezius (C, I)	Anterior deltoid, pectoralis major and minor, biceps brachii
	External humerus rotation	Infraspinatus, teres minor, posterior deltoid (C, I)	
Upper arm	Elbow extension	Triceps brachii (C, I)	Biceps brachii, brachialis, brachioradialis
Lower arm	Elbow extension	Anconeus (E, I)	
	Elbow supination	Supinator (C, I)	
Hand and fingers	Finger extension	Extensor digitorum, indicis, and digiti minimi; lumbricales manus; interossei dorsales (C, I)	
Neck (R)	Head rotation to right	Splenius capitus and cervicis, occipitals, upper trapezius (C, I)	Sternocleidomastoid
Neck (L)	Head rotation to right	Sternocleidomastoid (C, I, R)	Splenius capitus and cervicis, occipitals, upper trapezius

*Obturator externus and internus, gemellus superior and inferior, quadratus femoris, and piriformis.

C = concentric contraction, E = eccentric contraction, I = isometric contraction, R = relaxed.

Viparita Karani

Restorative Legs-Up-the-Wall Pose

[veep-uh-REE-tuh kuh-ruh-nee]

Viparita Karani means in the inverted or reversed position. Many yoga instructors, however, simply refer to this asana as the "Legs-Up-the-Wall" pose when using English terms.

DESCRIPTION

In this posture the student's torso is supine on the floor, while the legs are stretched up a wall. A bolster or blankets are often placed under the hips to lift the student's hips higher than the heart to loosen a tight low back. If props are not used then the sacrum is placed flat against the floor and the ischial tuberosities (sits bones) are pressed into the wall. This posture is often used as a modified inversion for menstruating women.

BENEFITS

- Helps relax low back
- Helps increase comfort and range for other forward bends
- Relieves menstrual discomfort

VERBAL CUES

- Place your mat perpendicular and flat on the floor against the wall.
- Lie on the outermost right edge of the mat on your right side in a fetal position. Press the bottom of your hips flat against the wall.
- Slowly roll your body onto your back so that you lie in the middle of your mat.
- Exhale as you straighten your legs and press them flat against the wall.
- With every exhalation feel your back and hips sink deeper into the floor.
- Breathe here and relax.

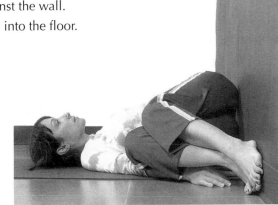

Starting position.

ADJUSTMENTS

hips—If the student's hips are not flat against the wall, then instruct the student to scoot the bottom back against the wall. If the student's hips are not flat against the floor, stand to the sides and press down on the soles of the feet. Another option is to place a blanket or bolster under the hips so that the student has more support.

shoulders—If the student's shoulders are up near the ears and rotated internally, then kneel above the student's head. Place your hands on the student's shoulders and gently press the shoulders away from the ears and against the floor.

MODIFICATIONS

tight hamstrings—If the student has difficulty straightening the knees, instruct the student to bend the knees slightly but to breathe and work to straighten the legs.

overly tight neck—If a student is so tight in the neck that he or she is unable to rest the back of the head on the floor, place pillows under the head to allow the student to relax.

KINEMATICS

Bolsters or blankets placed under the hips create more length in the low spine while providing support. In addition, the increase in the angle between the legs and torso allows those with tight hamstrings to find a comfortable position while keeping the knees straight.

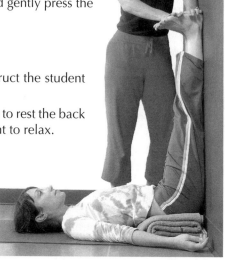

Adjustment: hips.

Viparita Karani

Body segment	Kinematics	Muscles released
Foot and toes	Neutral	
Lower leg	Neutral	
Thigh	Knee extension	Hamstrings, adductors
Hip and pelvis	Hip flexion	Gluteals
Torso	Spinal extension	
Shoulder	External rotation	
Upper arm	Elbow extension	
Lower arm	Wrist extension	
Hand and fingers	Neutral	
Neck	Extension	

The entire body is relaxed when properly in this posture, so no muscle contractions are listed.

Shavasana

Corpse Pose

[shuh-VAAH-suh-nuh]

Shava is the Sanskrit word for corpse. In this asana, the body resembles the stillness and detachment of an unmoving corpse.

DESCRIPTION

This supine pose is the quintessential finishing, resting, and restorative posture in which the student is reclining on the floor with the arms stretched beside the body. Because the nervous system is constantly bombarded with stimuli throughout the day and most people are distracted by unconscious, nonessential self-limiting thoughts (known as *vrtti*), the purpose of practicing Shavasana is to completely release all of the muscles of the body and to relax the mind into a meditative state. This posture may appear extremely simple because there is no movement in the body. Shavasana can, however, be one of the most challenging postures because it is much more difficult to relax the mind than it is to relax the body.

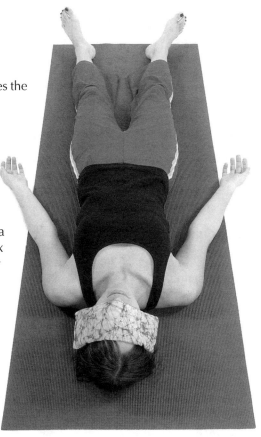

BENEFITS

- Relaxes both the mind and body after a more physical asana practice
- Allows for deep healing and relaxation leading to successful meditation
- Removes fatigue
- Valuable in increasing the psychoneuroimmunologic abilities of the body (see chapter 5)

VERBAL CUES

See appendix A for some sample relaxation scripts to help your students become completely relaxed into Shavasana.

Getting Into the Posture

- From a supine position, exhale and bring your knees to your chest and your head to your knees.
- Inhale and roll your back, shoulders, neck, and head onto the floor.
- Exhale and stretch your legs down onto the floor.
- Roll your shoulders open by bringing your palms up. Feel the upper corners of your shoulders press gently into the floor and settle your shoulder blades flat against the floor and your back.
- Relax your legs and hips, allowing your feet to roll to the outside. Feel your back sinking into your mat.
- Close your eyes and relax the muscles of your face.
- Allow your breath to flow in its natural pattern, no longer controlling it in any manner. Feel and visualize your breath as it flows over and through your body. With each breath allow your body and mind to sink deeper into relaxation. It is ideal to allow students at least five minutes of silent meditation time.

Bringing Students out of the Posture

- In the next few breaths, continue to focus on your breath and begin to notice your relaxed, recharged body.
- Start to gently move your wrists and ankles as you become more and more aware of your body. As that awareness builds, start to bring a little more movement into all of your limbs.

- When you feel comfortable and completely aware of your surroundings, begin to roll yourself to one side and continue to rest. Gradually and gently, when you feel ready, bring yourself back upright as we prepare to close our class.
- Namaste, Om Shanti.

ADJUSTMENTS

feet—Gently roll the student's feet externally.

arms—Rotate the arms externally so that the student's palms face upward.

shoulders—Kneeling above the student's head, place your hands on the shoulders and lightly press down and out to help the student relax more deeply.

neck—To lengthen the neck, cradle the base of the student's skull in your palm and lightly draw the head away from the shoulders.

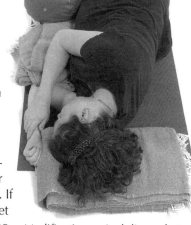

MODIFICATIONS

spinal discomfort—If the student has discomfort in the low back, instruct the student to bend the knees and place a bolster or a number of folded towels under the knees. Another possibility is to place a chair or fitness ball under the calves. If no props are available, instruct the student to bend the knees and move the feet as wide apart as is comfortable, and to let the knees roll together. This allows the student to rest without using any muscles.

Modification: spinal discomfort or pregnancy.

pregnancy—For pregnant women who feel uncomfortable lying on the back, have them roll to the left side in a restful fetal position. Place pillows or bolsters between the thighs and under the head for added comfort.

respiratory problems—If the student has difficulty lying on the back and breathing comfortably, place a bolster under the upper shoulders and head lifting the head higher than the chest.

KINEMATICS

Because all of the muscles are in a relaxed state, the kinematic chart illustrates the body's positioning in the pose.

Shavasana

Body segment	Kinematics
Foot and toes	Toe extension
Lower leg	Slight ankle plantar flexion
Thigh	Knee extension
Hip and pelvis	Femoral external rotation
	Hip extension
Torso	Spinal extension
Shoulder	Humerus external rotation, abduction
Upper arm	Elbow extension
Lower arm	Forearm supination
	Wrist extension
Hand and fingers	Finger extension
Neck	Neck extension

The entire body is relaxed when properly in this posture, so no muscle contractions are listed.

part 3

Structuring a Class

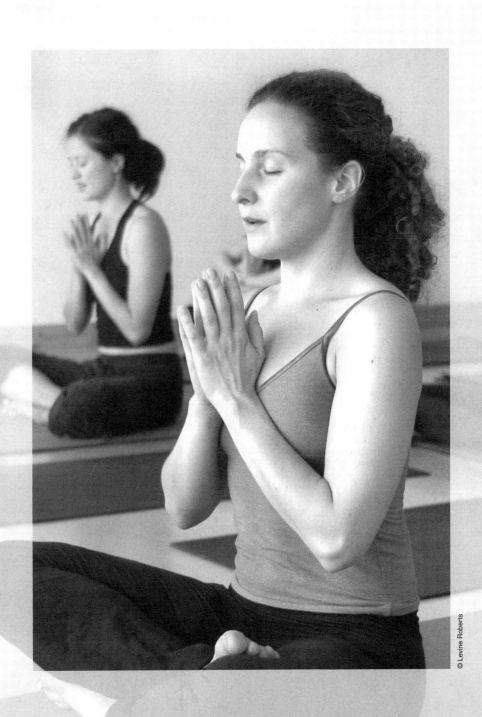

© Levine Roberts

chapter 12

Class Framework

Acomprehensive yoga class, like any other organized physical activity, follows a certain structure, which allows the class to flow. The class must be balanced and provide a variety of postures in a manner that facilitates harmony in the students' physical, mental, and spiritual well-being. Some hatha yoga styles such as Bikram and Ashtanga practice the same postures in the exact same progression each class session.

Just as yoga has many styles, many personality types make for effective yoga teachers. Some instructors plan a class with great detail and organization, down to such minute details as what song they will play during a particular asana, whereas other instructors simply wing it. Either way you must have a good repertoire and the ability to address the immediate and long-term needs of your class.

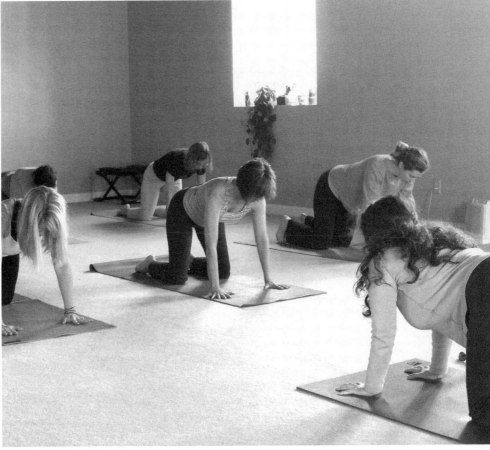

© Martha Work

Using the tools from chapter 2 regarding understanding your students' needs, you can apply the outlines in this chapter to create a workout formula and chart the progress of each workout for yourself or your students. From basic frameworks of a lesson plan for a generic or classical-eclectic hatha yoga class to more sophisticated and detailed class charts, examples are given to study and use literally or as inspiration.

Frameworks

A basic class framework is a vital yet somewhat superficial outline of a class. From a general concept to a more concrete example a class plan forms and, no matter how embellished or detailed, the basic framework is always there. Just as the foundation and frame of a house enable the rest of the house to be fabricated and complete so does a basic outline and lesson plan give form to a yoga-session strategy and allow it to unfold.

David Swenson, a well-known Ashtanga instructor, said that all of the series of Ashtanga hatha are structured like a sandwich: The warm-up and finishing poses are like the bread and the main workout is the filling for the sandwich. The warm-up and finishing poses are always the same for every series; only the workouts in between are different in each of the series.

A class framework also can be likened to a flight plan (table 12.1). The journey of a flight entails checking in with the control tower, which is like getting centered. Like the body's need to be warmed before it can go through more difficult poses, a plane's engine needs to warm up before it takes off. The flight itself could represent the workout, and the cool-down then is symbolized by the landing of the plane, which is gradual and often like Shavasana (Corpse Pose) may require the most skill.

Class Outline

In a yoga class, the basic framework consists of the following elements: a time for getting the mind and body centered, warming up the body, the main workout, the cool-down period, and the class closure. From this framework you can decide upon the goals of the class and the activities, rationales, and objectives to meet those goals. The asanas practiced and the pranayama you instruct are activities you offer to meet these goals. The following is a bare-bones class-structure outline that can be applied to almost any style of hatha yoga.

Centering

Getting centered is the time in class when students begin to prepare mentally for practice—a time to clear the mind of thoughts and to begin focusing within. To help your students move into this mindset, remind them to turn off their cell phones, move their belongings away from their practice space, and to slowly begin to let the outside world dissolve away. This portion of class is when atmosphere plays a big part in directing students to their practice. Playing music, if you choose to use it, softly in the background as students enter the room can set the calming mood before a word is spoken.

- **Asanas for centering:** Traditionally, Tadasana (Mountain Pose) is used to bring the focus of the mind into the body. By having the students focus on their balance and alignment, they begin to ignore outside distractions and eliminate the stresses of their minds. However, restorative-styled yoga classes generally begin in a seated position sometimes accompanied by chanting and still others start in Shavasana to help push away ordinary distractions.

Table 12.1   Flight Plan

	Getting centered (control tower pre-check flight)	Warm-up (start engine and idle)	Work out (flight or trip)	Cool-down (landing)
Asanas	Tadasana or easy sitting poses	Continue with Tadasana or Sun Salutations, maybe some basic poses	Standing poses, some seated—supine and prone—maybe some inversions (include spinal movement in all six directions)	Finishing poses, then Shavasana
Breathing	Durga breath (three part, "full," or ujjayi)	Same	Same	Passive and natural belly breathing

- **Breathing.** Breath work, or pranayama, is used in most forms of hatha yoga to help keep the mind focused within the body. In general, durga or ujjai breathing (chapter 4) is practiced to slow the mind and create a feeling of relaxation. The breath also helps to warm the body and prepare it for the rest of the class. Focused breathing alone brings the energetic channels into balance. The *ida* and the *pingala* are the main channels of the polar energies and become more balanced as the breathing evens out between the left and right nostrils and more fully throughout the body with a focused mind.

Physical Warm-Up

To prepare the muscles and joints for asana practice, the tissue needs to be moved and warmed to a certain degree. This rationale is the same for any other type of physical activity. Warm muscles are less apt to strain and tear. Additionally, when the body is warmed, students are generally more willing to completely open themselves throughout the remainder of class.

Sun Salutations are often used as a warm-up. Practiced slowly or rapidly, they bring increased circulation to the muscles and joints, which allows for more ease of movement and a decreased risk of injury in the rest of the workout. As was presented in chapter 6, the sequencing of the classical Sun Salutations allows the students to link the movements with the breath, which creates a deeper mental and physical connection.

In some styles of hatha yoga, teachers either do not implement Sun Salutations or at least do not introduce them until the second half of the class. In classes that do not practice Sun Salutations, the warm-up portion of the class focuses on utilizing the breath as a means to warm the body. In the case of Iyengar-style yoga, the practice begins with standing postures.

In other styles, where the Sun Salutations are practiced later in the class sequence, the salutations then serve as the second warm-up or more intense "summit" of the workout before coming down to the floor for cool-down. When the Sun Salutations are not in the middle or toward the end of class as just described, then some inversions and backbends serve as the summit in the routine, and there tend to be more standing postures presented and fewer seated poses overall.

Main Practice

The bulk of the class session consists of the workout, which is generally the most physically challenging

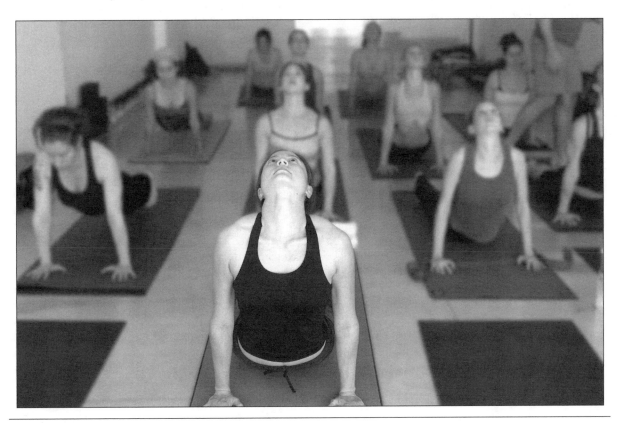

Lead your class through a warm-up such as Sun Salutations to help prepare the muscles and joints for the work to come.
© Levine Roberts

portion of the practice. This portion is where a variety of asanas are presented. Here, the muscles are warmed, the mind is focused, and the breath is flowing. Your students are now ready to deepen their practice—ready to open themselves to more complete lengthening and strengthening of their muscles and focusing of their minds.

Whether you are teaching an Ashtanga class or a gentle-yoga class, in order for the main practice to be well balanced, the asanas presented throughout the class should move the students' spines in all six directions in which the spine is able to move: forward, backward, laterally left, laterally right, rotated right, and rotated left. Postures in one direction should be followed by an oppositional or counterposture. For example, a forward-bending posture should be followed by a backward-bending posture and vice versa. After practicing a headstand or backbend, relaxing and stretching the spine in Balasana (Child's Pose) is appropriate in that it counters the intensity of the demanding effort of the previous asana.

Cool-Down

Asanas that are not as physically demanding work well near the end of class as part of the cool-down. Pranayama, eye exercises, or the like are good to practice when the mind is calm and still attentive and the body is comfortable and relaxed after a good workout.

Finishing asanas are those poses that are either very passive, thus facilitating the cooling-off period, or poses that require so much energy and stamina, such as the inversions, that only a few passive poses are practiced immediately afterwards. Many of the seated postures are restful and when practiced lower the heart rate and respiration as they move the mind into a more restful state.

Shavasana is the heart of yoga. The deep relaxation provided by this pose solidifies the body and mind into a restful state in which to recharge. Withdrawing the senses from the material world and excessive stimuli gives the nervous system a chance to relax and brings the rest of the systems back into a deeper balance.

When a student is able to release physical and mental tension, meditation then becomes almost automatic. The benefits of this relaxation include improved immune system function, an increase in will power and fitness levels, and a higher tolerance for outside stress factors. Conscious relaxation and meditation often is more healing or fortifying than sleep.

Sometimes students become so relaxed they actually fall asleep. (You can hear them snore!) But a true, deep relaxation occurs when a student can remain awake yet calm in body and mind. If you watch students' abdomens you can see their breath slowly and gently

rise and fall. Their hands and faces appear to have no tension and are calm and still. Often students will have a smile or words to share in appreciation of having been able to take the journey of your yoga class.

Class Closure

The class is considered finished by reviving and guiding students back to their bodies and bringing them back to a seated position. Many instructors use guided imagery to bring students back from their relaxed states. At this time, some instructors provide an inspirational reading or thought as a way of closing the class session. The classic closing gesture, which is also a salutation, is the chanting of "Om" and "Namaste."

Having a closure allows for a smooth transition from the yoga class to the next place a student is off to. It is a clear way of establishing that class is indeed over. And, although the work and activities on the mat have ended, the awareness and any other benefits gained during class can continue instead of being abruptly rolled up with the mat. Students can integrate relaxation more easily into their daily lives. A slow shift from class to "reality" also brings students back to the room if they ended up feeling spacey. Even a very brief closing is a way of saying, "Thank you and good-bye," thus showing your students you value the time and energy they have shared with you.

Lesson Plans and Class Descriptions

A lesson plan not only gives your class more structure and definition, but also it is quite useful for educating your students. The information in a lesson plan helps to keep you organized, explain your class to employers, and promote yourself and yoga in general. Eventually, teaching a class becomes second nature, but going through the process of writing a lesson plan can edify your understanding of yoga and how to teach and promote it.

One marketing spin many brochures include is the description of the class goals instead of a description of the class itself. All yoga classes share some wonderful goals in common. "Feel renewed and balanced in your body, mind, and spirit with the nurturing workout of our yoga journey" is a statement that can accurately describe the goal of almost any yoga class. These words explain expected or promised benefits rather than describing the class. This statement or others worded similarly are seen in many brochures, Web sites, and class catalogs. However, one would have no way of knowing if the workout is a gentle, passive class or an intense power class. Words that describe the style of a yoga workout and how it is taught include *alignment, mindfulness, breath awareness* or *attention, slow, fast, sustained, flowing, playful, serious, spontaneous, consistent, regimented, hot* or *heated, hands-on adjustments, meditative, strengthening, athletic.* Words such as *relaxing, rejuvenating,* and *therapeutic* are too nondescript as far as the style or methods of yoga that will be practiced. These concepts are important to keep in mind when composing a course outline, especially for a potential employer.

Measurable objectives of an ongoing yoga class are not always easy to list because the goals and ability of each student may be so different. The objectives can therefore be stated in relative terms, for example: "After 10 classes the student will be able to breathe at least two seconds longer on the inhalation and exhalation." Or, the objectives can be open ended: "After three weeks, with regular attendance of two classes a week, the student can expect to move further physically and to hold postures more comfortably for a longer period of time in at least three postures."

The rationale listed in a course outline or lesson plan is to justify and remind the instructor, students, or potential employer of the reasons behind practicing a particular technique. If the outline includes forward bends then the rationale could be "a counterpose for a previous back-bending posture." Another example might include listing a modification such as "Practicing Uttanasana (Intense Forward Bend) with bent knees." The rationale behind this statement is that practicing postures with bent knees is a way to alleviate tension in the low back.

Themes

Starting with a basic lesson plan and guideline, you can apply various themes and intensity levels. As part of the assessment on how she should teach the class, Kathy Lee asks for requests from her students. The most common requests are for postures that focus on the low back and neck and shoulders. While following a basic class plan, she integrates a number of postures that focus specifically on these areas. An attentive teacher also attempts to scrutinize the energy level of the class at large in order to pace the workout. Sometimes people do not recognize the possibilities or importance of focusing on the toes, abdomen, or elbows. Often what was meant as a clever remark by an unsuspecting student (such as, "Oh, I'd like to focus on my big toe.") ends up as a challenging workout.

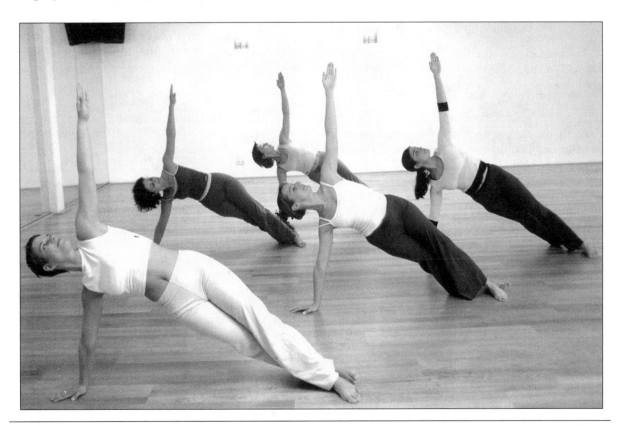

You can integrate students' requests for help in certain areas, such as overall body strengthening, into your lesson plans.

© Jumpfoto

The templates and outlines presented next are good guidelines, but keep in mind that all postures use many muscles and the overlap is unavoidable. Trying to isolate a muscle or body part in an asana is like trying to isolate a note when a chord is being played. Your muscles (your instruments) work together in concert as they express the poses. As a yoga teacher you can orchestrate a class routine to meet the needs and wishes of your students by being familiar with the proper biomechanics of postures and having rapport with your students.

Areas of Body Focus

After determining what your class will benefit from the most, use the examples described next to help you organize your class based on areas of the body. This is just a quick reference guide to asana categories. For more complete information see chapters 7 through 11, where each posture is described in detail.

Neck and Shoulders

- Utthita Trikonasana (Extended Triangle)
- Virabhadrasana I (Warrior I)
- Any asana with the arms overhead both during the warm-up and again later in the class
- Gomukhasana (Cow's Face) and passive neck positions such as rolling the head from shoulder to shoulder

Low Back

- Sun Salutations to warm up
- Any standing posture
- Side bends and twists and forward- and back-bending postures so that the spine is moved in six directions.
- Utthita Trikonasana
- Ardha Matsyendrasana (Half Lord of the Fishes)
- Uttanasana (Intense Forward Bend)
- Ushtrasana (Camel Pose)

Abdominals

- Focus on deep abdominal breathing
- Drawing the legs forward and backward during Sun Salutations instead of pushing off with the feet
- Navasana (Boat Pose)
- Utthita Chaturanga Dandasana (Plank Pose)
- Chaturanga Dandasana (Four-Limbs Staff Pose)
- Vasishthasana (Side Plank)

Hips

- Utthita Trikonasana
- Virabhadrasana II (Warrior II) with focus on frontal plane
- Natarajasana (King Dancer)
- Dhanurasana (Bow Pose)
- Parivrtta Trikonasana (Revolving Triangle Pose)
- Variations of Raja Kapotasana (Royal Pigeon Pose)

Hamstrings

- Utthita Trikonasana
- Parshvottanasana (Intense Side Stretch)
- All forward bends
- Hanumanasana (Forward-Splits Pose)
- Supta Padangusthasana (Reclining Hand-to-Toe Pose)

Calves

- Vrkshasana (Tree Pose) and other single-leg standing poses
- Virabhadrasana I
- Adho Mukha Shvanasana (Downward-Facing Dog) with emphasis on heels pressing down to floor, or placing the toes of one foot on the heel of the opposite foot

Chest Openers

- Bhujangasana (Cobra Pose)
- Urdvha Mukha Shvanasana (Upward-Facing Dog)
- Ushtrasana
- Setu Bandhasana (Bridge Pose)

Postures for Differing Energy Levels

To choose postures according to the energy levels, moods, and requests of students you can use the following as a general guide. However, remember that at any time all students can choose (consciously or unconsciously) to push themselves more or ease off on the energy they put into a posture.

The following asanas are listed from passive to more vigorous. Again, this is just a quick reference guide to asana categories. For more complete information see chapters 7 through 11, where each posture is described in detail.

Stamina and Endurance

- Tadasana (Mountain Pose)
- Utthita Trikonasana
- Virabhadrasanas
- Balancing poses: Utthita Hasta Padangusthasana (Extended Hand-to-Toe), single leg, and Bakasana (Crane Pose), arm balances
- Backbends: Urdhva Dhanurasana (Upward Bow Pose)
- Inversions: Salamba Shirshasana (Supported Headstand)

Twists

- Easy supine twists: Jathara Parivartanasana (Belly Twist), with knees bent
- Supported and seated twists: Ardha Matsyendrasana
- Standing twists
- Partner and assisted twists

Balancing

- Malasana (Basic Squat Pose)
- Inversions: Adho Mukha Vrkshasana (Handstand), unsupported
- One-legged standing poses: Vrkshasana or Garudasana (Eagle Pose)
- Pincha Mayurasana (Scorpion or Peacock Feather)

Inversions

- Forward bends: Uttanasana, Prasarita Padottanasana (Extended-Leg Forward Bend)
- Adho Mukha Shvanasana
- Salamba Sarvangasana (Supported Shoulderstand)
- Salamba Shirshasana
- Pincha Mayurasana

Forward Bends

- Supported by a chair, exercise ball, or the wall
- Uttanasana
- Paschimottanasana (Seated Forward Bend)
- Parshvottanasana

Backbends

- Supta Urdvha Dhanurasana (Restorative Backbend)
- Bhujangasana
- Setu Bandhasana
- Virabhadrasana I
- Ushtrasana
- Urdvha Dhanurasana (Full Backbend)

chapter 13

Sample Classes

Given the defining factors illustrated thus far in this text, how do you determine what asanas to include in a class when there are so many variables? Teaching yoga has many layers. One person needs to be reminded to breathe more, another student might need help with selecting the appropriate prop to use, and yet another will be best served by the softest touch on the head to cue the neck to relax away unconscious tension. As you multitask giving verbal cues, physical adjustments, and demonstrations you must also observe the level of comfort and ability of each of your students. Your lesson plan is like a map, and as the instructor you navigate the course and guide the students through their journey. You have a plan but you must remain ready to adapt your teaching based upon your observations. Having a foundation of postures for a lesson plan gives you bearings. This foundation also allows you the option to exploit the structure by using the examples presented here literally or making alterations if and when you are inspired to do so. Following are sample outlines for classes lasting 30, 60, and 90 minutes. The minutes noted beside each asana include the time it takes to bring the student into and out of the posture in a flowing manner with few or no pauses.

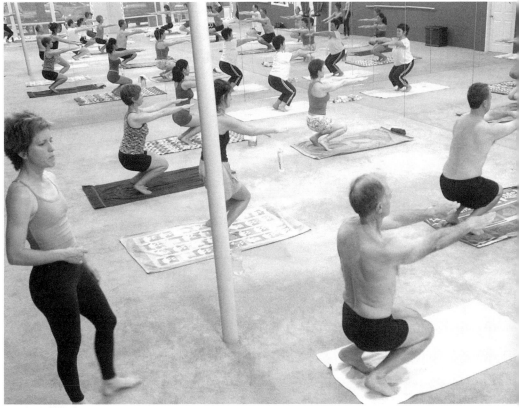
© davidsandersphotos.com

Sample 30-Minute Class

A 30-minute class is most likely the shortest class you might teach. Although the time frame is short, a 30-minute class can nicely introduce students to the basics of asana practice— learning the names of postures, getting used to the flow of a class, beginning to work on body awareness and alignment. This time frame is seen in many school physical education programs. The following outline illustrates foundational postures and an easy progression in which to introduce yoga to students.

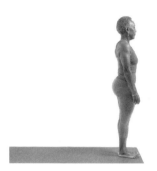

1 Tadasana; 1.5 minutes.

See Chapter 6

2 A Surya Namaskara series; 2 times for 1 minute each.

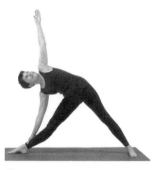

3 Utthita Trikonasana; right side 2 minutes.

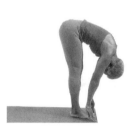

4 Uttanasana; 1 minute.

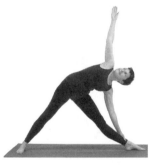

5 Utthita Trikonasana; left side 2 minutes.

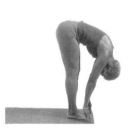

6 Uttanasana; 1 minute.

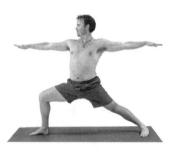

7 Virabhadrasana II; right side 1 minute.

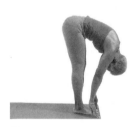

8 Uttanasana; 1 minute.

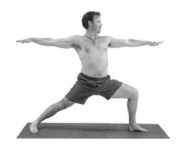

9 Virabhadrasana II; left side 1 minute.

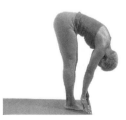

10 Uttanasana; 1 minute.

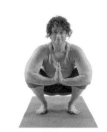

11 Malasana; 1 minute.

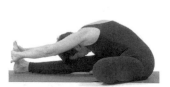

12 Janu Shirshasana; right side 1.5 minutes.

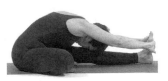

13 Janu Shirshasana; left side 1.5 minutes.

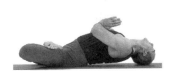

14 Matsyasana; 2 minutes.

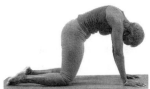

15 Durga-Go; 1.5 minutes.

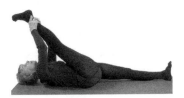

16 Supta Padangust-hasana; right side 1 minute.

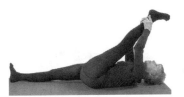

17 Supta Padangusthasana; left side 1 minute.

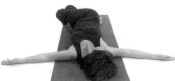

18 Jathara Parivartanasana; legs to left side 1 minute.

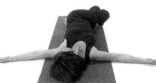

19 Jathara Parivartanasana; legs to right side 1 minute.

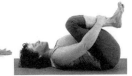

20 Knees to chest; 30 seconds.

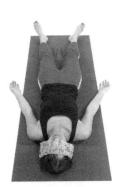

21 Shavasana; 4.5 minutes.

Sample 60-Minute Class

To expand a 30-minute basic class into a 60-minute class you can simply double the holding times in each posture, taking more time to focus on alignment and breathing. Or, the additional 30 minutes can allow you to add postures for variety. Most fitness and recreational facilities allot 60 minutes for their classes. The additional 30 minutes also allows you to walk through the class and provide necessary adjustments to students, especially in larger classes. As the students become more comfortable in the postures and their awareness, flexibility, and endurance increase, begin to add variety to the class by using different postures.

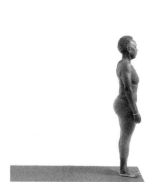

1 Tadasana; 3 minutes.

See
Chapter 6

2 A Surya Namaskara series; 2 times for 3 minutes each.

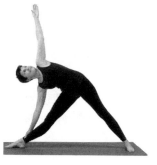

3 Utthita Trikonasana; right side 1.5 minutes.

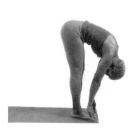

4 Uttanasana; 1 minute.

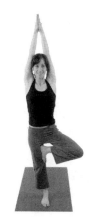

5 Vrkshasana; standing on right leg 2 minutes.

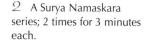

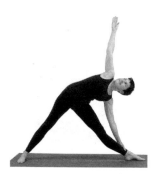

6 Utthita Trikonasana; left side 1.5 minutes.

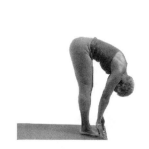

7 Uttanasana; 1 minute.

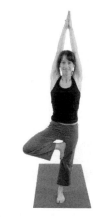

8 Vrkshasana; standing on left leg 2 minutes.

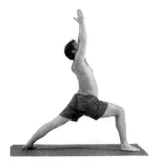

9 Virabhadrasana I; right side 1 minute.

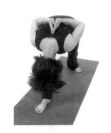

10 Parshvottanasana; right side 1 minute.

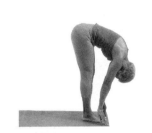

11 Uttanasana; 1 minute.

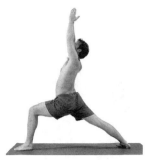

12 Virabhadrasana I; left side 1 minute.

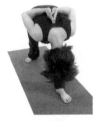

13 Parshvottanasana; left side 1 minute.

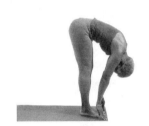

14 Uttanasana; 1 minute.

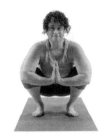

15 Malasana; 1 minute.

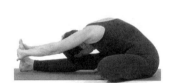

16 Janu Shirshasana; right side 1 minute.

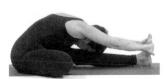

17 Janu Shirshasana; left side 1 minute.

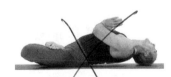

18 Matsyasana; 3 minutes.

seated spinal twist

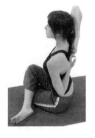

19 Gomukhasana; right side 1 minute.

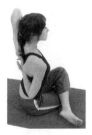

20 Gomukhasana; left side 1 minute.

(continued)

(Sample 60-Minute Class continued)

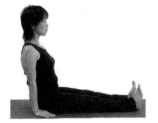

21 Dandasana with easy chin-to-chest stretch; 1 minute.

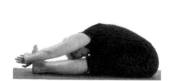

22 Paschimottanasana; 2 minutes.

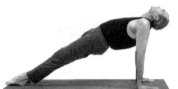

23 Purvottanasana; 1 minute.

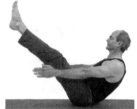

24 Navasana; 1.5 minutes.

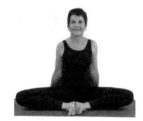

25 Baddha Konasana; 1 minute.

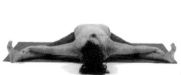

26 Upavishta Konasana; 1.5 minutes.

or turtle variation instead

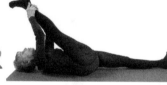

27 Supta Padangusthasana; right side 2 minutes.

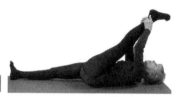

28 Supta Padangust-hasana; left side 2 minutes.

29 Jathara Parivartanasana; legs to left side 2 minutes.

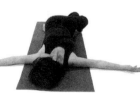

30 Jathara Parivartana-sana; legs to right side 2 minutes.

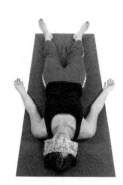

31 Shavasana; 12 minutes.

Sample 90-Minute Class

Many yoga studios and some fitness facilities allot 90 minutes for a class. This amount of time may seem daunting at first; however, the additional time allows for more creativity and time to practice postures that often require more hands-on help from the instructor such as Shirshasana and Sarvangasana.

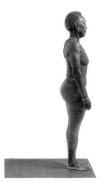

1 Tadasana; 3 minutes.

See
Chapter 6

2 A Surya Namaskara series; 4 times for 3 minutes each.

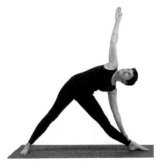

3 Utthita Trikonasana; left side 2 minutes.

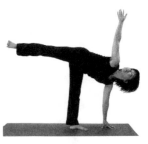

4 Ardha Chandrasana; left side 1.5 minutes.

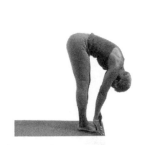

5 Uttanasana; 1 minute.

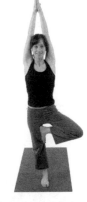

6 Vrkshasana; standing on right leg 2 minutes.

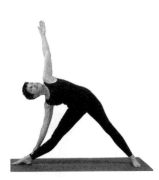

7 Utthita Trikonasana; right side 2 minutes.

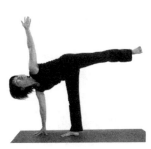

8 Ardha Chandrasana; right side 1.5 minutes.

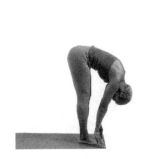

9 Uttanasana; 1 minute.

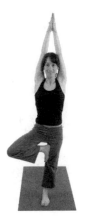

10 Vrkshasana; standing on left leg 2 minutes.

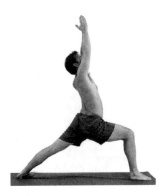

11 Virabhadrasana I; right side 1 minute.

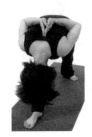

12 Parshvottanasana; right side 1 minute.

(continued)

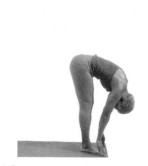

13   Uttanasana; 1 minute.

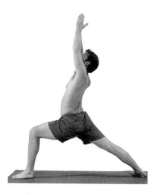

14   Virabhadrasana I; left side 1 minute.

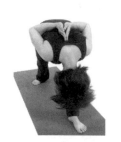

15   Parshvottanasana; left side 1 minute.

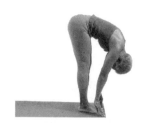

16   Uttanasana; 1 minute.

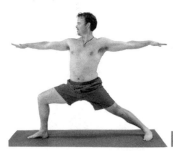

17   Virabhadrasana II; right side 1.5 minutes.

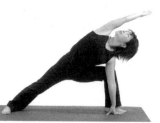

18   Utthita Parshvakonasana; left side 1 minute.

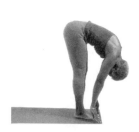

19   Uttanasana; 1 minute.

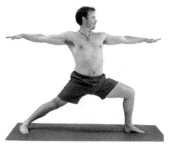

20   Virabhadrasana II; left side 1.5 minutes.

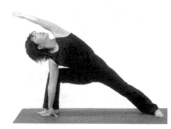

21   Utthita Parshvakonasana; right side 1 minute.

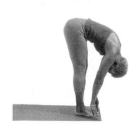

22   Uttanasana; 1 minute.

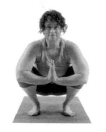

23   Malasana; 1 minute.

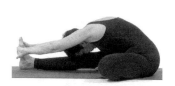

24   Janu Shirshasana; right side 1 minute.

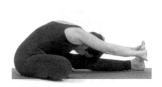

25   Janu Shirshasana; left side 1 minute.

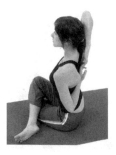

26   Gomukhasana; right side 1 minute.

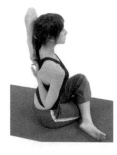

27   Gomukhasana; left side 1 minute.

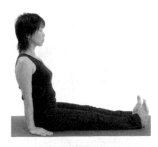

28   Dandasana with easy chin-to-chest stretch; 1 minute.

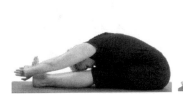

29 Paschimottanasana; 2 minutes.

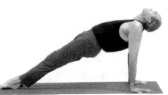

30 Purvottanasana; 1 minute.

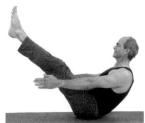

31 Navasana; 1.5 minutes.

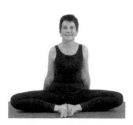

32 Baddha Konasana; 1 minute.

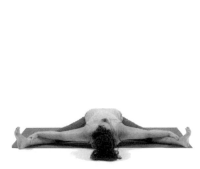

33 Upavistha Konasana; 1.5 minutes.

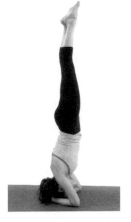

34 Salamba Shirshasana; 5 minutes.

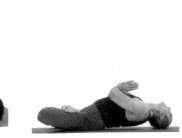

35 Salamba Sarvangasana; 5 minutes.

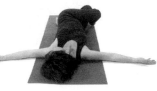

36 Matsyasana; 3 minutes

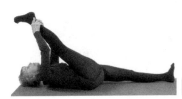

37 Supta Padangusthasana; right side 2 minutes.

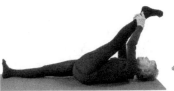

38 Supta Padangusthasana; left side 2 minutes.

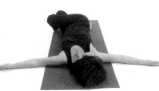

39 Jathara Parivartanasana; legs to left side 2 minutes.

40 Jathara Parivartanasana; legs to right side 2 minutes.

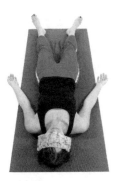

41 Shavasana; 15 minutes.

Sample Six-Week Course

To help give you ideas on how a series of classes with a limited time frame might progress, a detailed class outline for a six-week Introduction to Classical-Eclectic Hatha Yoga course is provided next. This sample course meets twice a week for 75 minutes and is a generic example intended for you to use as part of your own lesson plans if you desire.

1. Introduce yourself by name; and, if appropriate, hand out your email or business phone number. Break the ice just enough to establish that you are both nurturing and organized. Be humble, but still express authority in order to gain their trust. Here is a good example of an opening statement:

   "Namaste, or Salutations, my name is _____, and I will facilitate your class for the next six weeks. I am here to guide and support your practice and, more important, your discovery of how yoga may appeal to you. Please know and take comfort in the fact that I cannot do all the postures perfectly. I may briefly demonstrate poses as part of the learning process; however, the idea is not to do them exactly as I do them but rather to experiment and see how much your own body and mind can engage in the asanas while you are comfortably challenged."

2. Offer a brief explanation of what pace and style the class will follow during the next six weeks. If you are teaching a specific style of hatha such as Ashtanga or Iyengar, make sure this is clear to the students. Otherwise, the following sample introduction is for a classical-eclectic hatha class:

   "This class is a mind-body fitness class; therefore, I do not have time to go over much philosophy or meditation. However, in your handout (or on the white board) I have included a small list of resources for your further study if you are interested. Also, I invite you to take to heart the words of a great contemporary yoga master, Pattabhi Jois—'Yoga is 95 percent practice and only 5 percent theory.'

   "We will practice a really great foundational routine, and each week we will add a few variations and build on the strength, flexibility, and endurance you gained from previous sessions. The pace will be such that everyone can follow along as I see the need, or as you tell me, and I will assist you in modifying the postures to make them easier or more challenging as you wish."

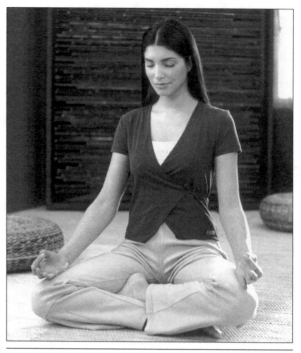

Many students may wish to experience the relaxation and calmness of mind that comes with meditating. You should inform your students whether or not you will be able to help guide them in this area, and if you will provide informational materials.

© Jumpfoto

3. In a handout or on a white board include the following information:

   - Your name and contact information if you are willing to provide it
   - Class syllabus (a sample syllabus appears in appendix C in an easy-to-copy form)
   - The word *Namaste* and its general meaning (loosely translated, "The Divine light within me salutes the Divine light within you")

   Although many yoga studios and athletic clubs offer classes of different styles and levels of intensity, the issue of a "beginning" versus "advanced" class is a very relative matter as most classes are multileveled, with students at every level of ability. The ideal plan is to teach a foundational workout and to build on it by adding variations to postures and gradually introducing new asanas. The provided syllabus in appendix C is a guideline only, and it is your responsibility to determine how to adjust the time spent on particular poses based on the ability, comfort, and requests of your students.

4. If appropriate, at the end of the course, have students fill out a brief class evaluation (a sample evaluation form is included in appendix C).

Week One: Foundation

Introduce breathing techniques, teach names of asanas, and practice basic postures.

- Teach the complete yogic breath, breathing in and out of the nose from the abdomen. Try having students breathe for four seconds in and four seconds out.
- Postures:
  - Tadasana
  - Basic Surya Namaskara, two rounds
  - Utthita Trikonasana
  - Uttanasana
  - Virabhadrasana II
  - Malasana
  - Janu Shirshasana
  - Marichyasana A
  - Durga-Go
  - Utthita Hasta Padangusthasana
  - Jathara Parivartanasana
  - 15 minutes of Shavasana with a mini guided progressive relaxation

Week Two: Expanding the Foundation of Balance

Work on increasing strength and focus.

- Review breathing while students are in Tadasana.
- Postures:
  - Tadasana
  - Surya Namaskara with variations of clasping the hands behind the back while lunging in the second round
  - Vrkshasana
  - Uttanasana
  - Utthita Trikonasana
  - Malasana
  - Janu Shirshasana
  - Marichyasana A
  - Paschimottansana
  - Padmasana (or sitting in any comfortable cross-legged position with easy neck stretches)
  - Durga-Go with alternating arm and leg extended
  - Supta Padangusthasana
  - Five breaths resting supine with knees bent while focusing on belly breaths and hands resting on the abdomen
  - Jathara Parivartanasana
  - 10 minutes of Shavasana with a mini guided relaxation

Week Three: Adding More Endurance to the Core Foundation

All asanas are held longer than in the previous classes.

- Tadasana, with focus on breathing: working to increase the complete yogic breath from a two- to a four-second inhalation and exhalation and then to a seven-second inhalation and seven-second exhalation
- Two Surya Namaskaras (the first with the hands lifted off the floor while in Bhujangasana; the second with the arms lifted overhead while kneeling in the lunge)
- Utthita Trikonasana (held longer by a few breaths)
- Uttanasana
- Virabhadrasana I
- Malasana (held longer, focusing on balance)
- Janu Shirshasana (held longer)
- Marichyasana A (held longer)
- Padmasana or variations, adding easy neck stretches
- Gomukhasana
- Supta Padangusthasana (held longer)
- Jathara Parivartanasana (work to extend legs)
- Shavasana (main focus is watching the breath)

Week Four: Adding More Variation to Poses

- Tadasana with focus on breathing: continuing to lengthen the time of inhalation and exhalation toward seven seconds each
- Two Surya Namaskaras: the first with Urdhva Mukha Shvanasana instead of Bhujangasana; the second with Adho Mukha Shvanasana with one leg lifted off the floor for 30 seconds, then the other leg lifted for the same amount of time.
- Parivrtta Trikonasana
- Uttanasana, focusing on finding the edge of the balance on the feet
- Virabhadrasana II with arm binding
- Malasana (held longer, focusing on balance)
- Janu Shirshasana (held longer)
- Deeper version of Marichyasana (B or C)
- Padmasana or variations, with easy neck stretches
- Gomukhasana, bending forward and backward from the hips for variation
- Supta Padangusthasana (after basic posture, extend the legs out to the side to open the hips further)
- Jathara Parivartanasana (work to extend legs)

- Shavasana (main focus is to be aware of the breath)

Week Five: Expanding the Practice

- Tadasana (centering longer)
- Two to three Surya Namaskaras (first one easy, the second two with variations to postures)
- Utthita Trikonasana
- Parivrtta Trikonasana
- Malasana
- Janu Shirshasana with a twist
- Paschimottanasana
- Gomukhasana
- Garudasana
- Upavishta Konasana (with variations of twisting or side bending)
- Baddha Konasana
- Supta Padangusthasana
- Setu Bandhasana
- Shavasana

Week Six: Review and Renew Postures

- Tadasana
- Surya Namaskaras
- Vrkshasana
- Utthita Trikonasana
- Uttanasana (with arm variations)
- Padottanasana
- Virabhadrasana II (side-lunge version)
- Utthita Parshvakonasana
- Malasana
- Janu Shirshasana
- Marichyasana A
- Paschimottanasana
- Durga-Go
- Dhanurasana
- Supta Padangusthasana
- Jathara Parivartanasana
- Shavasana (review abdominal breathing with hands on abdomen, mini guided relaxation)

Putting It All Together

The beginning of this book outlines the basic philosophical tenets and ancient lineage of yoga and provides answers to questions typically asked by students new to yoga practice— questions that you as their instructor should be able to answer. Following chapters provide information that will enable you to discover your own individual teaching and practice style to help you to connect with students to guide them to experience their innermost Selves through yoga. An overview of basic breathing techniques and how the body works to heal itself is provided so that you can create specialized classes that will reach most, if not all, of your students on some level. The asana chapters comprise detailed information on how to present 66 fundamental asanas, variations, and modifications with a kinematic breakdown of each. The final chapters pull together the information presented throughout the book into a usable format. The foundational postures of a basic workout are presented in a manner that shows examples of appropriate sequencing of postures. You have also been shown ways that allow you to teach your students to go beyond the "beginning" phase or awareness of yoga practice on to more "evolved" levels of practice. Examples of how to structure a 30-, 60-, or 90-minute class with variations of poses and routines to challenge and build on the foundational class structure or framework are provided as are sample goals, activities, rationales, and objectives. A sample six-week syllabus is provided as a reference and inspiration in planning your classes. Incorporating this information into your teaching repertoire will provide you with the tools to adapt your lesson plans and class routines to most any yoga teaching assignment, whether it is an adult education facility, a physical education class, a gym, or a yoga studio.

Table 13.1 brings together the elements outlined throughout this book as a whole and illustrates a sample class (with examples of asanas in order). The table also lists the physical and energetic effects of each asana. Considerations for students' Ayurvedic constitutions (the doshas of vata, pitta, and kapha explained on page 24), with cues that can be used as teaching tips, are also included with modifications and variations for each asana. By utilizing adjustments, props, and other modifications, every student in your class can reap personal and universal benefits in any structured yoga routine that you design.

Table 13.1 Asanas in a Sample Class

		Strengthens and stabilizes	Stretches and opens	Chakra emphasis	Remind Vata to:	Suggest or explain to Pitta:	Motivate Kapha to:	Adjustments and instructions	Variations and options	Plane and spinal direction
1	Tadasana	Whole body	Chest and trapezius	Muladhara	Use legs	Breath work	Lift chest	Arch and knee lifts, align hips, drop shoulders	Feet width, hands position (active/relaxed, overhead or by sides)	Neutral
2	Uttanasana	Feet, fronts of legs	Hamstring, back	Muladhara, svadishthana, manipura	Breathe into back area	Relax the belly, release the spine	Stay at edge	Relax head, lift knees	Bend knees, feet width	Forward bend
3	Lunge	Legs, abdomen	Hips, chest	Same as above plus anahata visuddha	Release knee out	Press back heel	Press arms more	Square hips, lower shoulders, lift chest	Kneeling, chair, wall, pigeon	Backward bend
4	Bhujangasana	Back (if active)	Chest	Svadishthana, manipura, anahata	Tuck tailbone	Open shoulders	Keep legs active	Drop shoulders, keep elbows in	More or less active, no arms, legs lifted	Backward bend
5	Adho Mukha Shvanasana	Arms, shoulders, back	Shoulders, upper/lower legs	Anahata, visuddha, ajna	Release head, rest if needed	Move hips up and back, lengthen spine	Push hands into floor	Roll shoulders open	Bend knees, one leg lifted	Neutral and forward bend
6	Utthita Trikonasana	Neck, back, hips	Hamstrings, hips, flank	Svadishthana, visuddha	Really use feet	Go over details	Find edge of balance	Hips—frontal plane, bottom shoulder relaxed, ribcage straight, feet working	Block, wall (flat and/or hands touching), kneeling, do one side more	Side bends
7	Vrkshasana	Hips, feet	Ribs	Muladhara, manipura	Reach tailbone downward	Try closing eyes	Lift arms with intensity	Hips—frontal plane, bottom shoulder relaxed, ribcage straight, feet working	Block, wall (flat and/or hands touching), kneeling, do one side more	Neutral
8	Virabhadrasana II	Hips, low back, legs, shoulders	Hips, knees	Same as lunge	Drop shoulders	Press through outer feet to open hips more	Keep arms active, chest open	Make sure knee is turned out, frontal plane, align torso	Wall, seated, add flank/parsva, arm support	Neutral
9	Malasana	Ankles, thighs if lowering actively	Hips, low back	Muladhara, svadishthana	Relax neck and shoulders	Keep knees apart, feet parallel	Try active variations	Heels down	Props, twist, wall	Neutral and forward bend
10	Janu Shirshasana	Back (when active)	Legs, spine	Same two as above plus manipura anahata	Relax shoulders down, breathe into it	Align hips and belly button toward straight leg	Lift front ribs forward, shoulders back	Level ribs, lower shoulders, roll out bent knees	Active/passive foot/hand position, bandhas	Forward bend, slight twist
11	Gomukhasana	Shoulders	Arms, triceps, shoulders	Anahata, visuddha	Lift chest	Arms in	Lift head	External rotation, drop shoulders	Strap, forward bend	Neutral
12	Salamba Shirshasana	Upper back, shoulders, neck, veins		Manipura, anahata, visuddha, ajna, sahasrara	Take it slow	Take it easy	Take it seriously	Elbows in, open chest, tuck pelvis	10-15+ minutes, twist, Lotus Pose	Neutral
13	Shavasana		Relaxes everything	Ajna	Let body dissolve or melt into breath	Visualize breath as white healing light	Progressive relaxation	Roll palms up, press shoulders down	Pillows, bolsters	Neutral

Poses 2 through 5 make up Sun Salutations.

Now that you have read this book, do not make the mistake of thinking that you have learned all that you can about teaching and practicing yoga! Continue to learn by making time for your personal practice, enrolling in workshops and conferences, and sharing ideas with fellow yoga instructors. May you and your students share the benefits of the wisdom you gain as you continue to practice and teach with awareness.

"The function of the teacher is indeed an affair of the transference of something, and not one of mere stimulation of the existing intellectual or other faculties in the taught."

Swami Vivekananda

Practice!

Namaste.

appendix A
Sample Relaxation Scripts

Even after a rigorous asana practice when students are completely ready to relax their bodies, many students have difficulty allowing their minds to come into the same state of relaxation. Left to their own devices, many students find themselves focusing on what comes next in their day. The following scripts are examples of ways you can guide your students into deeper states of relaxation as they settle into Shavasana.

Progressive Relaxation

- Breathe deeply into your left foot. Hold your breath and visualize it filling your entire left leg. Tense your left leg. Lift it off the ground slightly. Tense it still more. Exhale and completely relax your left leg and imagine it dissolving into the breath.

- [Repeat instructions for the right leg.]

- Breathe into your left hand. Spread your palm and fingers open wide. Now make a fist. Hold your breath in and visualize your arm filled with the breath. Lift your left arm and tense it a little more. Exhale and completely release your left arm and let it dissolve and become the healing white light of the breath.

- [Repeat instructions for the right arm.]

- Inhale as fully as you can into your belly and fill it like a balloon held to its fullest capacity. Hold your breath. Exhale through your mouth and deeply and completely relax.

- Now breathe into your ribcage, deeply filling your lungs in all directions. Expand your lungs and ribcage to their fullest capacity. Hold the breath. Exhale deeply and completely relax your

back and chest . . . [move down through the rest of the body].

Star Relaxation

- Visualize a blue (or gold or white) star flowing in through the crown of your head. Allow every skin cell, every muscle cell, and every bone and blood cell in this area to relax completely.

- [Wait a couple of breaths.]

- With the next breath flowing in, visualize the star penetrating deeper into the space behind your eyes and between your eyebrows.

- [Wait a couple of breaths.]

- As you breathe in again, continue to visualize the star moving down and spreading its light and energy throughout your whole body.

- [If you have the time, talk the students through every joint of the body.]

Belly-to-Universe Relaxation

- Feel your breath rise and fall gently in your belly. Visualize the breath as a sphere of white light about the size of a softball. Let this sphere of white light expand gradually with each breath.

- With your next inhalation, let the sphere expand to the size of your entire torso. Expand the healing white light of this sphere in all directions so that it moves not only through your body but beyond the boundaries of your body.

- Let your body and breath become one as you continue to expand this sphere of light with each breath. Allow the next breath in to expand the sphere into a bubble surrounding you and yet letting your body be completely one with the breath as you deeply relax.

- With every inhalation feel expansion, and with every exhalation feel even more deeply relaxed.

- In the next breath expand the sphere and your body to the size of the room . . . then the size of the building . . . then the city . . . the planet . . . the universe. Feel your whole body as one with the power and wisdom of the universe.

- [After 5 to 10 minutes guide the students back by saying something such as]: In the next few breaths, retaining that sense of expansion and limitlessness, gradually breathe yourself back into the perfect form of your rested and recharged body on the ground. In the next few breaths, begin to gently roll to one side and come up to sitting.

Tibetan Healing Breath Relaxation

- As your breath comes into your body, visualize and feel it as pure, healing white light. As the breath exits your body see it as smoky grey. Let the breath remove any last bits of tension, toxins, imbalances, or resistance, allowing you to deeply relax.

- As the breath is clearing and purifying your body, visualize and feel each breath as it exits your body turn from a smoky grey to only slightly grey until finally the exhaled breath is as clear and pure as the healing breath you inhale.

Yoga Resources

YOGA PERIODICALS

Yoga International

Himalayan International Institute
of Yoga Science and Philosophy of the USA
RR1 Box 1127
Honesdale, PA 18431-9706
570-253-5551; 800-822-4547
www.yimag.org

Yoga Journal

2054 University Avenue
Suite 600
Berkeley, CA 94704
www.yogajournal.com

Yogi Times Magazine

3226 Thatcher Avenue
Marina Del Rey, CA 90292
310-577-1611
www.yogitimes.com

INFORMATION ON SANSKRIT, AYURVEDA, ASHRAMS, AND OTHER IN-DEPTH YOGA PROGRAMS

American Institute of Vedic Studies

Books and correspondence courses on Ayurveda,
Jyotish, Vedas, and more
David Frawley
P.O. Box 8357
Santa Fe, NM 87504-8357
505-983-9385
www.vedanet.com

American Sanskrit Institute

Sanskrit classes and products
Vyaas Houston
980 Ridge Road
Brick, NJ 08724
732-840-4104; 800-459-4176
e-mail: sanskrit@sbcglobal.net
www.americansanskrit.com

Asana Names and the Language of Yoga (book and double CD)

Nicolai Bachman
Sanskrit Sounds
P.O. Box 4352
Santa Fe, NM 87502
505-670-2013
www.SanskritSounds.com

Ayurvedic Institute

Ayurvedic College and Treatments
Dr. Vasant Lad
11311 Menaul Boulevard
N.E. Albuquerque, NM
505-291-9698
www.ayurveda.com

International Sivananda Yoga Vendata Centers

www.sivananda.org

Swami Rama's Ashram

P.O. Pashulok
Ramnagar NE
Rishikesh, UP 249 203
India
91-135-431-485
www.bindu.org

Yoga Meditation of the Himalayan Tradition

www.swamij.com

Yogafinder

International site for finding yoga classes, retreats, teachers, workshops, and products www.yogafinder.com

USEFUL PUBLICATIONS

Coulter, H.D. 2001. *Anatomy of Hatha Yoga: A Manual for Students, Teachers, and Practitioners.* Honesdale, PA: Body and Breath, Inc.

Frankel, V.H. and M. Nordin. 1980. *Basic Biomechanic of the Skeletal System.* Philadelphia: Lea & Febiger.

Gray, H. 1974. *Gray's Anatomy.* Edited by T.P. Pick and R. Howden. Philadelphia: Running Press.

Kapit, W. and L.M. Elson. 2001. *The Anatomy Coloring Book*, 3rd ed. San Francisco: Benjamin Cummings.

Luttgens, K. and N. Hamilton. 2001. *Kinesiology: Scientific Basis of Human Motion*, 10th ed. New York: McGrawHill.

Motoyama, Hiroshi. 2001. *Theories of the Chakras: Bridge to Higher Consciousness.* New Delhi: New Age.

Swenson, D. 1999. *Ashtanga Yoga: The Practice Manual.* Austin, TX: Ashtanga Yoga Productions.

Tortora, G.J. 2002. *Principles of Anatomy & Physiology*, 10th ed. Indianapolis: Wiley.

YOGA ASSOCIATIONS AND SOCIETIES

Ashtanga Yoga Research Institute

www.ayri.org

British Yoga Teachers Association

10 Bromley Crescent
Ruislip Gardens
Mddx. HA4 6PG
01-895-470-883
www.yogateachers.org.uk

California Yoga Teachers Association

www.yogateachersassoc.org

Canadian Yoga Alliance

www.yoga.niagara.com/canadianyogicalliance. htm

European Yoga Council/European Yoga Alliance

http://fiy.yoganet.org/eurocouncil.html

Green Yoga Association

2340 Powell St. #141
Emeryville, CA 94608
888-659-7925
www.greenyoga.org

Himalayan International Institute of Yoga Science and Philosophy of the United States

www.himalayaninstitute.org

International Association of Black Yoga Teachers

P.O. Box 360922
Los Angeles CA 90036
213-833-6371
www.blackyogateachers.com

International Association of Yoga Therapists

P.O. Box 2513
Prescott, AZ 86302
928-541-0004
e-mail: mail@iayt.org
www.iayt.org

International Kundalini Yoga Teachers Association

3HO IKYTA
6 Narayan Court
Espanola, NM 87532
505-367-1313
www.kundaliniyoga.com

International Society of Yoga Education

519-352-8298; 877-407-9642
www.yogacertificationinternational.com

International Yoga Teachers Association (Australia)

www.iyta.org.au

Web site also provides contact information for the following countries:

Austria	Puerto Rico
Brazil	Singapore
Canada	South Africa
Germany	Spain
Greece	United Arab Emirates
Hong Kong	United Kingdom
India	Vietnam

Iyengar Yoga Association of the United Kingdom

www.iyengaryoga.org.uk

Lotus Yoga Teachers Association (Chicago)

1323 Cunant Court, Ste. #2
Lake in the Hills, IL 60156
847-658-1258
www.lotusyogateachers.com

North American Studio Alliance (NAMASTA)

NAMASTA
2313 Hastings Drive
Belmont, CA 94002-3317
877-626-2782
www.namasta.com

Yoga Alliance (USA)

7801 Old Branch Avenue, Ste. 400
Clinton, MD 20735
301-868-4700; 877-964-2255
www.yogaalliance.org

Yoga Education Society (San Diego County, CA)

www.yes4yoga.org

Yoga Teachers Association of Australia

0500-559-024
www.yogateachers.asn.au

YogaWell's Yoga Teacher Training Programs and Workshops

Institute of Progressive Therapies
2333 Camino del Rio South, Ste. 240
San Diego, CA 92108
619-460-7080
www.yogawell.com

RELATED INFORMATION FOR TRENDS IN THE FITNESS INDUSTRY

Aerobics and Fitness Association of America

15250 Ventura Boulevard, Ste. 200
Sherman Oaks, CA 91403
877-968-7263
www.afaa.com

American College of Sports Medicine (ACSM)

PO Box 1440
Indianapolis, IN 46206-1440
317-637-9200
www.acsm.org

American Council on Exercise

800-529-8227
www.acefitness.org

IDEA Health & Fitness Association

10455 Pacific Center Court
San Diego, CA 92121-4339
800-999-4332
Outside the U.S. and Canada 858-535-8979
www.ideafit.com

YOGA PRODUCTS AND DISTRIBUTORS

Blue Lotus Yoga Essentials

3120 Central Avenue
Albuquerque, NM 87106
505-268-9738
www.bluelotusyoga.com

Crescent Moon Yoga

1150 North Miller Street
Anaheim, CA 92806
www.crescentmoonyoga.com

Hugger-Mugger Yoga Products

Yoga gear, books, and CDs
3937 South 500 West
Salt Lake City, UT 84123
800-473-4888
www.huggermugger.com

Meditation Generation

4631 Noble Place
Parrish, FL 34219
www.MeditationGeneration.com

Tools for Yoga and Studio Yoga

Green Village Road #202
Madison, NJ 07940
888-648-9642
www.studioyoga.info

appendix C

Reproducibles

Self-Inquiry Questionnaire

Ask yourself the following questions. Write down your answers in a notebook or journal so that in the future you can look back on your responses to see how you may have evolved in your knowledge and applications. Be honest; no one but you will see your answers. The purpose of asking these questions is to increase your awareness—not to be right.

Note: Reading chapter 2 will give you a good idea of the relevance of your answers. If you would like a more detailed commentary of possible responses to the Self-Inquiry questions please contact the authors (www.yogawell.com) for more information.

1. Why do you want to teach yoga?
    a. money
    b. it is easier on my body than teaching aerobics, spin classes, or the like
    c. my boss told me to
    d. so I can get more yoga workouts
    e. other _____

2. How often do you practice yoga?
    a. the occasional conference or workshop
    b. an average of 30 minutes a day or more at home
    c. group classes at least twice a week
    d. work out with videos every once in awhile
    e. other _____

3. What is your motivation for practicing yoga?
    a. to meditate better
    b. to improve flexibility or strength
    c. to look good while I teach
    d. to deepen my understanding of the asanas
    e. other _____

4. How often do you meditate?
    a. have never tried it
    b. tried it but could not get into it
    c. every once in awhile
    d. at least two minutes a day
    e. other _____

5. What would you do if a student were to cry during or at the end of class?

    _____

    _____

6. What would be your response if a student asked to see you socially outside of class?

    _____

    _____

7. What would you do if a new student you had never met before rushed into the class 10 to 20 minutes late?

_____

_____

8. True or False: T/F

   a. I feel somewhat ashamed to teach yoga because I do not feel my
      body looks good enough in the poses.   _____

   b. I feel somewhat guilty because I teach yoga, yet I drink beer and
      eat meat.   _____

   c. If I needed to tell one of my yoga students to refrain from wearing a
      strong perfume because it is disturbing to other students I would be
      afraid of creating hurt feelings.   _____

   d. I do not care what my students think of me.   _____

   e. It is extremely important to maintain strict order in my classes.   _____

   f. It is important to me that my students like me.   _____

   g. I should know every student's medical history in order to teach them
      more safely.   _____

   h. All students automatically give consent to be physically adjusted by
      the fact they are in my class.   _____

9. What are the top qualities a yoga teacher should have?

_____

_____

From *Instructing Hatha Yoga* by Kathy Lee Kappmeier and Diane Ambrosini, 2006, Champaign, IL: Human Kinetics.

Yoga Class Evaluation Form

Rate the following on a scale of 1 to 4.
  1—unacceptable
  2—below average
  3—above average
  4—awesome

1. Punctuality (started and ended class on time)   1   2   3   4

2. Teaching voice:
    a. Volume   1   2   3   4
    b. Tone   1   2   3   4
    c. Pace   1   2   3   4
    d. Clarity of words and direction   1   2   3   4
    e. Ability to soothe   1   2   3   4

3. Trust (Did I feel the instructor knew what she or he was doing and saying so   1   2   3   4
    that I felt safe during the class?)

4. Attention to alignment   1   2   3   4

5. Focus (Did the instructor seem present and attentive?)   1   2   3   4

6. Inspiration (Did the instructor help you to feel motivated?)   1   2   3   4

7. Creativity (Did the instructor present the postures in a creative manner and   1   2   3   4
    use expressive words to describe, modify, or move you into
    the poses?)

8. Sense of flow   1   2   3   4

9. Use or mention of breath   1   2   3   4

10. Balance in overall sequence of the asanas (Did the routine include postures   1   2   3   4
    that moved the body in all directions? Was there a warm-up, peak(s), and a
    cool-down? Were counterposes presented?)

11. Approachability (Did I feel comfortable asking the instructor questions?)   1   2   3   4

12. Environment (Were there distractions such as noise, lighting, temperature?)   1   2   3   4

13. Comments:

    (What did you like the most and least? Write down any suggestions or miscellaneous comments.)

    _____

    _____

    _____

    _____

    _____

    _____

From *Instructing Hatha Yoga* by Kathy Lee Kappmeier and Diane Ambrosini, 2006, Champaign, IL: Human Kinetics.

Classical-Eclectic Hatha Course Syllabus

Overview of Class

Yoga is 6,000 years old! Yoga means "to yoke" or "to join." Yoga works to develop every human faculty (physical, emotional, mental, spiritual) to bring them together harmoniously. Yoga stretches, strengthens, tones, aligns, and improves the health of the body. Yoga enhances the awareness of the body and breath and can help a person to develop a state of mental calm and emotional stability. Yoga is a "discipline without dogma": It is not a religion.

Hatha yoga is the type of yoga most people are familiar with in the West. Hatha yoga is understood to include postures and breath. Types of hatha yoga include Ashtanga (aerobic flow series), Iyengar, Kundalini, Bikram, and so on. This class is classical-eclectic hatha and involves moving slowly and sinking deeper into the postures. The deeper into the posture you allow yourself to go the more advanced or deep the yoga practice.

Kindness and acceptance. Yoga is not competitive. Yoga is about quieting the mind and accepting the process. Students are taught to listen to and observe the body, rather than trying to force it toward reaching a goal. Yoga is about being kind to your body and accepting of where you are today.

Remember, your body is your vehicle, so honor it. You are also responsible to be kind to and accepting of others to create a positive and relaxing class environment.

General Policies

1. You may purchase a locker from the equipment room. The cost is $8 per semester.

2. You may store your personal items in the exercise room with the understanding that the instructor and the university cannot be responsible for any stolen or lost property.

3. Wear clothes that are nonrestrictive. Street clothes such as cargo pants or jeans will restrict your ability to participate fully.

4. You may bring or borrow a mat and a blanket each day.

Attendance and Participation Policies

1. Students are not permitted to work out until the instructor is present for safety reasons.

2. Please pick up your name card and place it by your yoga mat at the beginning of class! I will use them to take attendance and to remember names. Remaining cards are used to record absences.

3. Meditation/Breath Work/Relaxation will begin at 9:00 A.M., and movement instruction will begin 2 to 3 minutes after the hour. If you arrive late, please come in quietly from the back of the class and set up in the back of the room.

4. Students will be released at 45 minutes after the hour. If you must leave before that time, please get permission from the instructor before exercise begins. I will simply remind you to set up your mat near the back door so that leaving early will not be disruptive.

5. Please remember that leaving class without permission is a form of academic dishonesty.

Grading Policies (Subject to Change)

1. Ninety percent of your grade will be determined through attendance. The remaining part of your grade will be earned through assignments or quizzes.

2. If you miss 8 classes before the last week of class you will be automatically dropped.

3. No make-ups are permitted in this class. Excused absences are reserved for extreme cases and require documentation. Whether an absence is excused is at the discretion of the instructor. Excused absences do not have an impact on one's grade.

From *Instructing Hatha Yoga* by Kathy Lee Kappmeier and Diane Ambrosini, 2006, Champaign, IL: Human Kinetics.

The table demonstrates *only* how your grade is affected by absences. Remember, 10 percent of your grade will rely on other assignments.

Safety Warning

There are inherent risks of injury when a student participates in yoga. Students assume these risks when they are involved in this class.

Basic Safety Procedures

1. Students with preexisting conditions MUST clear their enrollment in yoga class with their primary healthcare provider before class begins.

2. If in ANY stretch you feel discomfort you should release immediately and with care. In addition, if at any time you choose to rest during class you can sit out for a pose and go into Balasana (Child's Pose), Shavasana (Corpse Pose), or lie down until you are ready to resume. Never attempt to do anything you are uncomfortable with. Listen to your body and speak with the instructor about possible modifications or substitutions.

3. Please listen carefully to instructions on technique. Correct technique works to ensure safety.

4. Notify instructor *immediately* if you or a classmate becomes injured or ill during class.

5. If you become overly tired, dizzy, or faint take a break from the exercise and sit or lie down. Make sure to let the instructor or a friend know you don't feel well so he or she can keep an eye on you. Please do not leave the room alone if you don't feel well. Take a buddy, and always report back.

Safety Modifications

Students with preexisting conditions must share in the responsibility to modify exercise to prevent injury. High blood pressure, glaucoma or detached retinas, disk problems in the neck or back, or pregnancy must be reported to the instructor because certain poses are contraindicated or can simply be modified.

- High blood pressure may demand that you keep the head above the heart level.
- Heart problems may decrease the duration that one should maintain a static pose.
- Glaucoma or detached retinas may make inversions (going upside down) dangerous.
- Disk problems in the neck or back may require that you keep the head in a neutral position rather than releasing it back.
- Pregnancy may require that you avoid inversions (going upside down). You may also need to part your legs during squats and forward bends. Do not place any pressure on your belly!

Special Needs

If you have any special needs or considerations, please see the instructor prior to beginning exercise in this class. If special needs or considerations arise during the course, notify the instructor immediately. Adaptations can be made.

How Your Grade Is Affected by Absences

Absences	Percent	Grade
0	100	A+
1	97.5	A
2	95	A
3	92.5	A
4	90	A-
5	87	B+
6	85	B
7	82	B-
8	78	C+
9	75	C

From *Instructing Hatha Yoga* by Kathy Lee Kappmeier and Diane Ambrosini, 2006, Champaign, IL: Human Kinetics.

Reprinted, by permission, from C. Robertson.

appendix D

Chapter Review Answers

Chapter 1

1. **Q: Approximately how old is yoga?**

   A: 6,000 years or older.

2. **Q: How would you define yoga in just a few sentences?**

   A: "Yoga is a discipline without a dogma." It is any path that unites or connects you to your spiritual realizations. There are infinite types of yoga but it is most often discovered or known by this modern Western society as a mind-body exercise (asanas and pranayama).

3. **Q: What are the four main types of yoga, and of which type is hatha yoga?**

   A: Karma, bhakti, jnana, and raja. Raja, often considered the true Ashtanga, is the type of yoga that includes hatha.

4. **Q: What is *Ashtanga* yoga?**

   A: Ashtanga means the eight limbs of yoga as outlined in the *Yoga Sutras*. There is a style of hatha yoga as taught by Pattabhi Jois that is referred to as "Ashtanga" or "the Ashtanga series."

5. **Q: How did Patanjali codify yoga practice in 200 to 300 B.C.?**

   A: He wrote the *Yoga Sutras*.

6. **Q: What well-known type of hatha yoga focuses on alignment, form, and the use of props?**

   A: Iyengar.

7. **Q: What are some of the most popular styles of hatha yoga practiced today?**

   A: Classical-eclectic hatha (including "Vinyasa flows"), Iyengar, Ashtanga series, Bikram, Restorative, Kundalini, and Perinatal, to name a few.

8. **Q: What are some issues facing modern yoga practitioners and what are some of the ways the needs of today's students and teachers are being met?**

   A: Hatha yoga alone is so vast and relative that it is challenging to create standards for teachers that allow the uninformed public, as well as instructors, to find a consistent level of education. Issues of safety, ethics, and career options in addition to the history and future of yoga are all hot topics in the field today.

9. **Q: What are the five categories outlined by the Yoga Alliance?**

   A: 1. Techniques 2. Teaching and Methodology 3. Anatomy and Physiology 4. Philosophy, Ethics, and Lifestyle 5. Practicum.

10. **Bonus Question: Explain the words *yamas*, *niyamas*, and *neti pot*.**

    A: Yamas (guidelines for ethical standards and moral conduct): Ahimsa; nonviolence, doing no harm. Satya; truthfulness. Asteya; not stealing. Bramacharya; moderation. Aparigrapha; not coveting and nonattachment.

    A: Niyamas (observances and disciplines): Saucha; cleanliness. Santosha; contentment or equanimity. Tapas; austerities. Svadhyaya; the study of spiritual scriptures. Isvara pranidhana; practicing awareness and surrender.

    A: A neti pot is a device used to wash the nasal passages as a daily ritual, like brushing your teeth.

Chapter 2

1. Q: What are the four Cs of teaching yoga?

   A: Connection, compassion, confidence, and commitment.

2. Q: What are the three basic types of learning styles?

   A: Visual, auditory, and kinesthetic.

3. Q: Which dosha is made up of air?

   A: Vata.

4. Q: Which type of student usually has trouble staying motivated?

   A: Kapha.

5. Q: List two things that students typically like and dislike about their instructors.

   A: Students like teachers who can motivate and connect with them. Students dislike instructors who are focused on themselves or express any negative comments at all. *See the Like and Dislike table in chapter 2 for more examples.*

6. Q: How is the word asana used as an acronym for teaching yoga?

   A: A = ahimsa (and ask), S = suggest, A = align, N = nurture, A = assess.

7. Q: True or False? There is a very strict code of ethics you are legally required to abide by as a professional yoga teacher.

   A: False.

8. Q: What aspects of your personal yoga practice will make you a better teacher?

   A: It is all relative. The key is that you are engaged in a personal yoga practice. *For more details on aspects and to explore your own answer review the Self-Inquiry Questionnaire in appendix C.*

9. Q: Define *ahimsa*.

   A: First and foremost, an aspect of the limbs of yoga; also "ahimsa" means causing no harm.

Chapter 3

1. Q: Why would yoga practitioners choose to wear white cotton or other natural fibers?

   A: To foster the electromagnetic field surrounding them during practice.

2. Q: What are three indispensable things when practicing yoga?

   A: Bare feet, comfortable clothing, and a proper yoga mat.

3. Q: How are blocks used?

   A: Blocks generally are used during standing postures to extend the reach of the arms toward the ground without causing undue strain in the hamstrings and back. They also may be used in the place of bolsters or blankets to provide more stable elevation when needed.

4. Q: What is the most important safety issue when physically adjusting your students?

   A: Remember to respect each student's body as if it were your own.

5. Q: How long should the average person wait after a meal before practicing yoga and why?

   A: A couple hours should pass before a yoga practice because the circulation and energy is needed for the practice.

6. Q: What is the ideal setting for a yoga class?

   A: A spacious, warm area free from outside distractions, with good ventilation and comfortable lighting.

7. Q: What temperature is generally considered the lowest acceptable for yoga?

   A: 76 degrees Fahrenheit (24 degrees Celsius).

8. Q: What are some pros and cons of using music while teaching yoga?

   A: Pros: Music can drown out other audible distractions; it can set the mood.

   Cons: Students may become dependent on music. Sometimes music itself can be distracting.

Chapter 4

1. Q: What is an epidemic in today's society that contributes to the high anxiety and stress suffered by many?

   A: Poor breathing.

2. Q: How can a student bypass the chatter in the mind and ego?

   A: By focusing on the breath.

3. Q: _____ can be triggered negatively through shallow, labored breathing or positively with smooth, flowing breaths, which stabilize thoughts and allow relaxation to set in.

   A: Emotions.

4. Q: Choppy, shallow breathing is associated with which nervous system?

A: The sympathetic nervous system, which activates the body for the fight-or-flight response.

5. Q: What is a type of breathing mentioned in a National Institute of Health report that when practiced can improve physical endurance?

A: Deep, slow, and through the nose.

6. Q: How many breaths per minute does the average human take?

A: 16 to 20.

7. Q: What are the three most common pranayama techniques taught in asana classes?

A: 1. Deep abdominal, 2. complete yogic breath, and 3. ujjayi breathing.

8. Q: What is nadi shodhana and what effect on the brain hemispheres does it have?

A: Alternate nostril breathing can activate and balance both hemispheres of the brain and therefore increase learning up to 500 percent.

9. Q: Which is usually better, to inhale or exhale, while entering Uttanasana (a forward bend)?

A: Exhale.

Chapter 5

1. Q: Define "safe" yoga instruction.

A: Safe instruction is where any touch or words from the teacher encourages the most accurate awareness in the students' minds in order to move energy, muscles, or bones in ways that don't result in injury.

2. Q: What is a *nadi?*

A: A nadi is an Ayurvedic term for an energy channel of the human body. Ayurveda is a sister science of yoga. The body has 72,000 nadis. These nadis are affected just as the physical body is during yoga. The nadis are connected to the chakras.

3. Q: What is *mula bandha* and with which chakra is it associated?

A: Mula bandha is the root lock and is like a kegel exercise. It strengthens the pelvic floor and the supporting structures of the urinary and genital systems. It also prevents energy leakage and imbalance, enabling the practi-

tioner to have greater endurance. The effects of mula bandha are felt primarily through the root chakra (muladhara).

4. Q: Is it advisable for a woman to practice yoga while menstruating?

A: Only the inversions are contraindicated for physical and energetic reasons. In fact, some asanas can help alleviate some monthly discomfort.

5. Q: What anatomical plane does Utthita Trikonasana (Extended Triangle) move through?

A: The frontal plane.

6. Q: What are the six directions the spine should move through in a balanced workout?

A: Forward, backward, twist to right, twist to left, side bend to right, side bend to left.

7. Q: Give examples of a few asanas that stimulate osteogenisis and create joint stability.

A: Any weight-bearing posture will promote bone strength. The standing and especially the balancing poses create and maintain joint stability of the hips, knees, and ankles. Asanas that demand work of the arms, such as Adho Mukha Shvanasana (Downard-Facing Dog), or variations of plank poses can build stability of the shoulder joints. Twists and inversions keep the spine strong and in alignment.

8. Q: What does it mean to "lift the knee caps"? Why, when, and how would you teach this?

A: Contraction of the quadriceps will raise the patella. This contraction is done to engage the leg muscles and energy more effectively as well as protect the knee joint from hyperextension. The best ways to teach this technique verbally are to say, "Lift your kneecaps" or "Flex your quads (front upper legs)." A great hands-on adjustment process is to very gently hold the sides of a student's kneecap and wiggle it (which can only be done if it is loose and therefore not lifted), then tap the student's quads.

9. Q: Which muscles in the torso are used to move into a standing forward bend, and what type of contraction is utilized? When entering into a standing backbend?

A: The spinal muscles, along with the hip extensors, utilize an eccentric contraction to move into a standing forward bend. The abdominal muscles eccentrically contract to move into a standing backbend.

10. **Q: What type of contraction is going on during the holding of most asanas?**

A: When holding an asana the muscles are often actively in an isometric contraction.

11. **Q: How long should asanas be held?**

A: In general, wait until 20 percent of your students have given up and come out of the asana; then begin to bring the class out of the posture and move on. Working one on one with a student you can use a scale of 1 to 10 and encourage the student to work at the 6 to 8 range in endurance with focus on good alignment, strength, and steady breathing.

12. **Q: Define what makes a yoga student more advanced.**

A: When students find they are happier being in a posture they initially did not like practicing, that is a far more profound achievement than improved flexibility. It is far more imperative for students to realize how to recognize areas of tension and weakness within the body so they can work on tailoring an asana to meet their needs ideally for balance versus striving for what they think the pose should look like. If students don't work with this principle, they are just doing gymnastics, not yoga.

glossary

anjali mudra [UHN-juh-lee muhd-RAAH]—Positioning of the hands, palms flat together, wrist hyperextended with the thumbs pressing against the chest. Also known as "prayer pose." Used in greetings and for centering in many asanas.

apana [uh-PAAH-nuh]—Energy that moves down and out of the body.

asanas [AHH-suh-nuh]—The physical postures of yoga. Translated literally means "to stay," "to be," "to sit;" a way to become seated in your higher consciousness.

ashram [AASH-rum]—A hermitage, yogic monastery, or nunnery.

Ayurveda [AAH-yoor-veh-duh]—The ancient, traditional healing system of India; a sister science of yoga.

bandha [BUHN-dhuh]—A lock; a physical technique to hold energy within the body and prevent its leakage.

Bikram [BEEK-rum]—Style of hatha yoga named after Bikram Choundhury. Sometimes referred to as "hot" yoga because it is practiced in a contained room at high temperature.

Buddha—The "enlightened one"; historical icon of spiritual practice originating from India around 200 to 300 B.C.

chakra [CHUK-ruhs]—A wheel or disk of energy. There are seven major chakras in the body located along the spine.

chitta [chit-TUH]—Means focused conscientiousness; a field of thought.

classical-eclectic hatha—A generic term for a style of yoga usually having ties to a Himalayan lineage. Incorporates classical ways of practicing asanas, such as the alignment of Iyengar or the flow of Ashtanga, while allowing for teacher interpretation and creativity.

concentric contraction—Muscular contraction where the muscle fibers shorten or move toward the midline. This action brings the ends of the muscles closer together, closing the angle of the joint that the muscle crosses.

coronal plane—A vertical plane that passes through the body from side to side, splitting the body into anterior (front) and posterior (back) parts. Also called frontal plane.

deep abdominal breathing—Method of breathing that emphasizes the expansion of breath using the diaphragm instead of the chest muscles.

deep external rotators—The piriformis, obturator internus and externus, superior and inferior gemellus, and quadratus femoris are six small muscles located in the posterior hip whose primary function is to externally rotate the femur and to stabilize the femur into the acetabulum.

dogma—An axiom or authoritative opinion.

dosha [DOH-shus]—Energies, elements, and constitutional types utilized in Ayurvedic medicine.

drishti [dr-EESH-tee]—Means "to see" and is derived from darsha, a term used in Ashtanga yoga, describing where to direct the gaze during asana practice.

eccentric contraction—Muscular contraction where the muscle fibers lengthen from a shortened state. The muscle fibers generally do not physically lengthen but act to resist against gravity or another external force.

energetic anatomy—The subtle energetic fields surrounding the body. The existence of this type of energy is somewhat measurable by patterns of electrical potential in cells.

external rotation—Rotation where the anterior (front) aspect of a body segment, such as the humerus (upper arm bone), turns away from the midline laterally.

frontal plane—A vertical plane that passes through the body from side to side, splitting the body into anterior (front) and posterior (back) parts. Also called coronal plane.

guru—A title for a special spiritual teacher or mentor. Literally translated as "dispeller of darkness."

horizontal plane—Plane passing horizontally through the body dividing it into upper and lower parts. Also called transverse plane.

ida [EEE-d-aah]—Energy channel, or nadi, that begins at the left nostril. It is also considered the channel of lunar energy.

isometric contraction—Muscular contraction where the muscle fibers remain the same length. Muscular tension exists without movement.

Iyengar—Style of hatha yoga named after B.K.S. Iyengar. This style emphasizes strict body alignment and utilizes props and adjustments for that purpose.

kapha [KUP-huh]—Ayurvedic constitutional dosha of earth and water.

karma [KAR-muh]—Means action, cause and effect. Karma yoga is selfless action for the good of others.

kinematics—Pertaining to the motions of body segments. In this text a table accompanies each asana, which illustrates the movement patterns of each body segment as they relate to that specific posture.

kinesiology—The study of (human) movement.

kinesthetic—Sensory understanding derived from movement.

kosha [KOH-shuhs]—Energetic layers or sheaths surrounding the body: annamaya, pranamaya, manomaya, jnanamaya, vijnanamaya, anandamaya.

Krishnamacharya [krish-NUH-maahch-AAR-yuh]—Renowned mentor and guru of both B.K.S. Iyengar and Pattabhi Jois.

Kundalini [KOOHN-duh-lee-nee]—Latent human potential energy coiled at the base of the spine. Also a yoga style stemming from Sikhism that involves dynamic movement, special pranayamas, and mantra chanting.

kyphosis [kai-FOH-sis]—Convex curve of the thoracic spine.

lordosis [lor-DOH-sis]—Concave curve of the lumbar spine.

meditation—The art of bringing the mind to a state beyond thought.

mudra [muhd-RAAH]—A seal; a sacred gesture of the hands or other body positioning that has a special effect on the body's energy.

nadi [NAAH-dee]—Energy channels within the body.

nadi shodhana [NAAH-dee SHOH-duh-nuh]—Translated as "scraping of the nadis." Alternate nostril breathing. Used to open and balance the nasal nadis (ida and pingala).

namaste or namaskar(a) [nuh-muh-STAY] [nuh-muhs-KAAH-ruh]—Variations of a salutation, or greeting. Often translated as "The light within me recognizes and bows to the light within you; together we are one in this light."

neti pot [neh-TEE]—A small cup with a spout, used to pour water into the nostrils in order to cleanse the sinuses.

neutral spine—Relaxed, natural curvature of the spine.

nirodha [NEER-owd-ha]—Ending or ceasing.

niyama [nee-YUH-muh]—Observances.

om—The ancient sound of the universe. The mantra-word is associated with infinite energy and blessings from the universe and beyond.

Patanjali [pa-TAHN-jah-lee]—Ancient sage credited with writing the *Yoga Sutras*.

Pattabhi Jois [puht-TAAH-bee JOY-ss]—Renowned master considered the father of Ashtanga hatha yoga.

perineum [per-ee-NEE-um]—Area between the anus and genitals.

pingala [peen-GUH-laah]—Energy channel, or nadi, that begins at the right nostril. It is also considered the channel of solar energy.

pitta [PEE-taah]—Ayurvedic constitutional dosha associated with fire.

power yoga—Generic term for a hybrid style of Ashtanga hatha yoga.

prana [PRAAH-naah]—The life force or energy inherent in the breath.

pronation—The inward (medial) rotation of the forearm where the thumbs point toward the body. Also, the internal rotation of the foot where the arch presses down toward the floor while standing.

prone—Position where the body is face down.

psychoneuroimmunology—The study of how the relationship between the mind and body affect overall health; most specifically relating to the endocrine system.

raja [RAAH-juh]—Royal or supreme.

sagittal plane—Vertical plane bisecting the body from front to back, dividing it into left and right parts.

samadhi [suh-MAAHD-hee]—Superconscious state of enlightenment. "Goal" of the eight limbs of Ashtanga.

Sanskrit—The earliest known Indo-European language. Ancient language in which yoga was originally taught.

scoliosis—Abnormal lateral curvature(s) of the spine.

Self—Refers to the aspects of one's being that are not connected with the ego. Generally referred to as "higher self", soul or spirit.

shanti [SHAAHN-teeh]—Divine peace. Also spelled "shantih."

supination—The outward (external) rotation of the forearm where the thumbs point away from the midline. Also, the external rotation of the foot where the lateral (little toe) side of the foot presses into the floor while standing.

supine—Body positioned face up.

sutra [SOOT-raah]—A thread, a verse of scripture.

traction—The expanded space gained in the skeletal structure; usually created by a pulling force such as a pulley in medical traction.

transverse plane—Plane passing horizontally through the body dividing it into upper and lower parts. Also called the horizontal plane.

udana [oo-DAH-nuh]—Upward moving force.

ujjayi [oo-JAAHY-ee]—Victory or surrender; a type of pranayama breathing involving air vibrating against the glottis and making a sound.

vata [VAAH-tuh]—The Ayurvedic constitutional dosha associated with air and ether.

vinyasa [vin-YAAH-suh]—The flow of asanas linked together in a series.

vritti [VRIT-tee]—Disturbances and distractions.

yamas [YAAUHH-muhs]—Guidelines for ethical standards and moral conduct.

Yoga Korunta [koh-ROON-tuh]—Ancient text discovered by Krishnamacharya and the basis of Ashtanga hatha yoga.

references and resources

Alter, M.J. 2004. *Science of Flexibility*, 3rd ed. Champaign, IL: Human Kinetics.

Barrett, J. 2004. Ethical Dilemma. *Yoga Journal* March/April: http://www.yogajournal.com/views/1211_1.cfm.

Basmajian, J.V., and C.J. De Luca. 1985. *Muscles Alive: Their Functions Revealed by Electromyography*, 5th ed. Baltimore: Williams & Wilkins.

Bauman, A. 2002. Is Yoga Enough to Keep You Fit? *Yoga Journal* September/October: http://www.yogajournal.com/practice/739_1.cfm.

Capouya, J. 2001. Real Men Do Yoga: 21 Star Athletes Reveal Their Secrets for Strength, Flexibility, and Peak Performance. *Yoga Journal* November: http://www.yogajournal.com/views/1081_1.cfm.

Desikachar, T.K.V. 1999. *The Heart of Yoga: Developing a Personal Practice*. Rochester, VT: Inner Traditions.

Desikachar, T.K.V., and R.H. Cravens. 2001. *Health, Healing, and Beyond: Yoga and the Living Tradition of Krishnamacharya*. New York: Aperture.

Dryden, G., and J. Vos. 2001. *The Learning Revolution: Visions of Education*. Stafford, United Kingdom: Network Educational.

Feuerstein, G. Ed. 2002. *Yoga Gems: A Treasury of Practical and Spiritual Wisdom from Ancient and Modern Masters*. New York: Bantam Books.

Issacs, N. 2003. Pumping Iron, Practicing Yoga. *Yoga Journal* August: http://www.yogajournal.com/views/1008_1.cfm.

Iyengar, B.K.S. 1979. *Light on Pranayama: The Yogic Art of Breathing*. New York: Crossroad General Interest.

Jois, K.P. 2002. *Yoga Mala*. New York: North Point Press.

Mayo Clinic Health Letter. 2003. Learn Better Breathing With Yoga. September: http://www.mayoclinic.org/news2003-sct/1935.html.

Swami Muktibodhananda. 1993. *Hatha Yoga Pradipika*. Munger, Bihar, India: Yoga Publications Trust.

Swenson, D. 1999. *Ashtanga Yoga: The Practice Manual*. Austin: Ashtanga Yoga Productions.

Viti, L. 2003. Tim Dwight. *Yogi Times*, October.

"Yoga in America" Market Survey (February 7, 2005), *Yoga Journal Press Release*, www.yogajournal.com.

about the authors

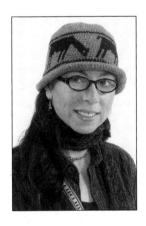

Kathy Lee Kappmeier has studied yoga in India and has more than 20 years of experience teaching yoga and training yoga teachers. She has given numerous workshops, retreats, and presentations both in the United States and abroad and has taught in a variety of venues, including public schools, hospitals, colleges, recreation centers, and sports medicine clinics. Intensely involved with the evolution, promotion, and direction of yoga education and standards, she has developed, directed, and appeared in numerous yoga videos, developed yoga programs, and founded YogaWell's Institute of Progressive Therapies in San Diego.

The former secretary of the Yoga Education Society, Ms. Kappmeier developed and coordinated a 1,000-hour course of study for holistic health practitioners at a vocational school. She received a BA in psychology and BS in physical therapy from the Union Institute & University in Cincinnati, and she received certifications in personal training, Tibetan Buddist psychology, and medical exercise. A registered yoga teacher through the Yoga Alliance, she is working on her PhD. In her spare time she enjoys creating art, riding her motorcycles, playing the Native American flute, and writing.

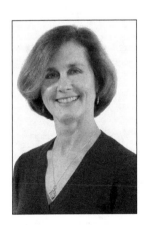

Diane M. Ambrosini earned an MA in physical education with an emphasis in kinesiology and biomechanics from San Diego State University. Her strong interest in movement science and the art of yoga led her to help expand the Institute of Progressive Therapies' Yoga Teacher Training programs by developing anatomy, physiology, and biomechanics components for continuing education workshops.

Ms. Ambrosini is registered with Yoga Alliance at the 500-hour teaching level. She is a partner in the Rancho San Diego Yoga Center and a member of Yoga Alliance, the Yoga Education Society, and the California Association for Health, Physical Education, Recreation and Dance. She is also a personal trainer and Pilates and fitness instructor. She enjoys hiking, camping, and gardening.

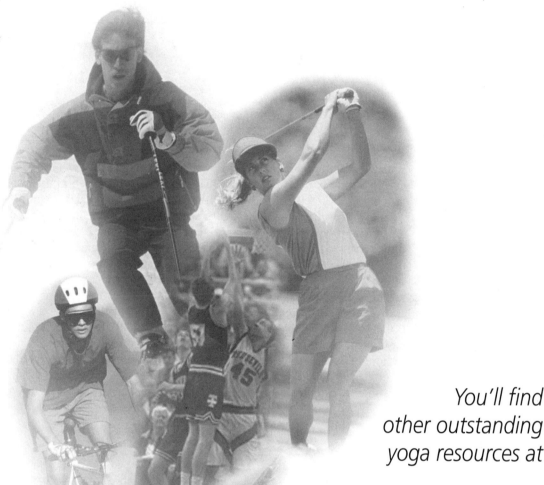